From Posts to Patterns

From Posts to Patterns

Using Social Media to Investigate Drivers of Population Health

Thu T. Nguyen
Quynh C. Nguyen
Shaniece Criss
Yulin Hswen

WILEY

Published by John Wiley & Sons, Inc., Hoboken, New Jersey.

Library of Congress Cataloging-in-Publication Data

Names: Nguyen, Thu T. author | Nguyen, Quynh C. author | Criss, Shaniece author | Hswen, Yulin author
Title: From posts to patterns : using social media to investigate drivers of population health / Thu T Nguyen, Quynh C Nguyen, Shaniece Criss, Yulin Hswen.
Description: Hoboken, New Jersey : Wiley, [2026] | Includes bibliographical references.
Identifiers: LCCN 2026003362 (print) | LCCN 2026003363 (ebook) | ISBN 9781394338375 paperback | ISBN 9781394338399 adobe pdf | ISBN 9781394338382 epub
Subjects: LCSH: Public health–Research–Methodology | Social media–Research | Social media in medicine
Classification: LCC RA440.85 .F75 2026 (print) | LCC RA440.85 (ebook)
LC record available at https://lccn.loc.gov/2026003362
LC ebook record available at https://lccn.loc.gov/2026003363

Cover Design: Wiley
Cover Images: Thu T. Nguyen, Olha Mykhaylyuk/Getty Images

Set in 10.5/14pt Warnock Pro by Straive, Pondicherry, India

DEDICATION

For Leal, Milo, Sebastian, Bella, and Hong—From Thu
For Yan, Finn, and Hong—From Quynh
For Demond, Sage, Christi, and Bill—From Shaniece
For Masi—From Yulin

CONTENTS

ABOUT THE AUTHORS

Dr. Thu T. Nguyen is an Associate Professor in the Department of Epidemiology and Biostatistics at the University of Maryland School of Public Health. As a social epidemiologist, she examines social drivers such as the social and built environment, educational attainment, and racial bias on population health. One area of focus has been using social media data with quantitative, qualitative, and artificial intelligence/machine learning methods to investigate temporal and geographic trends in discourse related to marginalized populations and implications for policy, hate crimes, and health. She is the principal investigator of several National Institutes of Health grants examining the impact of discrimination and racial bias on health using social media data. Her work also examines the positive impact of connection, communication, and community and cultural knowledge. Dr. Nguyen also leads the interdisciplinary research collaborative, Big Data for Health Equity (BD4HE). BD4HE is composed of faculty, trainees, and students from universities across the United States and is committed to advancing theories, methods, and findings related to the use of Big Data for health equity research. The group investigates the impact of the social, cultural, and built environment on health inequities and identifies levers for change. An overarching objective of the group is to provide a formal space for training, mentorship, and collaboration. Dr. Nguyen received her bachelor's degree in Human Biology from Stanford University, her Master of Science in Public Health (MSPH) in Epidemiology from the UNC Gillings School of Global Public Health, and her Doctor of Science (ScD) in Social Epidemiology from the Harvard T.H. Chan School of Public Health.

Dr. Quynh C. Nguyen is an intramural investigator at the National Institute of Nursing Research (NINR). Dr. Nguyen is a social epidemiologist who leverages technology and big data sources to investigate and address health disparities. She served as principal investigator of a career development grant and two R01 grants from the National Institutes of Health to pursue this research program. Specifically, she utilized geotagged Twitter data to characterize the neighborhood social environment and Google Street View data to characterize the neighborhood built environment. Currently, her team is building a question-and-answer chatbot for pregnant and parenting mothers and investigating predictors of fatal motor vehicle collisions using street view imagery and computer vision. Prior to joining NINR, Dr. Nguyen served on the faculty of the University of Maryland School of Public Health in the department of Epidemiology and Biostatistics and the University of Utah College of Health in the department of Health Promotion and Education. She received her bachelor's degree in Human Biology from Stanford University and master's and doctoral degrees in epidemiology from the UNC Gillings School of Global Public Health.

Dr. Shaniece Criss Criss is the Director of the Advocacy and Social Policy Master's Program and Associate Professor in the Health Sciences Department at Furman University in Greenville, SC. As a public health scholar and founding member of the Big Data for Health Equity Research (BD4HE) Collaborative, Dr. Criss utilizes qualitative research to examine how societal issues impact health and to advance health equity and health communication. Beyond academia, Dr. Criss serves as an elected city council member, where she founded the Youth Council Academy, a leadership initiative for middle school students. She also hosts Civically Grown, a leadership podcast reaching listeners in more than 25 countries. In addition, she serves on the board of a healthcare system that serves more than 1.2 million patients annually. As a public health practitioner, Dr. Criss served as the producer and host of a national television show for Guyana's Ministry of Health during her Peace Corps service. She also held positions at ICF International, Centers for Disease Control and Prevention, and CNN. Dr. Criss earned a Doctor of Science (ScD) degree from Harvard T.H. Chan School of Public Health, a Master of Public Administration from Harvard Kennedy School, a Master of Public Health from Emory University, and an undergraduate degree in communication from Oglethorpe University.

Dr. Yulin Hswen is an Associate Professor at the Artificial Intelligence Interdisciplinary Institute at Maryland, Computer, Mathematics and Natural Sciences, the Department of Epidemiology and Biostatistics, School of Public Health at the University of Maryland. She also serves as an Associate Editor at JAMA and JAMA+ AI where she hosts JAMA+ AI conversations. Dr. Hswen received her training as a social and computational epidemiologist at the Harvard T.H. Chan School of Public Health. Dr Hswen is a distinguished AI scholar and her research agenda focuses on developing novel artificial intelligence and multimodal analytic methodologies that integrate social media, clinical, imaging, environmental, and digital behavioral data to identify underlying and unseen factors that drive population health. Dr. Hswen has been at the forefront of public health social surveillance, where she has conducted internet based digital disease intelligence with validated methods used by the CDC, WHO, DHS, DOD, HHS, and EU. She is an expert in creating public facing digital platforms for public health, designed to engage the public and deliver real time information that drives meaningful societal change. Her publication record includes publications in top tier journals such as The New England Journal of Medicine, Journal of the American Medical Association, American Journal of Public Health, Science, Preventive Medicine, Journal of Medical Internet Research, npj Digital Medicine, Nature Human Behaviour, and Scientific Data, and her work has garnered national attention through features in The New York Times, ABC News, Bloomberg News, Nature, and The Wall Street Journal.

LIST OF CONTRIBUTORS

Amrutha S. Alibilli
Department of Epidemiology and Biostatistics
School of Public Health
University of Maryland
College Park
MD
USA

Shaniece Criss
Department of Health Sciences
Furman University
Greenville
SC
USA

Elizabeth Dennard
Department of Epidemiology and Biostatistics
School of Public Health
University of Maryland
College Park
MD
USA

Pankaj Dipankar
National Institute of Nursing Research (NINR)
National Institutes of Health (NIH)
Bethesda
MD
USA

Yulin Hswen
The Artificial Intelligence Interdisciplinary Institute at Maryland (AIM), College of Computer, Mathematical, and Natural Sciences (CMNS),
Department of Epidemiology and Biostatistics
School of Public Health
University of Maryland
College Park
MD
USA

Vidur Jain
Department of Epidemiology and Biostatistics
School of Public Health
University of Maryland
College Park
MD
USA

Katrina Makres
Department of Epidemiology and Biostatistics
School of Public Health
University of Maryland
College Park
MD
USA

Heran Mane
Department of Epidemiology and Biostatistics
School of Public Health
University of Maryland
College Park
MD
USA

Junaid S. Merchant
Department of Epidemiology and Biostatistics
School of Public Health
University of Maryland
College Park
MD
USA

Penchala Sai Priya Mullaputi
Department of Epidemiology and Biostatistics
School of Public Health
University of Maryland
College Park
MD
USA

Quynh C. Nguyen
National Institute of Nursing Research (NINR)
National Institutes of Health (NIH)
Bethesda
MD
USA

Thu T. Nguyen
Department of Epidemiology and Biostatistics
School of Public Health
University of Maryland
College Park
MD
USA

Diego Salazar
National Institute of Nursing Research (NINR)
National Institutes of Health (NIH)
Bethesda
MD
USA

Adwaith Santhosh
Department of Data Science,
College of Computer, Mathematical, and Natural Sciences
University of Maryland
College Park
MD
USA

Kyle Seelman
Department of Computer Science
University of Maryland
College Park
MD
USA

Alaa Sharaf
Department of Epidemiology and Biostatistics
School of Public Health
University of Maryland
College Park
MD
USA

Xiaoya Tang
Department of Electrical and Computer Engineering
University of Utah
Salt Lake City
UT
USA

Tolga Tasdizen
Department of Electrical and Computer Engineering
University of Utah
Salt Lake City
UT
USA

Yajie Xiong
Department of Sociology
University of Maryland
College Park
MD
USA

Xiaohe Yue
Department of Epidemiology and Biostatistics
School of Public Health
University of Maryland
College Park
MD
USA

POSITIONALITY STATEMENTS FOR THE AUTHORS

Thu T. Nguyen

As a social epidemiologist, I examine social drivers of population health. I am particularly interested in investigating issues related to marginalization and resilience. My interests first developed from personal experience, where I learned of the importance of social determinants of health. I immigrated to the United States from Vietnam when I was five with my twin sister and mother. My mom raised us as a single mom with less than a high-school education. Growing up, my mom worked as a waitress and then a flower shop owner. Our family benefited from social programs such as Medicaid and food stamps. I saw my mother's strength in keeping us safe, providing a home, and working hard with the limited resources she had. I also benefited from the love of my father, who, while an ocean away in Vietnam, showed me kindness and care. My childhood and my mother's example imparted upon me a sense of determination and persistence, which is essential in academia. I grew up in an area of California colloquially called "Silicon Valley" for the presence of numerous technology companies. This was an area of great innovation and even greater wealth disparities. My background gave me a firsthand understanding of how social factors such as poverty, immigration policy, race, ethnicity, education, and technology can impact health and sparked my lifelong interest in social epidemiology. I am a mother to two boys. I am also a wife, daughter, sister, friend, mentor, and scholar. I aspire to be a lifelong runner. Running reminds me to dream big and to create and find strength in the struggle.

Quynh C. Nguyen

Thu and I are twin sisters, and hence we share the background described above. Additionally, my perspectives have been shaped not only by the privilege of coming to the United States as a refugee but also by attending incredibly resourced institutions like Stanford University for my undergraduate degree in Human Biology (concentration in marginalized populations) and the University of North Carolina at Chapel Hill for my master's and doctoral degrees in Epidemiology (concentration in social epidemiology). As a graduate student at UNC, I benefited immensely from working with research teams implementing national, population-based health studies. When I transitioned to a faculty role, I continued to be interested in implementing national studies by leveraging existing big data sources such as social media data and Google Street View to measure neighborhood conditions across the United States. I am also a mother, wife, friend, and scholar focusing on the use of data science and artificial intelligence to examine and promote population health.

Shaniece Criss

As a public health scholar, I examine how social, cultural, and digital environments shape population health. As a Christian Black woman raised in the South, my faith and lived experiences ground my commitment to service, compassion, and advocacy while shaping my perspective and approach to research. My middle-class background and higher education provided opportunities and expanded my understanding of power and privilege, while I also witnessed health disparities within my community. These experiences deepened my understanding of how social systems and access shape health and opportunity.

I am a professor, elected official, wife, mother, former foster parent, and community leader. These roles shape how I engage with research, teaching, and communities. Through community-engaged qualitative research, I seek to center the experiences of those with lived experience. In the context of social media and population health, I am particularly interested in how digital communication environments influence trust, access to information, civic participation, and health outcomes across diverse communities.

Yulin Hswen

Studying at Harvard University was a defining moment in pushing myself to think bigger, challenge convention, and learn from some of the most influential minds in science and society. It was there that I recognized the immense power of online spaces and digital communities. The forums and platforms where people confessed fears, searched for belonging, debated ideas, and revealed hidden aspects of themselves were not trivial corners of the internet. They were living records of human behavior, emotion, vulnerability, and social change. That realization shaped my career. I saw that the digital world could become a powerful lens into the collective psyche of society, especially for populations whose voices are often ignored, stigmatized, or unseen in traditional systems. I believe people are often more honest online than anywhere else, and through multimodal analysis of language, images, behaviors, and interactions, we can better understand the forces shaping public health, belief systems, trust, fear, and identity. Social media is deeply imperfect, but it is also one of the most powerful and consequential infrastructures of modern life. It can distort truth and amplify harm; yet it can also expose injustice, democratize voices, and reveal societal shifts in real time. Understanding that tension has become central to my work. Beyond science, I am drawn to objects and spaces with history, craftsmanship, and emotional depth. I collect watches, French and Italian jewelry, art, and crystal from the eighteenth through twentieth centuries because they reflect eras of human ambition, beauty, and expression. I am inspired by intricacy and character, not sterility. Whether in research, design, or life itself, I believe meaning comes from passion, boldness, and a sense of purpose.

Amrutha S. Alibilli

As a first-generation Indian immigrant born in a small rural town in southeast India, my cultural heritage and diverse life experiences have transformed my worldview. Throughout my upbringing, I witnessed the stark realities of healthcare disparities, including long wait times and substandard treatment in the sole district government hospital for over 2.7 million residents in my birth town. These challenges became particularly poignant when my grandfather passed away, not from any disease, but due to the critical shortage of hospital beds during the height of the COVID-19 pandemic in India. Coupled with other profound healthcare experiences, these disparities catalyzed my aspiration to become a physician who upholds ethical integrity, safeguards patient rights, and advances health policy reform.

I represent many "firsts" in my family—the first to attend college in the United States and the first to pursue a medical career. The deeply ingrained gender roles in my family's ancestry have imparted a lasting impression upon me: my great-grandmother toiled under the scorching sun as an agricultural laborer, my grandmother was victim to a child marriage at the tender age of five, and my mother has remained a homemaker despite earning a B.S. in Mechanical Engineering. Considering my ancestral lineage deeply rooted in female homemakers, I aspire to shatter traditional gender stereotypes and become the first female healthcare professional in my family, dedicated to the pursuit of knowledge and the humble service of underserved populations.

This vision to serve a purpose greater than my own has driven me to serve diverse communities. Whether I am translating for Spanish patients at rural medical clinics, assisting terminally ill hospice patients, advancing social justice themes through Indian classical dance, or supporting peers with mental health challenges, I have strived to weave translational health research, public policy advocacy, and complementary dance therapy into a healthcare career rooted in humility, compassion, and holistic healing for all individuals.

Elizabeth Dennard

As an epidemiologist and graduate student, I acknowledge that my life experiences have shaped my worldview, research interests, and professional relationships. My positionality statement serves as an opportunity to be more aware of my own biases and ensure that my research is intentional while respecting those who are impacted by the topics addressed in this book. My primary research interests include the implementation of evidence-synthesis approaches and the examination of social determinants of health, food insecurity, and mental health outcomes among individuals who experience discrimination. As a cisgender woman of Irish and French descent, I recognize that my identity affords privileges in academic and professional spaces. Growing up in a predominantly rural, middle-class town about an hour south of Atlanta, Georgia, I was afforded access to education, housing, and a sense of security based on my perceived race and socioeconomic status. I was primarily raised by my mother, an educator and lifelong learner, who modeled resilience and went out of her way to make me feel safe, loved, and heard. With support from my mother and grandparents, I pursued educational and professional opportunities outside of the small town I grew up in, where I could assess health equity through a qualitative lens for the first time at the University of Georgia. After graduation, I accepted a fellowship at the Food and Drug Administration and pursued my MPH at the University of Maryland, where I realized I wanted to become a social epidemiologist. As a PhD student, these professional and academic opportunities serve as a constant reminder to always approach research with humility, openness, and a willingness to learn from others.

Pankaj Dipankar

I am a first-generation Indian immigrant from a small rural town in central India, known for its rich culture and heritage. I am currently working as a Postdoctoral Visiting Fellow at the National Institute of Nursing Research (NINR), NIH, under the mentorship of Dr. Quynh C. Nguyen. I was trained as an immunologist with a PhD from the Indian Institute of Technology Roorkee. My research combines biomedical sciences with advanced computational methods to address pressing health issues by leveraging machine learning, natural language processing, and computer vision to develop tools for early disease detection and to prevent adverse health outcomes. My work is motivated by a commitment to disparities-focused research and to using technology for meaningful public health impacts. My background is shaped by my journey through biotechnology, immunology, and computational health sciences, as well as my personal experiences navigating diverse academic and cultural settings. I earned a bachelor's degree in biotechnology from Punjab Technical University and a master's degree in biotechnology from Kumaon University. These experiences and perspectives continue to inform my research and reinforce my commitment to enhancing public health.

Vidur Jain

As a first-generation Indian American and a practicing Jain, my values of compassion, equity, and service deeply reflect and shape how I approach my work in public health. Growing up in New Jersey, I witnessed firsthand how chronic conditions like diabetes disproportionately affect communities of color, including my own family. These early experiences shaped my interest in health equity and taught me to think critically about the role of social factors in well-being. My background in data science and my personal connection to health disparities motivate me to continue exploring how technology can be better used to address these challenges. My work with youth-focused programs has shown me the power of education and empathy in creating long-term change. These efforts, along with my broader interests, remind me that meaningful solutions must center the voices and experiences of those most affected. As a student and researcher, I strive to approach every project with humility, curiosity, and a strong sense of purpose grounded in justice.

Katrina Makres

As a public health researcher, I have broadened my understanding of public health throughout the years by obtaining my MPH focused on health equity and spending the years analyzing public health data. My past and current experiences have an impact on my professional and personal life. I am a cis woman of Greek descent, born in Houston, Texas, and I moved throughout my childhood to various states and a different country. I grew up with three older brothers and often found myself in spaces where women were treated differently from men, shaping who I am today. I do recognize the privileges that I have been afforded due to my identity and socioeconomic status, and I try to ensure that my actions are focused on minimizing the gaps we see throughout our lives. I have also faced familial, mental, and physical health and financial hardships that greatly impact my life and how I view my day-to-day. I am a daughter, sister, godmother, aunt, friend, community member, mentor, and researcher. I bring my experiences and perspective to my work centered around public health research.

Heran Mane

I built my career at the intersection of service and analysis. After more than 10 years in the restaurant industry, rising from hostess to board of directors at a restaurant group, I saw firsthand how decisions live or die on the quality of the data behind them and how easily bias can creep in. In 2020, I made a deliberate and drastic pivot into data science and analysis. Since then, I've been applying my training across research programs in public health, using careful data cleaning, statistical reasoning, and reproducible workflows to uncover various factors that affect public health and communicate these findings clearly. What I loved most about hospitality included anticipating needs and delivering what people require before they ask, which still guides my work. My goal is to stay close to people while tackling problems with meaningful, measurable impact, helping stakeholders make fair, evidence-based decisions. Being black, a woman, and an immigrant, I understand very well the paths that were paved for me to build the life I have. That perspective fuels my goal to stay close to people, anticipating needs and delivering clarity, while doing work that carves out more paths for others to live fulfilling, equitable, and healthy lives.

Diego Salazar

I was born and grew up in Colombia, where my career began as a pharmacist, working closely with pediatric and oncology patients. Those early experiences taught me the weight of responsibility in every prescription and awakened my curiosity about how we could use clinical data to go beyond immediate care and prevent risks and improve outcomes. That curiosity led me to research, first through a Master's in Biological Sciences and later a PhD in Engineering at Universidad de Los Andes, where I explored how systems biology, causal inference, and machine learning could bring together different layers of complex data. Over time, I worked at the National Library of Medicine and the National Institute of Nursing Research, where I focused on applying language and computer vision models to clinical records and urban environments, always with the goal of understanding how social and structural factors shape health. Alongside research, I enjoy teaching, mentoring, and collaborating with people from different fields because I think science is enhanced when it is a collaborative endeavor between different communities.

Yajie Xiong

I am a sociology graduate student with a long-standing interest in health inequalities. This passion began during my undergraduate years and grew deeper after an unexpected but eye-opening experience with courses in epidemiology and public health. These classes show clear connections between the key concerns of sociology, like social determinants, power, and inequality, and the questions at the heart of public health. And I also noticed important differences in how each field approaches these issues, both in methods and in focus. These interdisciplinary experiences gave me a more comprehensive lens through which to understand how structural forces shape who gets sick, who stays well, and why.

My perspective is further shaped by witnessing social media's explosive role in health these years. We have observed how these spaces amplify or disrupt health inequity through digital divides and peer support networks. From this context, it is interesting to ask: Whose health stories dominate these platforms? Who are algorithmically silenced? And how might we leverage digital tools to expose rather than entrench systemic barriers?

Xiaohe Yue

Born in China and later moved to the United States for school, my experiences across two very different cultures have shaped a global perspective that I can bring to my work in public health. All the contrasts have raised my interest in understanding how social, environmental, and digital contexts can impact physical and mental well-being, especially for marginalized communities. Living through the COVID-19 pandemic, which some groups referred to as the "Wuhan virus" on social media, reminded me of the urgent need to confront racism and xenophobia in public discourse.

Therefore, I have tried to approach research projects with a focus on health disparities. With over five years of experience applying data science in academic research, I have developed skills in Python, R, database management, and machine learning. Practicing technical skills within public health enhances research impacts and provides more options in resolving real-world issues. In the future, I will continue leveraging my technical expertise and cross-cultural perspectives in research projects, creating more meaningful changes in public health.

PREFACE

Social media is a pervasive exposure that has influenced how people communicate, the information they receive, and their interactions and behaviors both online and offline. We now spend an extraordinary amount of time on social media. This digital realm has become a significant ecosystem where much of our lives unfold. Social media not only reflects but also shapes politics, stock markets, and behavior patterns, and, as studies have shown, can ultimately influence health and the direction of societies. Researchers interested in social determinants of health often focus on exposures at school, work, and home but can neglect our online environment. When we think of research, we narrowly think of randomized controlled trials, clinic-based studies, cohorts of study participants, and questionnaires. These traditional studies are time-consuming, expensive, and may have limited temporal and geographic granularity. Social media remains an underutilized data source and a poorly understood and characterized exposure. Social media data are continuously generated and shared worldwide. They can be used to collect information on events, emerging diseases, behaviors, and therapies closer to real time. As a source of inspiration and community building, as well as a place for misinformation, fear, and hate dissemination, social media can be both a tool for harm and good, and it is up to researchers, policymakers, and the public to understand and use its potential.

Audience

There are three intended audiences.

Public health researchers. This book aims to provide useful guidance, tools, and examples for researchers already conducting research using social media or researchers who are interested in learning how to use social media. The book walks through essential steps in data collection, preparation, analysis, and presentation. We will cover what has been accomplished with social media and important future directions. The book is written using non-jargon language, so people with and without technical expertise in data science can understand and use this resource.

Policymakers. Too often, research findings do not reach policy makers, organizations, or communities who can more directly impact change. Key findings from pivotal studies will be included, and implications from the current landscape of research for reducing health disparities will be presented. Policymakers will learn about both the benefits and harms of social media uncovered through research in this area.

Public. The public will learn about ways to be savvier and more intentional about the social media data they create, use, and are exposed to. The book covers ways in which social media can be used for expression, communication, activism, growth, and self-development.

CHAPTER 1

INTRODUCTION—USING SOCIAL MEDIA FOR HEALTH DISPARITIES RESEARCH

Quynh C. Nguyen[1], Pankaj Dipankar[1], Yajie Xiong[2], Katrina Makres[3], Diego Salazar[1], and Thu T. Nguyen[3]

[1]National Institute of Nursing Research (NINR), National Institutes of Health (NIH), Bethesda, MD, USA

[2]Department of Sociology, University of Maryland, College Park, MD, USA

[3]Department of Epidemiology and Biostatistics, School of Public Health, University of Maryland, College Park, MD, USA

Overview

Disparities in physical and mental health outcomes are impacted by a host of social, biological, and environmental factors. Health disparities research focuses on preventable adverse health outcomes that are influenced by the differential distribution of resources, opportunities, risks, and hazards. This chapter introduces health disparities research—where it has been and where it is headed. Additionally, it explores how social media data, platforms, and interventions can improve health for all. Finally, the chapter highlights key opportunities and pitfalls linked to the intersection of social media and health disparities research.

LEARNING OBJECTIVES

1. Introduce foundational concepts linked to social media use, social determinants of health (SDOH), and health disparities research
2. Provide a summary of how social media has been used to strengthen health disparities research
3. Highlight strengths and limitations of using social media data for health disparities research

Defining Social Determinants of Health

Social determinants of health (SDOH) include the conditions where people are born, live, learn, work, play, and age that impact a wide variety of health and quality-of-life outcomes (Health 2000). Healthy People 2030 highlights five key SDOH domains, including economic stability, education access and quality, healthcare access and quality, neighborhood and built environment, and the social and community context (Health 2000). Over the last few decades, health disparity research has illuminated stark and persistent differences in morbidity and mortality across numerous health outcomes by race and ethnicity, socioeconomic status, gender, and sexual orientation. These differences are further compounded by environmental factors like exposure to air pollution, noise pollution, violence, and unequal access to high-quality education, healthcare, and housing.

One key driver of health disparities includes identity-based discrimination, which refers to the unfair treatment of members of a social group based on prejudicial assumptions and beliefs (Braveman 2013). Forms of identity-based discrimination can occur at the individual or interpersonal level, where a person's conscious or unconscious biases influence their social perceptions and interactions with others. Discrimination can also occur at the structural or institutional level through discriminatory policies, laws, cultural norms, and the inequitable distribution of resources. Examples include residential segregation, including Jim Crow laws that were state and local statutes that enforced segregation, and restricted the purchase of housing units in the United States from 1877 to the mid-1960s (Hein 2019). While housing discrimination is no longer legal, many individuals of color continue to be concentrated in neighborhoods with fewer amenities and resources (e.g., recreational opportunities, high-quality schools) and greater exposure to environmental toxins and risks (Estien et al. 2024).

Discrimination is most commonly assessed at the individual level using self-reports of racial discrimination that are influenced by coping mechanisms (e.g., denial), personality traits (e.g., stigma consciousness and race-based rejection sensitivity), and dimensions of racial identity (e.g., internalized racism) (Nuru-Jeter et al. 2018). Assessing individual-level prejudice via self-reported attitudes has several limitations, including bias and self-censorship, which can compromise the validity of exposure assessments (Krieger and Sidney 1996; Nuru-Jeter et al. 2018). Forms of racism operate at the individual (internalized, personally mediated) and institutional level (Jones 2000). While self-reported individual experiences of discrimination provide valuable insights, they do not capture the broader social climate, which represents another dimension of racial bias that can perpetuate negative health outcomes across diverse populations. Therefore, relying solely on individual-level data may underestimate the overall impact of discrimination and racism on health. In this chapter, we present social media as an underutilized data source for exploring drivers of health disparities. In particular, social media data can be used to construct area-level measures of racial sentiment and bias and enable the examination of health effects of social environment characteristics on individual health outcomes.

Defining Health Disparities

The National Institute on Minority Health and Health Disparities defines health disparities as (NIMHD 2025):

> Health disparities are largely preventable health differences that adversely affect populations who experience greater challenges to optimal health and are closely linked with intergenerational social, economic, and/or environmental factors—primarily observed among racial and/or ethnic minority populations and/or low socioeconomic status (SES) groups. Health disparities may be observed in the risks, prevalence, or problems resulting from specific behaviors, as well as the incidence, prevalence, and mortality from conditions, diseases, and/or disorders. Health disparities also can be observed in health care access, quality, and utilization, and within the delivery of clinical care.

Social media can generate opportunities in promoting health. One opportunity includes the promotion and facilitation of access to health information. For example, hashtags such as #SaludTues or #PrEP4Love have promoted the dissemination of culturally relevant information on SDOH and the promotion of campaigns using a sex-positive approach to HIV prevention, respectively (Phillips et al. 2020; Ramirez et al. 2021). Social media can facilitate the work of public health professionals by increasing engagement with otherwise hard-to-reach populations, such as rural communities. These dynamics can be especially useful for people living with chronic diseases or mental health challenges, positioning social networks as key tools for recruiting participants into health promotion programs (Ndumbe-Eyoh and Mazzucco 2016; Gabarron et al. 2018). Support groups within online communities are strengthened by empowering members and generating a sense of belonging (Keim-Klärner et al. 2023). Additionally, social media offers opportunities for individuals to express solidarity in response to specific events or with other populations.

While social media often supports individual and community-level health promotion, it can also advance health by facilitating broader structural changes, such as inclusive policies and investment in underserved communities. Moreover, information collected through these platforms enables real-time public health insights across diverse communities (Ndumbe-Eyoh and Mazzucco 2016). For example, social media platforms can provide timely understanding of public sentiment to various policies and interventions, offering unique insights that can inform decisions about where and how to deploy resources (Yeung 2018).

While social media can generate opportunities and measurable positive impacts on health, it also presents unique challenges. One challenge lies in the limited access to technology and home broadband, a barrier that especially affects communities of low socioeconomic status and older adults (Welch et al. 2016; Rivera-Romero et al. 2022; Pew Research Center 2024a). For instance, only 57% of U.S. adults with household incomes less than $30,000 have home broadband internet (Pew Research Center 2024a). Only 70% of older adults (65 years or older) and 73% of those living in rural communities have access to home broadband or high-speed internet access (Pew Research Center 2024a). Compounding this challenge is the lack of digital literacy among social media users, which can make it difficult to understand and use information appropriately. This includes the inability to discern between reliable information sources, interpret specialized medical language, and apply information to their health contexts (Welch et al. 2016). The situation is further exacerbated when health messages are not designed with the cultural values, beliefs, or linguistic needs of the target audience in mind. In addition, misinformation represents another major obstacle, as it can undermine trust in public health authorities, encourage harmful health behaviors, and perpetuate the spread of inaccurate information (Ryan and Kushalnagar 2018). Even well-intentioned messages can contribute to health inequities if they do not consider key factors such as SDOH, cultural beliefs of the audience, or barriers related to technology access and digital literacy (Ndumbe-Eyoh and Mazzucco 2016; Qureshi 2016). It is recommended that social media efforts be designed in an inclusive and culturally sensitive manner to minimize these risks and promote health for communities (Qureshi 2016).

Defining Social Media

Social media encompasses a broad array of technologies that enable people to create and share information in virtual communities and social networks (Tufts University Communications 2013; Ahmed et al. 2019). One key aspect of social media is the ability to "allow for the creation and exchange of user-generated content" (Kaplan and Haenlein 2010). Major social media platforms include Instagram, Facebook, X (formerly Twitter), YouTube, TikTok, WhatsApp, and WeChat. According to 2024 data from the Pew Research Center, 85% of U.S. adults have used YouTube, and 70% have used Facebook (Pew Research Center 2024b). About half of U.S. adults use Instagram, and smaller proportions use Pinterest, TikTok, WhatsApp, and X.

Usage of various social media platforms varies by age, gender, level of education, culture, and political party affiliation. For example, 51% of U.S. adult women have used Pinterest compared to only 19% of men (Pew Research Center 2024b). Additionally, social media usage often decreases with age, with 93% of adults aged 18–29 years report having used YouTube compared to 65% of those aged 65 years and older (Pew Research Center 2024b). For Instagram, Snapchat, and TikTok, the majority of are adults under 30 years of age (Gottfried 2024). Facebook, LinkedIn, and WhatsApp are exceptions to this age trend, with the highest usage reported by those in the middle of the age distribution (aged 30–49 years; Gottfried 2024; Pew Research Center 2024b). Concurrent usage of multiple social media platforms is more frequently reported by those under 30 years of age, with the majority (78%) using at least five social media platforms compared to 53% of those aged 30–49, 30% of those aged 50–64, and only 8% of those aged 65 years and older (Gottfried 2024). Additionally, social media usage often increases with one's level of education. This jump in platform usage is greatest for LinkedIn, with 54% of users having attained a college education or greater. However, this pattern is reversed for Snapchat and TikTok, which have higher proportions of individuals with a high school education compared to those with college education or greater (28% vs. 22% for Snapchat and 37% vs. 26% for TikTok; Pew Research Center 2024b). Additionally, these platforms rely on algorithms to curate content for users, so they are more likely to consume content based on their online activity, demographic attributes, and social connections.

Opportunities for the Incorporation of Social Media into Health Research

Social media offers researchers an efficient and cost-effective way to collect large and diverse sets of public health data. These data sources offer a unique opportunity to evaluate racial sentiment at the population level. Cultural values, beliefs, and attitudes expressed on these platforms not only reflect but also influence public norms and behaviors (Albarracin and Shavitt 2018; Radwan 2022). Unlike traditional survey methods, which can be expensive, time-intensive, and prone to self-report bias, social media provides a space where individuals can share a wide range of perspectives, including those related to race and identity (Amodio et al. 2003; Quillian 2006; Rosenman et al. 2011). Moreover, other studies indicate that the perceived anonymity of online environments often encourages individuals to express views they might withhold in face-to-face interactions, thus potentially allowing for a more candid understanding of what people truly believe (Suler 2004). This positions social media as a valuable tool for examining sensitive topics such as race-related conversations and identity-based discrimination. Additionally, Chapter 7 provides more detail about measuring cultural racism using social media data.

Examining Intersectionality

Health disparities are interconnected. Intersectionality—which emerged from Black feminist scholarship and posits that inequalities and life experiences are shaped by interlocking power structures and systems of marginalization (Crenshaw 1989; Collins 1990)—allows for a multiaxis analysis of disparities and discrimination (Cho et al. 2013). Each set of intersecting identities has a varied set of advantages and disadvantages. These identities vary across time and place and shape exposures, risks, and resources that impact health outcomes (Bowleg 2021, 2008). This approach underscores the need to understand disparities beyond single categories of race or gender and instead view them as overlapping systems influencing lived experience and health.

CASE STUDY 1. APPLYING INTERSECTIONALITY LENS TO HEALTH DISPARITIES RESEARCH

In health disparities research, there is growing recognition of the importance of examining how intersecting social identities impact health outcomes. Although intersectional theory has been well-articulated, there remains a relative scarcity of quantitative methods to investigate intersectionality using empirical data. Evans and colleagues applied the Intersectional Multilevel Analysis of Individual Heterogeneity and Discriminatory Accuracy (I-MAIHDA), a methodological innovation that offers social epidemiologists a theory-informed and statistically rigorous framework for quantifying intersectional health inequities and assessing their temporal dynamics. Traditionally, intersectionality research has relied on single-level models incorporating fixed interaction terms (Evans et al. 2023, 2024). However, as more social dimensions are included, these models become increasingly complex and less interpretable. Additionally, small sample sizes within certain intersectional strata may yield unstable estimates. I-MAIHDA addresses these limitations by employing a two-level multilevel random effects model where individual observations (level 1) are nested within intersectional strata (level 2). These strata are defined by all possible combinations of sociodemographic variables under examination. By leveraging the inherent properties of multilevel modeling, such as relative parsimony and precision-weighted effect estimates, this approach enhances the interpretability and robustness of study findings (Evans et al. 2023, 2024).

Using data from the 2017–2021 Youth Risk Behavior Surveillance System (YRBSS), researchers applied logistic I-MAIHDA with random effects to estimate intersectional inequities in suicidal ideation among U.S. high school students based on race, sexual orientation, and gender. Over the five-year period, 18.5% of adolescents reported suicidal ideation in the previous year (Merchant et al. 2025). Rates increased from 16.9% in 2017 to 20.9% in 2021. Heterosexual boys, across all racial groups, reported the lowest levels of suicidal ideation, followed by heterosexual girls. Conversely, bisexual girls (all races), White and Multi-race/Other lesbian girls, and White and Multi-race/Other bisexual boys exhibited the highest rates of suicidal ideation. Before 2020, substantial inequities in suicidal ideation were evident, ranging from 9.8% to 12.7% among heterosexual boys to over 50% among bisexual Multi-race/Other and White girls. Findings also suggested a general worsening of teen mental health over time, particularly among racial and sexual minorities.

Despite the growing crisis in youth mental health in the United States, especially among teen girls, sexual minorities, and certain racial groups, much of the literature is limited in its sociohistorical scope and typically focuses on singular demographic dimensions such as race and gender disparities. Consequently, how overarching sociopolitical factors, state-level policies, and public attitudes relate to intersectional changes in mental health outcomes remains unclear. To address these gaps, a study by Nguyen and colleagues integrated self-reported mental health and social identity data from the CDC YRBSS, state-level LGBTQ+ policy indices, and social media-derived measures of racial sentiment. I-MAIHDA was then applied to calculate precision-weighted estimates of suicidal ideation and suicide attempts at the intersection of six race/ethnicities, four sexual orientations, and two genders across five YRBSS surveys collected biennially from 2015 to 2023 (240 independent samples;Nguyen et al., 2026). The contextual/policy variables (four Census regions, five levels of state-level LGBTQ+ policy, and quartiles of state-level negative racial sentiment) were modeled as random coefficients.

Findings revealed that teen girls and sexual minorities reliably reported worse mental health outcomes compared to boys and heterosexual study participants. However, nuanced intersectional patterns emerged by race, year, and state-level context. Anti-LGBTQ+ policies demonstrated strong associations with suicidal ideation rates, such that teens in states with the worst (most oppressive) compared to best (most protective) LGBTQ+ policies consistently reported higher rates of ideation and exhibited greater inequities across all years compared to teens in states with more protective policies. For example, in 2015, 49% of White bisexual girls in the best-policy states reported suicidal ideation compared to 58% of their counterparts in the worst-policy states. However, suicide attempts were more strongly associated with social-media derived measures of negative racial sentiment. In 2021, teens in states with the most negative racial sentiment consistently had the highest suicide attempt rates, even among the lowest-ranked strata. For instance, suicide attempt rates among Asian heterosexual boys reached 9.2% in the highest sentiment quartile compared to 3.5% in the lowest. While suicidal ideation rates were similar across racial groups, Black, Hispanic, and Other race teens reported substantially higher suicide attempt rates (Nguyen et al., 2026).

These findings highlight the urgent need for more intersectional analyses in teen mental health research. By documenting how multiple, overlapping identities, along with structural and cultural forces influence suicidal ideation and behaviors, the study provides critical insights into the evolving mental health crisis among marginalized adolescents in the United States. Collectively, these observed trends underscore the need for more culturally responsive and policy-informed mental health strategies that address the structural and sociopolitical forces shaping youth suicidality.

Pitfalls for the Incorporation of Social Media into Health Research

Social media, like other forms of self-reported data, can be susceptible to several potential biases. However, it is worth noting that these systematic biases also apply to other observational and experimental studies alike. We will discuss three systematic biases: selection bias, information bias, and confounding bias.

Selection Bias: Selection bias is a distortion in the measure of association (e.g., odds ratio, risk ratio, and risk difference) due to sample selection that does not accurately reflect our target population. People on social media might be substantially different from the full population of interest and selection bias may be at play for certain analyses due to social media platform accessibility and user characteristics. For example, estimating the population prevalence of the flu or certain health conditions or health symptoms might be difficult without adjustment for differences in the compositional characteristics of social media users and the population or community to which the researcher aims to generalize. However, even if social media data cannot replace census measures, estimates derived from social media might still provide useful, albeit noisy, data on certain phenomena. Selection bias may be attenuated if researchers control for sociodemographics, which may require additional data collection and weighting procedures. For instance, researchers from the University of Michigan, Georgetown University, and Social Science Research Solutions conducted a nationally representative survey asking U.S. adults about their sociodemographics and whether they have a personal social media account. Then, they implemented a model-based small area estimation approach to estimate the prevalence and corresponding characteristics of Twitter users at the state level (Jackson et al. 2021). Finally, another way to mitigate selection bias includes using social media data from multiple platforms to increase representativeness and reduce overreliance on data from a single platform.

Information Bias: Information bias is characterized by systematic deviations from the truth arising from errors in data collection, recall, or handling of data. Information bias can occur from inaccuracies in measurement due to faulty equipment (e.g., a portable blood pressure monitor that has lower accuracy compared to the gold standard pressure meter), vague or confusing wording of survey questions, social desirability bias (i.e., tendency of a participant to provide an answer they think will be viewed favorably), interviewer bias (i.e., when the expectations of the interviewer interfere with the judgment of the interviewee), and many other measurement-related issues that can introduce bias. Information bias occurs when measures that the researcher uses do not fully map onto the concept or phenomenon they wish to measure. Using social media data in research may require measurement development for online data sources many of us were not traditionally trained to work with. For example, validated metrics such as the Everyday Discrimination Scale have not yet been developed for social media data. Hence, researchers may need to engage in further measurement development and validation. In addition, constructing a measure from social media data may entail working at the intersection of multiple fields. For instance, using techniques for natural language processing, developed from computer science, combined with scale development from the social sciences, may offer a well-informed approach. Social media-derived indicators can then be validated against previously established gold standards. A study by Kim and colleagues compared a depression classifier using social media text against the Patient Health Questionnaire-9 (PHQ-9) and found moderate accuracy levels (Kim et al. 2022). One important consideration is to clearly distinguish the measure and the concept it is trying to capture. In social sciences, there are theoretical concepts like a trait, behavior, opinion, and emotion that are conceptually distinct from the measure itself. Making this distinction between the concept and the measure allows researchers to evaluate the relationship between the concept and the measure in different ways using metrics such as validity, reliability, and precision as well as bias (Ladd et al. 2020).

Reliability: Reliability is the consistency with which a measure assesses a particular construct. Reliability can also be conceptualized as measurement error, where reliability equals the true variance of the construct divided by the total variance of the measure. A reliable measure produces the same score or classification each time it assesses the same phenomenon.

Construct Validity: Construct validity refers to the extent to which a measure accurately represents the theoretical construct it is intended to assess. It is typically evaluated qualitatively through expert judgment and theoretical grounding. A measure may demonstrate high reliability yet still lack construct validity if it systematically captures a construct different from that intended by the researcher (Ladd et al. 2020).

Confounding Bias: Confounding is another type of systematic bias that applies to observational studies. This bias can occur when another characteristic is correlated with both the exposure variable (or independent variable of interest) and the health outcome variable. To illustrate, if the exposure of interest is multivitamin use and the health outcome is overall mortality, a confounder could be other health behaviors commonly observed among people taking multivitamins (such as diet quality and physical activity). These health behaviors can influence mortality outcomes. In social media and health disparities research, one could examine state-level negative racial sentiment and adverse birth outcomes, where potential confounders could be state-level policies that support and promote maternal and child health outcomes. States with more negative racial sentiment may also have fewer maternal and child health safety net programs. Identifying and adjusting for potential confounders in social media research is challenging because many of the relevant contextual variables, such as policy and government investments, are not directly observable on social media platforms. Researchers may need to integrate data from external sources to mitigate confounding.

Misinformation/Disinformation: Social media platforms offer opportunities for individuals and organizations to share news, information, updates, and opinions. Nonetheless, with this increased ease of spreading information also comes the ease of spreading misinformation or disinformation. According to a 2024 Pew Report, 54% of Americans say they get at least some of their news from social media platforms (Liedke and St. Aubin 2024). While platform fact-checking and X's Community Notes, where people on X collaboratively add context to potentially misleading posts, provide some guardrails against inaccuracies, misinformation, conspiracy theories, and fake news reports are still commonplace. A 2021 study examining misinformation across various health topics on X found that the level of misinformation can reach upward of 87% for some topics. For example, misinformation on vaccines was most common at 43%, followed by noncommunicable diseases, especially cancer at 40%, nutrition and eating disorders at 36%, and various medical treatments at 30% (Suarez-Lledo and Alvarez-Galvez 2021).

Bots: Bots can be used to post messages thousands of times to incite dissent and controversy, and sometimes to further a particular agenda. A study conducted by Broniatowski and colleagues examined the behavior of bots ("accounts that automate content promotion") and trolls ("individuals who misrepresent their identities with the intention of promoting discord") in the context of vaccine debates. They found that bots disseminated anti-vaccine messages and trolls promoted discord and amplified both sides (Broniatowski et al. 2018). Advances in artificial intelligence have further enabled fake content to appear legitimate. High-quality, realistic fake images and videos have been used to fuel the spread of misinformation, propaganda, discourse, and to harass and blackmail individuals (Rana et al. 2022). Bots are not only a threat to individuals' understanding but may also skew social media research findings. Researchers should consider using bot-detection tools or metadata-based analyses to detect and examine the influence of automated accounts on the collected data. However, whether to filter out bots depends on the research question. Exposure to messages by automated bots may be relevant to include in analyses.

Misrepresentation: People online have the ability to misrepresent or distort their online identity. This includes instances where some users may lie about their demographic details and use certain words that represent different cultures. Users can also misrepresent their ideals and point of view to increase engagement and subsequent monetary gain. For example, on X, people can join the Creator Revenue Sharing Program, which gives them a verified account—a blue checkmark by their name—and allows them to get paid as people interact with their posts (X 2024). As controversial content has been seen as a driver for engagement, many users post this type of content, regardless of their true beliefs, to increase their payouts (Williams 2024). This could lead to a collection of posts that may not truly represent people's views or identities while directly impacting social media research data.

KEY POINTS AND TAKEAWAYS

Define Social Media, Social Determinants of Health (SDOH), and Health Disparities

SDOH are social, economic, and environmental factors that influence health outcomes. Advancing health for everyone involves removing barriers to health and ensuring access to health opportunities. Social media plays a role in shaping public perceptions, spreading health information, and offering insights into health disparities.

Discuss Potential Ways Social Media Is Used for SDOH and Health Disparities Research

Social media platforms provide real-time data on public sentiment, racial biases, and discussions linked to numerous health outcomes. Researchers use sentiment analyses, hashtag tracking, and geospatial mapping to study health disparities and systemic inequities. Social media platforms are also used in public health campaigns and community outreach to improve access.

Examine the Strengths and Limitations of Using Social Media for Health Disparities Research

Strengths:

- **Social Media Is a Powerful Tool for Health Disparities Research:** Digital discourse provides unfiltered insights into public perspectives that may be otherwise inaccessible through traditional research methods. Researchers can leverage these large-scale platforms to better understand social climates and address health inequities.
- **Social Media Can Facilitate Health Interventions:** Online campaigns, support groups, and public health initiatives have proven effective in expanding healthcare access, empowering marginalized communities, and promoting healthier behaviors. Social media serves as a bridge between public health organizations and the communities they aim to support.

Limitations:

- **Challenges such as Misinformation and Bias Must Be Addressed:** While social media democratizes information, it also facilitates the spread of misinformation and discrimination, influencing public perceptions and health decisions. Digital literacy gaps and selection bias in platform usage can further distort research findings, requiring careful mitigation strategies.

Conclusion

Social media is transforming health disparities research by providing real-time insights into public attitudes, health disparities, and SDOH. It has opened new avenues for community engagement, public health interventions, and advocacy, allowing researchers and policymakers to better understand and address systemic inequities. However, using social media in health research presents unique challenges. Selection bias, the spread of misinformation, and gaps in digital literacy can distort findings and widen disparities if not carefully addressed. To fully harness the potential of social media, researchers must refine data collection strategies, integrate social media insights with traditional health research methods, and develop culturally inclusive interventions that effectively reach and benefit diverse communities. Despite these challenges, social media remains a powerful and evolving tool for advancing health. By leveraging its strengths while mitigating risks, public health professionals can create more informed, equitable, and impactful strategies, ensuring that everyone, regardless of background, has the opportunity to achieve better health outcomes.

References

Ahmed, Y. A., Ahmad, M. N., Ahmad, N., & Zakaria, N. H. (2019). Social media for knowledge-sharing: a systematic literature review. *Telematics and Informatics, 37*(37), 72–112. doi:10.1016/j.tele.2018.01.015

Albarracin, D., & Shavitt, S. (2018). Attitudes and attitude change. *Annual Review of Psychology, 69*(1), 299–327. Annual Reviews. www.annualreviews.org/doi/10.1146/annurev-psych-122216-011911. doi:10.1146/annurev-psych-122216-011911

Amodio, D. M., Harmon-Jones, E., & Devine, P. G. (2003). Individual differences in the activation and control of affective race bias as assessed by startle eyeblink response and self-report. *Journal of Personality and Social Psychology, 84*(4), 738–753. doi:10.1037/0022-3514.84.4.738

Bowleg, L. (2008). When Black + Lesbian + Woman ≠ Black Lesbian Woman: the methodological challenges of qualitative and quantitative intersectionality research. *Sex Roles, 59*(5–6), 312–325.

Bowleg, L. (2021). Evolving intersectionality within public health: from analysis to action. *American Journal of Public Health, 111*(1), 88–90. ajph.aphapublications.org/doi/full/10.2105/AJPH.2020.306031. doi:10.2105/ajph.2020.306031

Braveman, P. (2013). What is health equity: and how does a life-course approach take us further toward it? *Maternal and Child Health Journal, 18*(2), 366–372. doi:10.1007/s10995-013-1226-9

Broniatowski, D. A., Jamison, A. M., Qi, S., L, A. K., Chen, T., Benton, A., Quinn, S. C., & Dredze, M. (2018). Weaponized health communication: Twitter bots and Russian trolls amplify the vaccine debate. *American Journal of Public Health, 108*(10), 1378–1384. ajph.aphapublications.org/doi/10.2105/AJPH.2018.304567. doi:10.2105/ajph.2018.304567

Cho, S., Crenshaw, K. W., & McCall, L. (2013). Toward a field of intersectionality studies: theory, applications, and praxis. *Signs: Journal of Women in Culture and Society, 38*(4), 785–810. doi:10.1086/669608

Collins, P. H. (1990). *Black Feminist Thought* (pp. 221–238). Routledge.

Crenshaw, K. (1989). Demarginalizing the intersection of race and sex: a black feminist critique of antidiscrimination doctrine, feminist theory, and antiracist politics [1989]. *Feminist Legal Theory, 1989*(1), 57–80. www.taylorfrancis.com/books/e/9780429500480/chapters/10.4324/9780429500480-5. doi:10.4324/9780429500480-5

Estien, C. O., Wilkinson, C. E., Morello-Frosch, R., & Schell, C. J. (2024). Historical redlining is associated with disparities in environmental quality across

California. *Environmental Science and Technology Letters, 11*(2), 54–59. doi:10.1021/acs.estlett.3c00870

Evans, C. R., Nieves, C. I., Erickson, N., & Borrell, L. N. (2023). Intersectional inequities in the birthweight gap between twin and singleton births: a random effects MAIHDA analysis of 2012–2018 New York City birth data. *Social Science & Medicine, 331,* 116063. doi:10.1016/j.socscimed.2023.116063

Evans, C. R., Leckie, G., Subramanian, S. V., Bell, A., & Merlo, J. (2024). A tutorial for conducting intersectional multilevel analysis of individual heterogeneity and discriminatory accuracy (MAIHDA). *SSM – Population Health, 26,* 101664. doi:10.1016/j.ssmph.2024.101664

Gabarron, E., Årsand, E., & Wynn, R. (2018). Social media use in interventions for diabetes: rapid evidence-based review. *Journal of Medical Internet Research, 20*(8), e10303. doi:10.2196/10303

Georgetown University, SSRS, and University of Michigan (2021). MOSAIC: Twitter state estimates [Dataset]. *Measuring Online Social Attitudes and Information Collaborative (MOSAIC).* portals.mdi.georgetown.edu/public/mosaic/MOSAIC-Twitter-State-Estimates.

Gottfried, J. (2024). Americans' social media use. *Pew Research Center.* www.pewresearch.org/internet/2024/01/31/americans-social-media-use/ (accessed 10 January 2026).

Health (2000). Homepage. *Health.* www.health.com/ (accessed 7 November 2025).

Hein, W. (2019. repository.law.umich.edu/mlr/vol118/iss2/5/??utm_source=repository.law.umich.edu%2Fmlr%2Fvol118%2Fiss2%2F5/?&utm_medium=PDF&utm_campaign=PDFCoverPages). The new housing segregation: the Jim crow effects of crime-free housing ordinances. *Michigan Law Review,* (118.2). doi:10.36644/mlr.118.2

Jackson, M., et al. (2021). *Understanding Who Uses Twitter State Level Estimates of Those on Twitter MOSAIC Methods Brief* (accessed 15 October 2025).

Jones, C. P. (2000). Levels of racism: a theoretic framework and a gardener's tale. *American Public Health Association, 90*(8), 1212–1215. doi:10.2105/ajph.90.8.1212. PMID: 10936998; PMCID: PMC1446334

Kaplan, A. M., & Haenlein, M. (2010). Users of the world, unite! The challenges and opportunities of social media. *Business Horizons, 53*(1), 59–68. www.sciencedirect.com/science/article/abs/pii/S0007681309001232. doi:10.1016/j.bushor.2009.09.003

Keim-Klärner, S., Adebahr, P., Brandt, S., et al. (2023). Social inequality, social networks, and health: a scoping review of research on health inequalities from a social network perspective. *International Journal for Equity in Health, 22*(1). doi:10.1186/s12939-023-01876-9

Kim, N. H., Kim, J. M., Park, D. M., Ji, S. R., & Kim, J. W. (2022). Analysis of depression in social media texts through the Patient Health Questionnaire-9 and natural language processing. *Digital Health, 8,* 205520762211142. doi:10.1177/20552076221114204

Krieger, N., & Sidney, S. (1996). Racial discrimination and blood pressure: the CARDIA study of young Black and White adults. *American Journal of Public Health, 86*(10), 1370–1378. doi:10.2105/ajph.86.10.1370

Ladd, J., Ryan, R., Singh, L. et al. (2020). *Measurement considerations for quantitative social science research using social media data.* https://www.zotero.org/google-docs/?bLfdpZ. 10.31234/osf.io/ga6nc (accessed 13 October 2025).

Liedke, J. and Christopher, S.A. (2024). Social media and news fact sheet. *Pew Research Center*, www.pewresearch.org/journalism/fact-sheet/social-media-and-news-fact-sheet/ (accessed 20 October 2025).

Merchant, J. S., Nguyen, T. T., Makres, K., & Evans, C. R. (2025). Intersectional inequities in suicide ideation by race, sexual orientation, and gender among U.S. high school students in the pre and post 2020 waves of the YRBSS: an application of random effects intersectional MAIHDA. *American Journal of Epidemiology*, kwaf114. Epub ahead of print. PMID: 40462348. doi:10.1093/aje/kwaf114

Ndumbe-Eyoh, S., & Mazzucco, A. (2016). Social media, knowledge translation, and action on the social determinants of health and health equity: a survey of public health practices. *Journal of Public Health Policy, 37*(S2), 249–259. doi:10.1057/s41271-016-0042-z

NIMHD (2025). What are health disparities?https://www.nimhd.nih.gov/about/what-are-health-disparities#:~:text=Health%20disparities%20are%20largely%20preventable,populations%20that%20experience%20health%20disparities (accessed 13 October 2025).

Nuru-Jeter, A. M., Michaels, E. K., Thomas, M. D., Reeves, A. N., Thorpe, R. J., Jr., & LaVeist, T. A. (2018). Relative roles of race versus socioeconomic position in studies of health inequalities: a matter of interpretation. *Annual Review of Public Health, 39*(1), 169–188. doi:10.1146/annurev-publhealth-040617-014230

Pew Research Center (2024a). Internet/Broadband fact sheet. *Pew Research Center: Internet, Science & Tech, Pew Research Center*. www.pewresearch.org/internet/fact-sheet/internet-broadband/ (accessed 10 October 2025).

Pew Research Center 2024b. Social media fact sheet. *Pew Research Center*. www.pewresearch.org/internet/fact-sheet/social-media/ (accessed 10 October 2025).

Phillips, G., et al. (2020). PrEP4Love. *JAIDS Journal of Acquired Immune Deficiency Syndromes, 83*(5), 450–456. doi:10.1097/qai.0000000000002297

Quillian, L. (2006). New approaches to understanding racial prejudice and discrimination. *Annual Review of Sociology, 32*(1), 299–328. doi:10.1146/annurev.soc.32.061604.123132

Qureshi, S. (2016). Creating a better world with information and communication technologies: health equity. *Information Technology for Development, 22*(1), 1–14. doi:10.1080/02681102.2015.1121585. (accessed 4 March 2020)

Radwan, M. (2022, www.nature.com/articles/s41599-022-01268-4). Effect of social media usage on the cultural identity of rural people: a case study of Bamha village, Egypt. *Humanities and Social Sciences Communications, 9*(1). doi:10.1057/s41599-022-01268-4

Ramirez, A. G., Aguilar, R. P., Merck, A., Despres, C., Sukumaran, P., Cantu-Pawlik, S., & Chalela, P. (2021). Use of #SaludTues tweetchats for the dissemination of culturally relevant information on Latino health equity: exploratory case study. *JMIR Public Health and Surveillance, 7*(3), e21266. doi:10.2196/21266. (accessed 25 June 2022).

Rana, M. S., Nobi, M. N., Murali, B., & Sung, A. H. (2022). Deepfake detection: a systematic literature review. *IEEE Access, 10*, 25494–25513. doi:10.1109/access.2022.3154404

Rivera-Romero, O., et al. (2022). Social media, digital health literacy, and digital ethics in the light of health equity. *Yearbook of Medical Informatics, 31*(1). doi:10.1055/s-0042-1742503

Robert, V. T., & Hill, L. G. (2011). Measuring bias in self-reported data. *International Journal of Behavioural and Healthcare Research*, *2*(4), 320–332. pmc.ncbi.nlm.nih.gov/articles/PMC4224297. doi:10.1504/ijbhr.2011.043414

Ryan, C., & Kushalnagar, P. (2018). Towards health equity: deaf adults' engagement in social e-health activities and e-communication with health care providers. *Journal of Health Communication*, *23*(9), 836–841. www.ncbi.nlm.nih.gov/pmc/articles/PMC6290250/. doi:10.1080/10810730.2018.1527875

Suarez-Lledo, V., & Alvarez-Galvez, J. (2021). Prevalence of health misinformation in social media: a systematic review. *Journal of Medical Internet Research*, *23*(1), e17187. doi:10.2196/17187

Suler, J. (2004). The online disinhibition effect. *CyberPsychology & Behavior*, *7*(3), 321–326. www.researchgate.net/publication/8451443_The_Online_Disinhibition_Effect. doi:10.1089/1094931041291295

Tufts University Communications (2013). Policy for official social media accounts. *Communications*. communications.tufts.edu/policies-guidelines/tuftssocialmediapolicy/.

Welch, V., Petkovic, J., Pardo, J. P., Rader, T., & Tugwell, P. (2016). Interactive social media interventions to promote health equity: an overview of reviews. *Health Promotion and Chronic Disease Prevention in Canada: Research, Policy and Practice*, *36*(4), 63–75, www.ncbi.nlm.nih.gov/pmc/articles/PMC4964231/. doi:10.24095/hpcdp.36.4.01

Williams, Z. (2024). Racism, misogyny, lies: how did X become so full of hatred? And is it ethical to keep using it? *The Guardian*. www.theguardian.com/technology/article/2024/sep/05/racism-misogyny-lies-how-did-x-become-so-full-of-hatred-and-is-it-ethical-to-keep-using-it

X (2024). Creator revenue sharing | X help. *X.com*. help.x.com/en/using-x/creator-revenue-sharing.

Yeung, D. (2018). Social media as a catalyst for policy action and social change for health and well-being: viewpoint. *Journal of Medical Internet Research*, *20*(3), e94. https://www.jmir.org/2018/3/e94. doi:10.2196/jmir.8508

CHAPTER 2

EMERGENCE OF SOCIAL MEDIA PLATFORMS

Thu T. Nguyen[1], Heran Mane[1], Xiaohe Yue[1], Penchala Sai Priya Mullaputi[1], Elizabeth Dennard[1], Amrutha S. Alibilli[1], Katrina Makres[1], Vidur Jain[1], and Shaniece Criss[2]

[1]Department of Epidemiology and Biostatistics, School of Public Health, University of Maryland, College Park, MD, USA

[2]Department of Health Sciences, Furman University, Greenville, SC, USA

LEARNING OBJECTIVES

1. Provide an overview of social media platforms and changes in use over time
2. Discuss types of engagement and drivers of engagement
3. Discuss experiences of navigating the online environment

Overview of Major Social Media Platforms

Social Media Changes Over Time

Since the advent of social media and digital information sharing, the popularity, functionality, and purpose of various platforms have evolved significantly. Social media is no longer limited to sharing personal updates with family and friends. Instead, it encompasses a broad ecosystem of personalized content, professional content creators, and highly curated information flows shaped by intermediaries such as search engines, internet service providers, content aggregators, and algorithms (Stamenković and Živadinović 2022). As users spend increasing amounts of time online, businesses have leveraged these platforms to target consumers more directly, contributing to a growth in online spending (Shahbaznezhad et al. 2022). Embedded within this transformation is the rise of participatory culture, characterized by users' ability to comment, download, and resend information (Stamenković and Živadinović 2022). This culture, enabled by the rapid development of new communication technologies, has fundamentally redefined the relationship between media producers and consumers. Users have shifted from being the "passive observers of content" to "active participants" and "co-creators of content," exerting influence through interactivity with media.

The transformation of digital communication began with the launch of the World Wide Web in 1989, originally designed for scientific information exchange. Its release to the public catalyzed a global shift in how information is shared and consumed across geographic boundaries (CERN 2025). A milestone came in 1997 with Six Degrees, the first modern social-networking site (Boyd and Ellison 2007). Since then, continuous innovation has made social media central to digital life. This section traces the historical development of social media by examining the rise of key platforms, their evolving features, and changes in user demographics, the foundation for understanding social media's expanding role in communication and consumer behavior.

The Early Pioneers

Classmates.com

Classmates.com, one of the earliest online networking platforms, was developed by Randy Conrads, a former Boeing engineer, in 1995. Having been raised in a military family, Conrads was acutely aware of the difficulties of maintaining social connections. He created Classmates as a way to help U.S.-based high school alumni remain connected, thereby laying the foundational groundwork for future advancements in online social networking. Surviving the rise of new competitors, Classmates continues to serve millions of users in a mixed freemium business model, offering both free and paid services within the platform (Classmates 2010).

Six Degrees

In 1997, a short-lived concept called Six Degrees was introduced based on "Six Degrees of Separation," a theory popularized by Stanley Milgram (1967). The theory suggests that any two individuals in the world can be connected through a chain of "a friend of a friend," linked by a degree of six or fewer networks of connections. Six Degrees, widely credited as the trailblazer of modern-day social media, enabled users to create personal profiles, build, and track their social networks. This feature allowed users not only to interact with their own contacts but also to engage with their contacts' connections and form interest-based groups. Although Six Degrees quickly amassed over a million users, it struggled with scalability and user retention, eventually ceasing operations in 2001. However, its core features and underlying concept became hallmarks of future social-networking platforms (Boyd and Ellison 2007).

Friendster

The early 2000s marked a significant acceleration in the growth of social media. In 2002, Friendster was launched with the aim of connecting users through mutual acquaintances and shared interests. Similar to Six Degrees, it offered profile creation, messaging, and features that provided information on events and topics of interest to users. While Friendster enjoyed rapid initial growth and popularity, it was soon plagued by technical issues. These performance issues, coupled with the emergence of rival competitors such as MySpace and Facebook, led Friendster to lose significant market share and eventually to its shutdown in 2015 (Boyd and Ellison 2007).

MySpace

Launched publicly in August 2003, MySpace became the most prominent social networking platform by the mid-2000s. It distinguished itself through highly customizable profile features, allowing users to modify their profiles using HTML and CSS, embed music and videos, maintain personal blogs and backgrounds, allowing users to turn their profile pages into digital reflections of their identities and fostering a culture that promoted self-expression. This made MySpace especially popular among teenagers, underground subcultures, and musicians (Boyd 2008; Lenhart 2009; Britannica 2025). MySpace was instrumental in shaping the early stages of "digital celebrity" culture. Artists and public figures could create profiles to upload content and interact with fans, ushering in a new era of engagement and visibility (Shklovski and Boyd 2006). Additionally, aspiring artists also leveraged the platform to share their work, engage with audiences, and grow their following. This facilitated the development of parasocial relationships, in which users developed one-sided connections or attachments to a media figure. By 2006, MySpace had become the most visited social media site in the United States (NPR, 2006). However, its dominance was short-lived, as users began migrating to new, more streamlined sites, most notably Facebook. Although MySpace remains operational, its influence and user base have waned significantly in the face of a more competitive and dynamic social media ecosystem.

The Rise of Modern-Day Social Media

The 2000s marked a pivotal period for the proliferation of social media platforms and mobile technologies. The release of the iPhone in 2007 and Android devices in 2008, supported by increasingly accessible Wi-Fi infrastructure, marked a watershed moment that significantly altered how people connected and accessed information (Teodorescu et al. 2023). This smartphone evolution fueled the growth of mobile applications, driving both the emergence of new social media platforms and the transition of existing online networks into mobile apps (Tilson et al. 2012). Previously, digital communication often required returning home to send an email, make a phone call, or transmit a fax. In contrast, mobile internet access enabled instantaneous communication and interaction, fundamentally changing how individuals engage with one another. Smartphones allow users to connect with friends, families, employees and employers, politicians and constituents, sellers and buyers, strangers with shared interests, celebrities and fans, effectively placing social networks in the palm of their hands (Marwick and Boyd 2011). This transition marks a crucial period in the history of social media as it continues to evolve toward mobile applications. The launch of Facebook and YouTube mobile applications in 2007 and 2008 solidified social media's dominance in the mobile era. Facebook

Launched in 2004, Facebook emerged during a time when niche platforms like MySpace dominated the digital landscape. Initially restricted to Harvard students, Facebook soon expanded to other universities and eventually opened to the general public. The company values transparency with limited user anonymity to foster peer-to-peer connections. Several early features contributed to Facebook's widespread appeal. Status updates enabled real-time self-disclosures, and elements like the "poke" feature, which offered a unique way to engage with friends and new connections, fostered a sense of intimacy and playfulness, contributing to Facebook's early success and popularity. Other features, such as photo sharing, group creation, liking posts, and tagging, further promoted the platform's widespread popularity. Furthermore, Facebook provided an unprecedented opportunity for direct consumer engagement, allowing businesses to market products and services directly to users (Hall 2025). In 2006, the company released its Application Programming Interface (API), allowing developers to enhance the platform and improve the user experience. Over time, Facebook evolved into one of the most globally used platforms, attracting over three billion annual users (Statista 2025). Approximately 70% of U.S. adults report using the platform, with disproportionately higher usage among older adults and women compared to other platforms (Pew Research Center 2024; Schaeffer 2024).

Reddit

Founded in 2005 as a news-sharing website, Reddit has evolved into a prominent platform for social commentary and community discussion. Formerly characterized as the "front page of the Internet," Reddit is the seventh-most-visited website in the world, with approximately 5.14 billion monthly visits (Semrush 2025). In contrast to platforms like X and Instagram, Reddit is structured around anonymous, community-oriented topical discussions. Its features include upvoting and downvoting posts, posting anonymously, and aggregating content through subreddits, which are topic-specific communities within Reddit where users discuss and share contents related to particular interests. Despite its community-content focus, the platform has introduced various features for user personalization and identity recognition, including customizable avatars and achievement badges (Sondhi 2025). The Reddit user base is demographically diverse, with approximately 44% of users aged 18–29 years, a predominantly male user base (60%), and 58% residing in the United States (Duarte 2025).

X (Formerly Twitter)

Originally launched in 2006 as Twitter and rebranded to X in 2023, the platform continues to excel in real-time communication with global audiences and serves as a critical venue for health discussions (Karami et al. 2020). Twitter began as a micro-blogging site with a 140-character text limit. These posts, now called "tweets," offered concise updates and quickly attracted a broad user base that included bloggers, tech enthusiasts, and other individuals. The platform introduced several innovations to engage users, including retweets, hashtags, and trending topics. These features enabled real-time categorization of content and facilitated dynamic conversations around unfolding events (Pardes 2017). In 2017, Twitter expanded its character limit from 140 to 280, allowing for more expansive user expression while maintaining the principles of brevity that the platform was established upon. With its rebranding to X in 2023, the platform signified its desire to expand beyond a micro-blogging platform to a more all-inclusive app (Ivanova 2023). X remains a central hub for real-time digital communication, attracting media, political users, celebrities, and niche communities with a historical demographic trend toward younger, male users (Wojcik and Hughes 2019). Approximately 33% of X posts from U.S. adults involve political content, underscoring the platform's political reach (Bestvater et al. 2024). As text-based platforms matured and saturated the digital space, a new wave of visually driven networks emerged, redefining how users share and engage with content and ushering in the next stage of social-media evolution.

Expansion into the Visual Era

YouTube

Launched in 2005, YouTube has become the most widely used video-sharing platform, hosting an immense repository of user-generated health content (Osman et al. 2022). It enables users to engage with multimedia content through sharing, editing, and commenting (AppLogic Networks 2025). Its intuitive user interface and feedback features allow it to be used for a myriad of purposes, from hosting educational webinars to promoting public awareness about diverse topics (Curran et al. 2020). The platform saw explosive growth during the COVID-19 pandemic, as global lockdowns heightened online engagement. However, YouTube also became a significant vector for misinformation. A 2020 study found that approximately 27.5% of COVID-19-related videos contained misinformation, reaching millions of viewers worldwide (Li et al. 2020). Thus, YouTube remains a ripe site for the proliferation of misinformation, and if unchecked, has the potential to significantly undermine evidence-based public knowledge and discourse. YouTube users encompass all age groups, with 90% of teens using the platform and approximately 54% male users (Anderson et al. 2023; Ceci 2025). Given its widespread reach and influence, YouTube plays a complex and powerful role in shaping public understanding, particularly during public health crises. However, it is important to note that the spread and amplification of misinformation applies to all major social media platforms as well.

Pinterest

By 2010, social media had become fully integrated into everyday life, and visual content was emerging as a defining feature of digital platforms. Pinterest launched in 2010 and made publicly available in 2012, quickly gaining traction as a visually oriented platform. It functions as a virtual pinboard, enabling users to save and organize images related to products, inspiration, and creative ideas, particularly within domains such as fashion, design, cooking, and hobbies. While Pinterest may not be considered a traditional social media platform with a focus on direct messaging, it still provides a robust environment for user interaction and boasts 570 million monthly active users that interact with each other's pins, with a notable skew toward a female user base in the United States (Auxier and Anderson 2021).

Instagram

Another visual-centric application, Instagram, was introduced in 2010. It centers on visual storytelling and has become a key platform where influencers, including health professionals, shape narratives, beliefs, and behaviors (Pretorius et al. 2022; Amon et al. 2024). Its dynamic evolution has been marked by the integration of multimodal content. Originally launched as a photo-sharing app, Instagram expanded its offerings by incorporating video content in 2013, shortly after the release of Twitter's Vine (Thompson 2013). The addition of Stories and Reels to its interactive, engaging user interface attracted diverse users. Acquired by Meta in 2012, Instagram has become a popular social media platform among younger, female users, and it is now dominated by content creators and influencers (Meta 2012). Instagram's algorithm-driven feed and influencer ecosystem have made Instagram a powerful hub for lifestyle, health, and wellness content. The platform's visual emphasis allows for the rapid spread of both inspiration and misinformation, positioning it as a key player in the ongoing evolution of digital communication (Rogers 2021). However, research has revealed negative effects: Instagram use has been linked to higher body dissatisfaction and social comparison among female adolescents, revealing its potential adverse impact on mental health (Pedalino and Camerini 2022).

Snapchat

Snapchat, originally launched as Picaboo in 2011, emerged as an influential visual platform. The key concept of the application centered on the sharing of photos and videos that disappeared after a short period, appealing to a desire for ephemeral content sharing and communication (Bayer et al. 2016). Distinctive features such as augmented-reality filters and Bitmojis (personalized emoji avatars) helped the platform distinguish itself from other social media networks. In 2013, the introduction of Stories further boosted its popularity among users and heralded the era of the selfie phenomena (Piwek and Joinson 2016). This innovation later inspired other platforms like Facebook and Instagram to implement similar ephemeral story formats, especially after Meta's offer to purchase Snapchat was declined (Rusli and MacMillan 2013). Compared to other social media platforms, Snapchat has a higher proportion of younger individuals, with about 65% of the user base being between 18 and 29 years old (Sidoti et al. 2024).

TikTok

TikTok, launched in 2016, has rapidly gained global prominence as a short-form video platform. It offers a highly engaging format for sharing content, including public health messages related to chronic disease, mental health, and other public health topics (Zenone et al. 2021; McCashin and Murphy 2023; O'Donnell et al. 2023; Zehrung and Chen 2024). There has been a rapid growth of health and wellness content on TikTok, highlighting its potential as a vehicle for health communication (Sattora et al. 2024). Notably, the most active 25% of U.S.-TikTok users generate 98% of all content, underscoring the significant influence of a relatively small group of creators (Bestvater et al. 2024). Approximately 56% of individuals aged 18–34 years report using the platform, drawn in by its viral short-form videos propelled by a powerful, algorithm-driven feed (Bestvater et al. 2024).

Truth Social

In 2022, Donald Trump launched Truth Social in response to being suspended from platforms such as Twitter (now X) and Facebook in the wake of the January 6th Capitol uprising (Alba et al. 2022). These suspensions have since been lifted. Truth Social offers many familiar features of mainstream social media, such as creating profiles, connecting with other users, and exchanging comments and messages. What sets this platform apart, according to Donald Trump, is his stated commitment to "true freedom of speech" without fear of censorship despite its policy prohibiting content that "disparages, tarnishes or otherwise harms the backers of the site" (Colvin 2021).

Bluesky

BlueSky was first announced in 2019 as an initiative branching out of Twitter before becoming an independent company in 2021. By 2023, BlueSky became an invitation-only microblogging platform during its open beta testing phase and managed to attract over 1 million users. In February 2024, BlueSky announced its public launch and subsequently experienced a surge in users signing onto the platform (Marquit 2025). Although many of the core user-facing features BlueSky offers are similar to its predecessor Twitter, it differentiates itself through its emphasis on openness and decentralization. This structure gives users greater control over their own algorithms and thus empowers them to customize their content feeds. Additionally, BlueSky's commitment to transparency and user empowerment is highlighted by its emphasis on platform interoperability, and it aims to build a service that exists in a wider ecosystem, enabling users across different platforms to interact seamlessly, provided they adopt compatible protocols such as the Authenticated Transfer (AT) protocol, BlueSky's open communication network (Bluesky 2025). BlueSky's focus on transparency and user empowerment highlights a potential shift in the social networking paradigm from invisible algorithms toward a more user-driven and decentralized system.

Other Platforms

Beyond the major platforms discussed above, numerous other services, both established and emerging, have contributed to the broader social media ecosystem. Companies are leveraging existing technologies and finding new ways to reach their target audience and gain market share. Messaging applications such as Meta's WhatsApp, Telegram, and Signal have expanded their functionalities to include social media-like features, such as group creation, broadcast channels, and community hubs, further blurring the line between text messages and public social interaction. These messaging apps have gained wide popularity due to their focus on security and privacy through end-to-end encryption.

In addition, other services like gaming platforms and newly emerging virtual environments are redefining online networking and communication. For example, Twitch, which launched in 2011, is primarily known as a live streaming platform, where gamers broadcast themselves in real time while playing. Although its popularity stems from gaming, Twitch offers other types of content sharing, ranging from live music and sports commentary to everyday lifestyle streams. Platforms like Twitch continue to blur the boundaries between traditional entertainment and personal interaction, fostering more intimate connections with friends and strangers alike, and have been cementing themselves as true challengers of traditional social media markets.

Meanwhile, companies such as Meta are experimenting with immersive digital futures. In 2021, Meta announced The Metaverse, a virtual reality (VR) environment, accessed through VR headsets or glasses, which extends social interaction into three-dimensional, simulated worlds (Meta 2021). Through such technologies, users can transcend the limitations of everyday life and engage in novel, immersive forms of community, entertainment, and interaction.

The history of social media is constantly evolving and adapting, driven by emerging technologies and the desire to reach broader audiences quickly. This dynamic landscape continues to reshape society in profound ways, both beneficial and concerning. These platforms illustrate the power of the digital landscape and the unique opportunities they provide to advance health communication and promote health for all by leveraging diverse formats, algorithms, and creative approaches to engage global audiences effectively (Fung et al. 2020). However, their potential to proliferate harmful and inaccurate health information must not be overlooked (Chan et al. 2021; Osman et al. 2022; Oh 2023; Allen et al. 2024; Ittefaq 2024). As digital platforms continue to expand their reach and capabilities, it is critical to approach their influence with both optimism and caution, recognizing their ability to either reinforce or undermine public well-being. Understanding the evolution of these platforms sets the stage for examining how they function today, particularly how their design features shape user interactivity and engagement.

Interactivity and User Engagement

Interactivity

Interactivity is a core feature of social media platforms, defined by their capacity to enable users to engage with, influence, and shape content while expressing personal identity. As noted by Stamenković and Živadinovic, this dynamic contributes to a broader "culture of simulation" in which users explore and project their individuality within digital environments (Stamenković and Živadinović 2022). Jensen defines interactivity as "a measure of the media's potential ability to let the user exert influence on the content and/or form of the mediated communication" (Stamenković and Živadinović 2022). In addition, interactivity plays a critical role in shaping communication patterns and user behavior online. It not only determines how messages are communicated but also influences users' behaviors and attitudes (Qiao 2019; Sreejesh et al. 2020). As a buildable process, past interactions influence future ones, creating evolving layers of engagement over time (Qiao 2019).

A deeper examination of interactivity reveals that social media supports interactivity in various formats: user-platform, user-user, and user-organization (Stamenković and Živadinović 2022). The extent to which these systems support these interactions is described as functional interactivity (Qiao 2019; Stamenković and Živadinović 2022). How users interact with each other and with an organization can be divided into different levels and described based on interaction type. Most social media platforms fall within the middle level of interaction, where common activities, such as sharing, commenting, and liking, are influenced by the content itself, individual characteristics, and social dimensions (Stamenković and Živadinović 2022). Furthermore, users' perceived interactivity, their sense of connectedness to the platform, others, and organizations play a key role (Xu et al. 2018). Those with higher levels of interactivity are more likely to use social media in the future (Xu et al. 2018). Building on these foundational concepts, Qiao (2019) categorizes interactivity based on level and type, reflecting both the richness of the interaction and the nature of exchange across platforms (Tables 2.1–2.2).

Types of User Engagement

Users' engagement on social media is typically categorized as either active or passive. Active engagement includes behaviors such as liking, commenting, sharing, and posting, while passive engagement refers to noninteractive behaviors like scrolling, viewing, or reading content without further involvement (Shahbaznezhad et al. 2022). Engagement is understood as a multidimensional construct, involving the feelings, experiences, and

Table 2.1 Levels of Interactivity on Social Media (Qiao 2019 / Online Journal of Communication and Media Technologies)

Level	Description
Lowest	Simple exchange of textual information. Examples: blogs and projects
Middle	Incorporation of multimedia content beyond text. Examples: Facebook and Instagram
Highest	Immersive interactions simulating face-to-face communication. Examples: Metaverse and Roblox

Table 2.2 Type of Interactivity on Social Media (Qiao 2019 / Online Journal of Communication and Media Technologies)

Type of interactivity	Description
Medium-based	Exchange of texts, links, photos, videos, etc between users/organizations.
Conversation-based	Dialogue that includes belief expression and opinion sharing between users/organizations.
Process-based	Deepened interaction, typically between organizations and users, developed through prior exchanges.

thoughts that people have—their state of mind—while using the platform, which can change over time (Smith and Gallicano 2015; Syrdal and Briggs 2018; Voorveld et al. 2018; Trunfio and Rossi 2021). There is ongoing scholarly debate over whether engagement is inherently unidirectional, reflecting one-way consumption or bidirectional, involving dynamic, reciprocal exchange (Smith and Gallicano 2015).

According to Qiao (2019), social media engagement encompasses both participation and socialization. Participation is quantifiable through metrics such as likes, comments, and posts, while socialization refers to the emotional content and interpersonal aspects of user activity (Qiao 2019). These dimensions are often employed to measure a social media platform's effectiveness and usability (Voorveld et al. 2018). Yet, previous studies have struggled to clearly distinguish between one's usage online and the emotional involvement associated with digital participation (Smith and Gallicano 2015). Platform design and social context also shape engagement (Di Gangi and Wasko 2016; Voorveld et al. 2018). When platforms are perceived as relaxing or entertaining, engagement levels tend to be higher (Voorveld et al. 2018).

Engagement can also be characterized by levels of user involvement, consumption, contribution, or creation (Trunfio and Rossi 2021). Consumption reflects the most passive form of engagement, limited to content viewing and reading without interaction (Trunfio and Rossi 2021). Users categorized as contributors engage in peer-to-peer interactions; they are actively engaging in social media and are deemed active participants (Van Asperen et al. 2018; Trunfio and Rossi 2021). At the highest level, creation involves producing and sharing original contents, such as posts, videos, or other user-generated media. These varying levels of engagement help illustrate the layered complexity of user interaction across social media ecosystems. While interactivity defines the structural affordances of platforms, user engagement captures how individuals actually participate within these digital spaces, reflecting their motivations, emotions, and degrees of involvement.

Factors Influencing User Engagement

User engagement on social media, manifested through actions such as liking, sharing, or commenting, is influenced by more than individual preference. Rather, it arises from a complex interplay of emotional stimuli, sociocultural context, and the structural design of digital platforms. Audience responses are contingent not only on the informational content itself, but also on the manner and timing of its presentation, the visibility of peer engagement, and the affective responses it elicits. A comprehensive understanding of why certain posts garner attention while others do not requires an examination of the converging emotional, social, and technological dimensions that shape interaction in digital environments.

One of the most consistently influential determinants of user engagement is emotional appeal, particularly as shaped by content framing. Narratives that are emotionally charged, especially those that evoke fear, empathy, or outrage, tend to generate stronger and more widespread reactions. For example, Hosseini and Staab (2023) found that emotionally negative misinformation was significantly more likely to be shared and replied to than content framed in neutral or positive terms. Moreover, the emotional tone embedded in these claims was frequently reflected in user replies, indicating a feedback loop that amplifies interaction and suggests the presence of emotional contagion. This pattern is particularly salient during periods of real-world crisis or disruption, when emotional and informational demands intersect. The COVID-19 pandemic offers a compelling illustration. According to Sievers et al. (2021), migration-related discourse on Twitter intensified during the early months of the pandemic. The report highlights that this surge occurred alongside rising incidents of xenophobia and discrimination directed at migrant communities, underscoring how moments of crisis can amplify emotionally charged discourse and mobilize online engagement. In moments of social disruption, including pandemics, natural disasters, or political upheaval, digital content often becomes both emotionally charged and time-sensitive, leading to greater amplification and intensified interaction.

In addition to emotional and contextual factors, personal and identity relevance also plays a central role in shaping user engagement on social media. Content that reflects a user's immediate needs or life circumstances often prompts more deliberate and goal-oriented interaction. For instance, a student who has recently lost a part-time job may be more inclined to engage with an Instagram post advertising emergency financial aid, as it directly addresses their current challenges. In such cases, personal relevance transforms social media from a space of passive consumption into one of purposeful engagement, guided by lived experience and practical necessity. Similarly, users are more likely to interact with content that aligns with their social identities, values, or collective histories. When a member of a marginalized community is harmed or targeted, such as in incidents of racial violence or anti-LGBTQ+ attacks, others within that community often respond with heightened engagement. For example, Brown et al. (2017) demonstrate this through the #SayHerName movement, where Twitter users identifying with the affected community mobilized tweeting and retweeting in response to police violence against Black women. This collective responsiveness is rooted in a shared sense of vulnerability and a need to assert or defend group identity. In such moments, identity relevance renders content a focal point for solidarity, prompting users to comment, share, and mobilize as a form of communal affirmation and resistance.

While identity and personal relevance are key motivators, they operate alongside broader social and technological dynamics that guide how engagement unfolds on digital platforms. User engagement on social media is rarely an isolated act; rather, it emerges from the interplay of social norms, spatial context, and platform architecture. Social media platforms function as relational spaces, where individuals often look to their peers to determine which content merits attention (Bakshy et al. 2012). This fosters mimicry of visible behaviors such as liking, sharing, or commenting, especially when content displays indicators of popularity such as high likes. These visible signals generate bandwagon effects, whereby content accrues engagement not solely due to its inherent quality, but because it appears socially endorsed. Platform algorithms reinforce these patterns by prioritizing already-popular posts, thereby amplifying existing trends and further embedding dominant forms of engagement (Carnovalini et al. 2025). This socially mediated interaction intensifies when content possesses local relevance. Geographic context significantly influences what users perceive as meaningful or urgent, particularly during periods of public disruption. Content that reflects region-specific conditions, such as local policies, health measures, or community events, often garners higher engagement. Empirical research by Xu et al. (2024) found that geographic co-location between public health experts (PHEs) and the public markedly increased engagement, particularly in discussions about masking and school closures. In such cases, geographic proximity enhances both emotional resonance and perceived immediacy, prompting users to engage more readily with content that speaks directly to their lived environments.

Technological advancements and platform design further enable and accelerate these behaviors. Features such as Instagram's "Poll" and "Question" stickers that are interactive tools in Stories that let users ask questions or gather opinions from their followers, encourage participatory behavior by making engagement simple and direct. Similarly, TikTok's duet and stitch tools allow users to either respond side by side to an existing video (duet) or incorporate a segment of another user's video into their own (stitch), fostering creative collaboration and visibility. These interactive elements lower the barriers to participation by making engagement quick, playful, and publicly visible. These interactive elements invite users to respond not only because of the content itself, but because of how accessible and socially rewarding the act of engagement has become.

Ultimately, user engagement on social media is shaped not solely by content, but by a convergence of social connection, context, and platform design. Emotional triggers, identity relevance, social influence, and technological affordances operate in concert to influence digital participation. Understanding this layered process reveals not only how users engage but also why such engagement carries significance in shaping online discourse and collective behavior. To fully grasp these implications, it is essential to explore how users experience social media, both positively and negatively, within their daily lives.

Navigating the Online Environment

Navigating the online environment requires critical thinking skills and social media literacy, particularly within the context of health disparities research. Social media literacy encompasses numerous skills, ranging from analytical to social to emotional, that empower users to engage with others responsibly online. Media literacy requires an understanding of the deep interconnectedness between digital and physical spaces, an essential perspective for navigating complex online environments and exposures (Polanco-Levicán and Salvo-Garrido 2022). While social media platforms can foster community-based support, knowledge sharing, and provide educational tools for combating misinformation, they simultaneously serve as spaces where users encounter identity-based harassment and discrimination. Online racism is frequently more overt than in-person forms, which are often characterized by microaggressions, stereotype-based assumptions, and coded language that subtly reinforces racial biases (Eschmann and Patton 2025). Openly hateful rhetoric is prevalent in a variety of online contexts, including video games and anonymous comments on social media. For example, an exploratory qualitative study by Criss et al. (2021) aimed to understand Twitter users' lived experiences with race and racism and explore user perceptions of how these experiences impacted their health and well-being. Study participants described overt and subtle forms of racism on Twitter, particularly targeted at Black and Latinx folks, which fueled online echo chambers, where similar views were amplified by other Twitter users (Criss et al. 2021). Additionally, participants noted negative mental, emotional, and physical health outcomes linked to online experiences of racism. Participants employed numerous tactics to navigate this online environment by blocking users, actively engaging in empowering content, and reducing Twitter use overall.

CASE STUDY 1. NAVIGATING IDENTITY IN DIGITAL SPACES

A study by Criss et al. (2025) examined how positive and negative interactions on digital platforms varied by respondent race, ethnicity, gender, sexual orientation, and religion. This exploratory qualitative study involved six focus groups. Participants (n =51) discussed their experiences related to platform engagement, social connectedness, identity-based interactions, and forms of online protection. While many acknowledged the potential of digital platforms to support self-expression and community-building, they also highlighted persistent identity-based discrimination, harassment, and exclusion that negatively impacted their well-being. Individuals of color reported numerous experiences of general hostility, identity-based discrimination, and racial homophily, a tendency for people to form relationships with others of the same racial group. Additionally, respondents who engaged in online gaming reported platform-specific racial discrimination in the form of racial slurs, colorism, and limited character customization options online.

Female gamers also reported a lack of female character customization and representation online. They described feeling unsafe while using gaming platforms and employed numerous security measures (e.g., gender homophily, silencing microphones, altering clothing, and minimizing self-expression) to reduce gender-based discrimination. Members of the LGBTQIA+ community reported frequent fetishization, harassment, and discrimination online, which led them to adopt security measures to conceal their sexual identity. Others noted that few social-media and gaming platforms promoted inclusivity or served as sources of empowerment for LGBTQIA+ users. Respondents also emphasized that factors such as religious affiliation, education level, socioeconomic status, and language influenced their unique online experiences. Ultimately, these findings highlight a need for future research exploring the impact of intersectionality and identity-based discrimination on physical and mental health outcomes among social media users and gamers, which has not received adequate attention across the literature. To protect social media users and gamers from identity-based discrimination, platforms could employ stronger anti-discrimination policies and moderation tools to mitigate negative experiences in real time. Additionally, collaboration with mental health professionals and organizations could also provide in-app resources tailored to users' diverse needs. Finally, promoting digital literacy and user education could help mitigate negative online experiences and the perpetuation of identity-based discrimination. While these identity-based experiences underscore the complexity of navigating digital spaces, a related inquiry considers how such interactions influence both individual and community health outcomes.

CASE STUDY 2. COMPLEXITIES OF CONNECTION

Another study by Criss et al. (2026) explored the health implications, risks, and strategies for self-protection, and safeguarding community members, when using social media and online gaming platforms. This qualitative study offers a nuanced understanding of how digital environments influence mental and physical health outcomes across diverse populations. Digitally active respondents ($n = 51$) reported both positive and negative health outcomes linked to social media and gaming platform use. Positive mental health effects included overall mood improvement, enhanced creativity, and improved social connectedness. Numerous participants noted that social media use elevated mood, combatted existing symptoms of depression and anxiety, and improved their intellectual and self-regulatory abilities. Positive physical health effects included access to health-related information and increased motivation to work out and improve personal dietary behaviors. Common negative mental health effects included decreased life satisfaction, increased addiction, social comparison, and interference with professional opportunities and personal relationships, while negative physical effects from prolonged social media use included eye strain, body aches, and insomnia. Finally, study participants highlighted the importance of personal and community-based protection strategies, including privacy settings and bystander intervention, but emphasized that platforms must do more to ensure user safety.

While online experiences can foster a sense of community and promote positive health outcomes, many platforms contribute to the perpetuation of identity-based discrimination and isolation, which can exacerbate negative health outcomes among marginalized individuals. In response to online threats and attacks, respondents employed numerous techniques to protect themselves and community members. Personal protection strategies included restricting account access, filtering, blocking, using private accounts, managing friend lists, and banning. Additionally, participants regulated content exposure by reducing time spent on social media platforms and avoiding known abusive online spaces. Some users reported that bystander intervention to protect other users from identity-based discrimination helped create a safer online environment. Ultimately, participants emphasized that digital platforms bear significant responsibility in safeguarding users. These findings underscore the dual nature of digital spaces, as arenas for both connection and creativity, as well as sites of discrimination and health harms, particularly for marginalized and identity-based communities.

Future Directions in Social Media Research

Geolocation and Demographic Analysis

Geolocation and demographic data extracted from social media offer significant opportunities for advancing public health research. When combined with external datasets such as census records, environmental factors, or health outcomes, these data enhance the contextual understanding of population-level health dynamics. For example, Nguyen et al. (2020, 2023) examined state-level racial sentiment and incidence of adverse birth outcomes. However, the availability and quality of such metadata are often limited. Geolocation tags may be sparse, inconsistently structured, or restricted due to privacy constraints.

In addition to analyses with geolocated data, researchers have developed demographic inference models to estimate user attributes such as age, gender, race, and socioeconomic status. These models draw from language patterns, user profile details, behavior, and network features to predict personal attributes. For example, He and colleagues (2023) demonstrated the use of brand-following behavior on Twitter to infer socioeconomic status. Their model was validated using a combination of Facebook advertising audience statistics, Twitter profile data, and survey sample responses. Similarly, some models can predict race based on name databases, profile images, self-descriptions, or linguistic cues (Chen et al. 2021). While these techniques expand analytic potential, they also introduce potential biases, particularly if the models are trained on non-representative datasets.

One key challenge in this area is the lack of high-quality training data and standardized evaluation frameworks for demographic prediction models. Without verified ground-truth data, it is difficult to train and evaluate model accuracy or detect systematic bias. This challenge is especially concerning when predictions involve sensitive attributes such as race or financial status, as inaccuracies can reinforce existing social inequities or negative stereotypes. For example, Fosch-Villaronga et al. (2021) highlight how gender prediction models on social media can misclassify users' gender, which can deepen existing biases. The authors advocate for the development of inclusive algorithms and diverse training datasets.

Ethical considerations are central to geolocation and demographic research. Inferring sensitive demographic information raises concerns about user consent, privacy, and potential misuse. Many users are unaware that their data may be used in research, and traditional notions of informed consent may not adequately address the passive nature of data collection in digital spaces. Ethical frameworks must evolve to account for these challenges, ensuring that social media data are used in ways that minimize harm and promote health for all.

Toward Integrated Multiplatform Research

Contemporary social media users engage with diverse platforms for distinct purposes, underscoring the importance of developing analytical approaches suited to multiple environments. For instance, individuals may use X to follow breaking news and public announcements, TikTok and Instagram for personal storytelling, Reddit for in-depth discussions, and Facebook to stay connected with friends, family, and community trends. Emerging platforms such as Bluesky, Mastodon, and Threads are also gaining traction, further expanding the digital ecosystem and offering new frontiers for public health research. Recent scholarship underscores the importance of this platform diversity. For instance, Lim et al. (2022) examined how young adults access and evaluate health information across platforms. Their findings indicate that young people frequently encounter health-related content from their friends or news sources through Facebook, while they prefer YouTube for its video-based learning format, which facilitates easier comprehension. Each platform is shaped by its unique user demographics, platform cultures, content moderation policies, and communication norms. These factors influence how health-related content is produced, shared, and received, necessitating platform-sensitive analytical approaches.

Research focused on a single-platform offers practical advantages, particularly in terms of consistent data structure and streamlined data collection. Such studies are often methodologically simpler and useful for platform-specific questions, such as evaluating a platform's functionality or moderation algorithms (e.g., Facebook's hate speech detection algorithm or reporting features) or examining community networking within a particular platform. However, single-platform analyses may introduce platform-specific bias that does not reflect broader public perceptions.

In contrast, multiplatform analyses provide a more comprehensive view by capturing diverse communicative modalities, including text, images, and videos. This approach enables researchers to observe a wider array of user behaviors and minimizes dependence on the affordances or biases of any single platform. For example, X provides metadata such as geolocation, which is often not available on other social media platforms' public APIs. By comparing data across platforms, researchers can identify cross-platform trends and gain access to a more diverse and representative sample of users. As social media ecosystems continue to diversify, developing robust multiplatform strategies will facilitate future research.

KEY POINTS AND TAKEAWAYS

- **Overview of social media platforms and changes in use over time.**
  Social media has transformed from early digital gathering spaces like Six Degrees and MySpace into multifunctional ecosystems such as Facebook, TikTok, and Reddit. This evolution, fueled by mobile technology and changing user expectations, has shifted platforms from simple networking tools to hubs for activism, commerce, public health messaging, and real-time information exchange. The rise of emerging platforms like BlueSky signals growing user demand for decentralization, transparency, and autonomy in digital interactions.
- **Types of engagement and drivers of engagement.**
  Engagement on social media exists along a spectrum shaped by a complex interplay of personal relevance, emotional intensity, and platform-specific affordances. Features such as TikTok duets or Instagram polls invite direct interaction, while algorithmic systems reinforce and amplify popular content. These dynamics help explain what compels users to like, comment, reshare, or simply observe and reveal how attention is captured, retained, and transformed into influence.
- **Experiences of navigating the online environment.**
  Users, especially those from marginalized backgrounds, may find affirmation, community, and voice, but also encounter harassment, misinformation, and exclusion. Navigation of these risks often involves platform-specific strategies like muting, blocking, or disengaging entirely. Such experiences are not evenly distributed; they are shaped by identity, algorithmic design, and moderation practices, highlighting that equitable participation demands not only access but also safety, transparency, and accountability.

Conclusion

Social media platforms have become integral to how individuals connect, express identity, and engage with pressing public issues. As these platforms evolve from early message boards to sophisticated, algorithm-driven ecosystems, they have not only transformed patterns of communication but also introduced new opportunities and challenges for researchers and practitioners in public health. Understanding user engagement requires more than tracking likes or shares; it demands a critical examination of how design features, social context, and user identities interact to shape behavior and discourse. This chapter provided a historical and conceptual overview of platform evolution, unpacked the complex drivers of engagement, and examined how users experience and navigate online environments. By foregrounding both the affordances and the risks of digital participation, especially for marginalized communities, it underscores the need for health disparities research and platform accountability. As social media continues to shift, so too must our frameworks for understanding it, ensuring they remain responsive to technological change, user needs, and broader social dynamics.

References

Ahmed, S. (2023). Navigating the maze: deepfakes, cognitive ability, and social media news skepticism. *New Media & Society, 25*(5), 1108–1129. doi:10.1177/14614448211019198

Alba, D., Koeze, E., and Silver, J. (2022). Trump's banishment from Facebook and Twitter: a timeline. *The New York Times*. www.nytimes.com/2022/05/10/technology/trump-social-media-ban-timeline.html (accessed 15 October 2025).

Allen, J., Watts, D. J., & Rand, D. G. (2024). Quantifying the impact of misinformation and vaccine-skeptical content on Facebook. *Science, 384*(6699), eadk3451. doi:10.1126/science.adk3451

Amnesty International (2019). 'The Great Hack': Cambridge Analytica is just the tip of the iceberg. *Amnesty International*. https://www.amnesty.org/en/latest/news/2019/07/the-great-hack-facebook-cambridge-analytica/ (accessed 15 October 2025).

Amon, K. L., Brunner, M., & Campbell, A. J. (2024). The reel health care professionals of Instagram: a systematic review. *Cyberpsychology, Behavior and Social Networking, 27*(3), 172–186. doi:10.1089/cyber.2023.0311

Anderson, M., Faverio, M., and Gottfried, J. (2023). Teens, social media and technology 2023. *Pew Research Center*. https://www.pewresearch.org/internet/2023/12/11/teens-social-media-and-technology-2023/ (accessed 3 October 2025)

AppLogic Networks (2025). The 2025 Global Internet Phenomena Report. https://www.applogicnetworks.com/phenomena (accessed 1 October 2025).

Auxier, B. and Anderson, M. (2021). Social media use in 2021. *Pew Research Center*. https://www.pewresearch.org/internet/2021/04/07/social-media-use-in-2021/ (accessed 1 October 2025).

Bakshy, E., Rosenn, I., Marlow, C., & Adamic, L. (2012). The role of social networks in information diffusion (No. arXiv:1201.4145). *arXiv*. doi:10.48550/arXiv.1201.4145

Bayer, J. B., Ellison, N. B., Schoenebeck, S. Y., & Falk, E. B. (2016). Sharing the small moments: ephemeral social interaction on Snapchat. *Information, Communication & Society, 19*(7), 956–977. doi:10.1080/1369118X.2015.1084349

Bestvater, S., Shah, S., Rivero, G., and Smith, A. (2024). How U.S. Adults use TikTok. *Pew Research Center*. https://www.pewresearch.org/internet/2024/02/22/how-u-s-adults-use-tiktok/ (accessed 10 September 2025).

Bluesky (2025). The AT protocol. https://docs.bsky.app/docs/advanced-guides/atproto (accessed 1 November 2025).

Boyd, D. (2008). Why youth (Heart) social network sites: the role of networked publics in teenage social life. *ResearchGate*. https://www.researchgate.net/publication/230854767_Why_Youth_Heart_Social_Network_Sites_The_Role_of_Networked_Publics_in_Teenage_Social_Life (accessed 1 November 2025).

Boyd, D. M., & Ellison, N. B. (2007). Social network sites: definition, history, and scholarship. *Journal of Computer-Mediated Communication, 13*(1), 210–230. doi:10.1111/j.1083-6101.2007.00393.x

Britannica (2025). Myspace: website, history, creators, & facts. https://www.britannica.com/topic/Myspace (accessed 1 November 2025).

Brown, M., Ray, R., Summers, E., & Fraistat, N. (2017). #Sayhername: a case study of intersectional social media activism. *Ethnic and Racial Studies, 40*(11), 1831–1846. doi:10.1080/01419870.2017.1334934

Carnovalini, F., Rodà, A., & Wiggins, G. A. (2025). Popularity bias in recommender systems: the search for fairness in the long tail. *Information, 16*(2), 151. doi:10.3390/info16020151

Ceci, L. (2025). Distribution of YouTube users worldwide as of February 2025, by gender. *Statista*. https://www.statista.com/statistics/1287032/distribution-youtube-users-gender/ (accessed 10 September 2025).

CERN (2025). A short history of the web. *CERN*. https://home.cern/science/computing/birth-web/short-history-web.

Chan, C., Sounderajah, V., Daniels, E., Acharya, A., Clarke, J., Yalamanchili, S., Normahani, P., Markar, S., Ashrafian, H., & Darzi, A. (2021). The reliability and quality of YouTube videos as a source of public health information regarding COVID-19 vaccination: cross-sectional study. *JMIR Public Health and Surveillance, 7*(7), e29942. doi:10.2196/29942

Chen, J., & Wang, Y. (2021). Social media use for health purposes: systematic review. *Journal of Medical Internet Research, 23*(5), e17917. doi:10.2196/17917

Chen, X., Wang, Y., Agichtein, E., & Wang, F. (2021). A comparative study of demographic attribute inference in Twitter. *Proceedings of the International AAAI Conference on Web and Social Media, 9*(1), 590–593. doi:10.1609/icwsm.v9i1.14656

Classmates (2010). About us. *Classmates.Com*. https://content.classmates.com/k/W/a/0/1270758312039.pdf (accessed 1 October 2025).

Colvin, J. (2021). Trump says he's launching a new media company with its own social media platform. *PBS News*. https://www.pbs.org/newshour/politics/trump-says-hes-launching-a-new-media-company-with-its-own-social-media-platform (accessed 1 October 2025).

Congress.gov (2018). Social media adoption by members of congress: trends and congressional considerations. https://www.congress.gov/crs-product/R45337 (accessed 1 October 2025).

Criss (2025). *Navigating identity in digital spaces: An exploratory study of social engagement and interactions* (accessed 15 September 2025).

Criss, S., Michaels, E. K., Solomon, K., Allen, A. M., & Nguyen, T. T. (2021). Twitter fingers and echo chambers: exploring expressions and experiences of online racism using Twitter. *Journal of Racial and Ethnic Health Disparities, 8*(5), 1322–1331. doi:10.1007/s40615-020-00894-5

Criss, S., Kim, H., Xiong, Y., Dennard, E., Nayreau, D. D., Bharadwaj, V., Helsel, E., Jain, V., Lau, S., Alibilli, A., Gonzales, S. M., & Nguyen, T. T. (2025). Navigating identity in digital spaces: an exploratory study of social engagement and interactions. *Social Sciences & Humanities Open, 12,* 102033. doi:10.1016/j.ssaho.2025.102033

Criss S, Xiong Y, Dennard E, Kim H, Nayreau DD, Bharadwaj V, Helsel E, Jain V, Lau S, Alibilli S, Gonzales SM, Hswen Y, Nguyen TT. (2026). Complexities of Connection: Understanding Health, Risk, and Safety on Social Media [Unpublished manuscript]. Department of Health Sciences, Furman University.

Curran, V., Simmons, K., Matthews, L., Fleet, L., Gustafson, D. L., Fairbridge, N. A., & Xu, X. (2020). YouTube as an educational resource in medical education: a scoping review. *Medical Science Educator, 30*(4), 1775–1782. doi:10.1007/s40670-020-01016-w

Di Gangi, P. M., & Wasko, M. M. (2016). Social media engagement theory: exploring the influence of user engagement on social media usage. *Journal of Organizational and End User Computing, 28*(2), 53–73. doi:10.4018/JOEUC.2016040104

Dixon, S.J. (2024). Number of monthly active Facebook users worldwide as of 4th quarter 2023. *Statista.* https://www.statista.com/statistics/264810/number-of-monthly-active-facebook-users-worldwide/.

Duarte, F. (2025). Reddit user age, gender, & demographics (2025). *Exploding Topics.* https://explodingtopics.com/blog/reddit-users (accessed 1 October 2025).

Eschmann, R., & Patton, D. U. (2025). Introduction to the section on race, racism, and digital media. In D. A. Christakis & L. Hale (Eds.), *Handbook of Children and Screens: Digital Media, Development, and Well-Being from Birth Through Adolescence* (pp. 263–267). Springer Nature Switzerland. doi:10.1007/978-3-031-69362-5_36

Fosch-Villaronga, E., Poulsen, A., Søraa, R. A., & Custers, B. H. M. (2021). A little bird told me your gender: gender inferences in social media. *Information Processing & Management, 58*(3), ISSN 0306-4573. doi:10.1016/j.ipm.2021.102541

Fung, I. C.-H., Blankenship, E. B., Ahweyevu, J. O., Cooper, L. K., Duke, C. H., Carswell, S. L., Jackson, A. M., Jenkins, J. C., Duncan, E. A., Liang, H., Fu, K.-W., & Tse, Z. T. H. (2020). Public health implications of image-based social media: a systematic review of Instagram, Pinterest, Tumblr, and Flickr. *The Permanente Journal, 24*(18), 307. doi:10.7812/TPP/18.307

Georgacopoulos, C. and Mores, G. (2020). How fake news affected the 2016 Presidential election. *LSU Fight Fake News.* https://faculty.lsu.edu/fakenews/elections/sixteen.php (accessed 20 October 2025).

Ghahramani, A., de Courten, M., & Prokofieva, M. (2022). The potential of social media in health promotion beyond creating awareness: an integrative review. *BMC Public Health, 22*(1), 2402. doi:10.1186/s12889-022-14885-0

Gilmour, J., Machin, T., Brownlow, C., & Jeffries, C. (2020). Facebook-based social support and health: a systematic review. *Psychology of Popular Media, 9*(3), 328–346. doi:10.1037/ppm0000246

Gire, S. (2014). The role of social media in the Arab spring. *Pangaea Journal.* https://sites.stedwards.edu/pangaea/the-role-of-social-media-in-the-arab-spring/ (accessed 20 October 2025)

Hall, M. (2025). Facebook social network. *Britannica Money.* https://www.britannica.com/money/Facebook (accessed 20 October 2025).

He, Y., & Tsvetkova, M. (2023). A method for estimating individual socioeconomic status of Twitter users. *Sociological Methods & Research, 54*(1), 38–73. doi:10.1177/00491241231168665

Hosseini, A. S. and Staab, S. (2023). Emotional framing in the spreading of false and true claims. 10.48550/ARXIV.2303.16733 (accessed 1 October 2025).

Ittefaq, M. (2024). "It Frustrates Me Beyond Words That I Can't Fix that": health misinformation correction on Facebook during COVID-19. *Health Communication, 39*(12), 2647–2657. doi:10.1080/10410236.2023.2282279

Ivanova, I. (2023). Twitter is now X. Here's what that means. *CBS News.* https://www.cbsnews.com/news/twitter-rebrand-x-name-change-elon-musk-what-it-means/ (accessed 20 October 2025).

Jacob, S. (2023). Vine — The history of social media. *Medium.* https://medium.com/@jacobls/vine-the-history-of-social-media-79d645f3d956 (accessed 15 October 2025).

Jha, A., Lin, L., & Savoia, E. (2016). The use of social media by state health departments in the US: analyzing health communication through Facebook. *Journal of Community Health, 41*(1), 174–179. doi:10.1007/s10900-015-0083-4

Karami, A., Lundy, M., Webb, F., & Dwivedi, Y. (2020). Twitter and research: a systematic literature review through text mining. *IEEE Access, 8,* 67698–67717. doi:10.1109/ACCESS.2020.2983656

Lenhart, A. (2009). Main findings. *Pew Research Center.* https://www.pewresearch.org/internet/2009/01/14/main-findings-13/ (accessed 15 October 2025).

Li, H. O.-Y., Bailey, A., Huynh, D., & Chan, J. (2020). YouTube as a source of information on COVID-19: a pandemic of misinformation? *BMJ Global Health, 5*(5). doi:10.1136/bmjgh-2020-002604

Lim, M. S. C., Molenaar, A., Brennan, L., Reid, M., & T, M. C. (2022). Young adults' use of different social media platforms for health information: insights from web-based conversations. *Journal of Medical Internet Research, 24*(1), e23656. doi:10.2196/23656. PMID: 35040796; PMCID: PMC8808344

Marquit, M. (2025). Britannica money. *Bluesky Social Media Platform.* https://www.britannica.com/money/Bluesky (accessed 1 October 2025).

Marwick, A., & Boyd, D. (2011). To see and be seen: celebrity practice on Twitter. *Convergence: The International Journal of Research into New Media Technologies, 17*(2), 139–158. doi:10.1177/1354856510394539

McCashin, D., & Murphy, C. M. (2023). Using TikTok for public and youth mental health – a systematic review and content analysis. *Clinical Child Psychology and Psychiatry, 28*(1), 279–306. doi:10.1177/13591045221106608

Meta (2012). Facebook to acquire instagram. *Meta Newsroom.* https://about.fb.com/news/2012/04/facebook-to-acquire-instagram/ (accessed 13 October 2025).

Meta (2021). Building the metaverse responsibly. *Meta.* https://about.fb.com/news/2021/09/building-the-metaverse-responsibly/ (accessed 13 October 2025).

Milgram, S. (1967). The small-world problem. *Psychology Today, 1*(1). https://snap.stanford.edu/class/cs224w-readings/milgram67smallworld.pdf

Nguyen, T. T., Adams, N., Huang, D., Glymour, M. M., Allen, A. M., & Nguyen, Q. C. (2020). The association between state-level racial attitudes assessed from Twitter data and adverse birth outcomes: observational study. *JMIR Public Health and Surveillance, 6*(3), e17103. doi:10.2196/17103. PubMed PMID: 32298232

Nguyen, T. T., Merchant, J. S., Criss, S., Makres, K., Gowda, K. N., Mane, H., Yue, X., Hswen, Y., Glymour, M. M., Nguyen, Q. C., & Allen, A. M. (2023). Examining twitter-derived negative racial sentiment as indicators of cultural racism: observational associations with preterm birth and low birth weight among a multiracial sample of mothers, 2011-2021. *Journal of Medical Internet Research, 25*, e44990. doi:10.2196/44990. PMID: 37115602; PMCID: PMC10182466

O'Donnell, N., Jerin, S. I., & Mu, D. (2023). Using TikTok to educate, influence, or inspire? A content analysis of health-related EduTok videos. *Journal of Health Communication, 28*(8), 539–551. doi:10.1080/10810730.2023.2234866

Oh, S.-W. (2023). YouTube, health information, and health literacy. *Korean Journal of Family Medicine, 44*(6), 301–302. doi:10.4082/kjfm.44.6E

Oremus, W. (2024). Bluesky, a trendy rival to X, finally opens to the public. *The Washington Post.* https://www.washingtonpost.com/technology/2024/02/06/bluesky-launch-public-jay-graber/ (accessed 20 October 2025)

Osman, W., Mohamed, F., Elhassan, M., & Shoufan, A. (2022). Is YouTube a reliable source of health-related information? A systematic review. *BMC Medical Education, 22*(1), 382. doi:10.1186/s12909-022-03446-z

Pardes, A. (2017). As Twitter doubles its character count, a brief history of their many changes. *Wired.* https://www.wired.com/story/a-brief-history-of-the-ever-expanding-tweet/ (accessed 20 October 2025).

Pedalino, F., & Camerini, A.-L. (2022). Instagram use and body dissatisfaction: the mediating role of upward social comparison with peers and influencers among young females. *International Journal of Environmental Research and Public Health, 19*(3), 1543. doi:10.3390/ijerph19031543

Pew Research Center (2024). Social media fact sheet. *Pew Research Center.* https://www.pewresearch.org/internet/fact-sheet/social-media/ (accessed 20 October 2025).

Piwek, L., & Joinson, A. (2016). "What do they snapchat about?" Patterns of use in time-limited instant messaging service. *Computers in Human Behavior, 54*, 358–367. doi:10.1016/j.chb.2015.08.026

Polanco-Levicán, K., & Salvo-Garrido, S. (2022). Understanding social media literacy: a systematic review of the concept and its competences. *International Journal of Environmental Research and Public Health, 19*(14), 8807. doi:10.3390/ijerph19148807

Pretorius, C., McCashin, D., & Coyle, D. (2022). Mental health professionals as influencers on TikTok and Instagram: what role do they play in mental health literacy and help-seeking? *Internet Interventions, 30*, 100591. doi:10.1016/j.invent.2022.100591

Qiao, F. (2019). Conceptualizing interactivity on social media and exploring the effects of interactivity on consumers' engagement with online social-interactions. *Online Journal of Communication and Media Technologies, 9*(3), e201913. doi:10.29333/ojcmt/5781

Rogers, R. (2021). Visual media analysis for Instagram and other online platforms. *Big Data & Society, 8*(1). doi:10.1177/20539517211022370

Rusli, E. M. and MacMillan, D. (2013). Snapchat spurned $3 billion acquisition offer from Facebook. *The Wall Street Journal.* https://www.wsj.com/articles/

BL-DGB-30794?gaa_at=eafs&gaa_n=ASWzDAgaaAq5HxStHYqaaWcyQqVBfO-T_nqqNVjl8IliR98TcX_cSjrNQDVsbJDIg58%3D&gaa_ts=684af011&gaa_sig=lXaBqHS5s6I-waNjwpb0lU7zjWdMJk2aS3LktCNwY-IFg9BT1mBhuLZ78u-BOZyF-1Cxw_Rx39mO2sC4l1cpUQ%3D%3D (accessed 20 October 2025).

Sattora, E. A., Ganeles, B. C., Pierce, M. E., & Wong, R. (2024). Research on health topics communicated through TikTok: a systematic review of the literature. *Journalism and Media, 5*(3), 1395–1412. https://www.mdpi.com/2673-5172/5/3/88

Schaeffer, K. (2024). 5 facts about how Americans use Facebook, two decades after its launch. *Pew Research Center.* https://www.pewresearch.org/short-reads/2024/02/02/5-facts-about-how-americans-use-facebook-two-decades-after-its-launch/ (accessed 3 September 2025).

Semrush (2025). Reddit.com: website traffic, ranking, and analytics. *Semrush.* https://www.semrush.com/website/reddit.com/overview/ (accessed 3 September 2025).

Shahbaznezhad, H., Dolan, R., & Rashidirad, M. (2022). The role of social media content format and platform in users' engagement behavior. *Journal of Interactive Marketing, 53*(1), 47–65. SagePub. doi:10.1016/j.intmar.2020.05.001

Shklovski, I. and Boyd, D. (2006). Music as cultural glue: supporting bands and fans on MySpace. *ResearchGate.* https://www.researchgate.net/publication/253458606_Music_as_Cultural_Glue_Supporting_Bands_and_Fans_on_MySpace (accessed 3 September 2025).

Sidoti, O., Dawson, W., Gelles-Watnick, R., et al. (2024). Social media fact sheet. *Pew Research Center.* https://www.pewresearch.org/internet/fact-sheet/social-media/ (accessed 3 September 2025).

Sievers, N., Rango, M., Rowe, F., et al. (2021). Sentiment towards migration during COVID-19: what Twitter data can tell us. *International Organization for Migration (IOM).* https://publications.iom.int/books/sentiment-towards-migration-during-covid-19-what-twitter-data-can-tell-us (accessed 3 September 2025).

Smith, B. G., & Gallicano, T. D. (2015). Terms of engagement: analyzing public engagement with organizations through social media. *Computers in Human Behavior, 53,* 82–90. doi:10.1016/j.chb.2015.05.060

Sondhi, P. (2025). The evolution of reddit profiles. *Agile Insider.* https://medium.com/agileinsider/the-evolution-of-reddit-profiles-c1060ebf2ba7 (accessed 3 September 2025).

Sreejesh, S., Paul, J., Strong, C., & Pius, J. (2020). Consumer response towards social media advertising: effect of media interactivity, its conditions and the underlying mechanism. *International Journal of Information Management, 54,* 102155. doi:10.1016/j.ijinfomgt.2020.102155

Stamenković, I., & Živadinović, T. Đ. (2022). Social media and interactivity from users' perspective. *Applied Media Studies Journal, 3*(2), 21–36. https://msae.rs/index.php/home/article/view/44

Statista. (2025). Facebook - Statistics & Facts. Statista. https://www.statista.com/topics/751/facebook/#topicOverview [Access date: September 3, 2025]

Syrdal, H. A., & Briggs, E. (2018). Engagement with social media content: a qualitative exploration. *Journal of Marketing Theory and Practice, 26*(1–2), 4–22. doi:10.1080/10696679.2017.1389243

Teodorescu, C. A., Durnoi, A., & Vargas, V. (2023). The rise of the mobile internet: tracing the evolution of portable devices. *Proceedings of the International Conference on Business Excellence, 17*(1), 1645–1654. doi:10.2478/picbe-2023-0147

Thompson, C. (2013). Facebook's Instagram Launches Short-Video Product. CNBC. https://www.cnbc.com/2013/06/20/facebooks-instagram-launches-shortvideo-product.html

Tilson, D., Sorensen, C., & Lyytinen, K. (2012). Change and control paradoxes in mobile infrastructure innovation: the Android and iOS mobile operating systems cases. *2012 45th Hawaii International Conference on System Sciences*, 1324–1333. doi:10.1109/HICSS.2012.149

Trunfio, M., & Rossi, S. (2021). Conceptualising and measuring social media engagement: a systematic literature review. *Italian Journal of Marketing, 2021*(3), 267–292. doi:10.1007/s43039-021-00035-8

Van Asperen, M., De Rooij, P., & Dijkmans, C. (2018). Engagement-based loyalty: the effects of social media engagement on customer loyalty in the travel industry. *International Journal of Hospitality & Tourism Administration, 19*(1), 78–94. doi:10.1080/15256480.2017.1305313

Voorveld, H. A. M., Van Noort, G., Muntinga, D. G., & Bronner, F. (2018). Engagement with social media and social media advertising: the differentiating role of platform type. *Journal of Advertising, 47*(1), 38–54. doi:10.1080/00913367.2017.1405754

Wojcik, S.and Hughes, A. (2019). Key takeaways from our new study of how Americans use Twitter. *Pew Research Center*. https://www.pewresearch.org/short-reads/2019/04/24/key-takeaways-from-our-new-study-of-how-americans-use-twitter/ (accessed 9 September 2025).

Xu, P., Raschid, L., & Frias-Martinez, V. (2024). *Does geo-co-location matter? A case study of public health conversations during COVID-19. (No. arXiv:2405.17710). arXiv*. doi:10.48550/arXiv.2405.17710 (accessed 9 September 2025)

Xu, X., Yao, Z., & Sun, Q. (2018). Social media environments effect on perceived interactivity: an empirical investigation from WeChat moments. *Online Information Review, 43*(2), 239–255. doi:10.1108/OIR-12-2016-0344

Yo, J., Minetti, K., Williams, G., & Taylor, P. (2025). Blame the robot: Writing challenges in theage of AI [Unpublished manuscript]. Department of English, University of Virginia.

Zehrung, R.F. and Chen, Y. (2024). Self-expression and sharing around chronic illness on TikTok. *AMIA Annual Symposium Proceedings, 2023*, 1334–1343. https://www.ncbi.nlm.nih.gov/pmc/articles/PMC10785898/ (accessed 9 September 2025).

Zenone, M., Ow, N., & Barbic, S. (2021). TikTok and public health: a proposed research agenda. *BMJ Global Health, 6*(11), e007648. doi:10.1136/bmjgh-2021-007648

CHAPTER 3

SOCIAL MEDIA DATA COLLECTION, CLEANING, AND PROCESSING BY PLATFORM (X, FACEBOOK, INSTAGRAM, REDDIT, AND BLUESKY)

Heran Mane[1], Xiaohe Yue[1], Penchala Sai Priya Mullaputi[1], Adwaith Santhosh[2], Vidur Jain[1], Kyle Seelman[3], Quynh C. Nguyen[4], and Thu T. Nguyen[1]

[1]Department of Epidemiology and Biostatistics, School of Public Health, University of Maryland, College Park, MD, USA

[2]Department of Data Science, College of Computer, Mathematical, and Natural Sciences, University of Maryland, College Park, MD, USA

[3]Department of Computer Science, University of Maryland, College Park, MD, USA

[4]National Institute of Nursing Research (NINR), National Institutes of Health (NIH), Bethesda, MD, USA

Overview

Social media data offer unparalleled opportunities to examine pressing public health issues in real time, from vaccine misinformation and health policy debates to public sentiment around mental health initiatives. However, the landscape is dynamic and constantly evolving. Platforms such as X (formerly Twitter), Facebook, Instagram, TikTok, and Reddit differ in their data access policies, user demographics, cultural norms, and content formats. In this chapter, we explore how these factors affect the utility of each platform for public health research. We also examine their relative strengths and limitations when studying specific populations and health questions. Additionally, we offer guidance on collecting, cleaning, and processing social media data, addressing both the challenges and opportunities associated with different platforms. The chapter begins by outlining the preparatory steps for launching a social media research project.

LEARNING OBJECTIVES

1. Outline the key steps involved in collecting, cleaning, processing, and analyzing social media data for public health research
2. Address platform-specific considerations in data acquisition, access policies, and technical constraints
3. Provide practical coding guidance and recommend relevant tools and resources

This includes formulating research questions, defining data collection purposes, identifying relevant data sources, and understanding data structures. Key considerations include platforms' policies, data-scraping techniques, storage capabilities, and project timelines. We also emphasize the importance of recognizing potential biases that may arise during the data collection process.

The chapter outlines the essential steps in data collection, preparation, analysis, and presentation. Figure 3.1 presents a high-level overview of key considerations that inform each stage of the social media data pipeline. Recommended steps include creating a clear plan for data capture, defining selection criteria (e.g., data types, platform languages, geographic location, and time windows), and addressing data security, compliance, and ethical considerations. The chapter then addresses the practical aspects of data acquisition, highlighting commonly used software tools, Application Programming Interfaces (APIs), and libraries designed for web scraping and data extraction. Given that many platforms support multiple access modalities, choosing a suitable technique is key to ensuring efficiency and alignment with research goals. Once a collection strategy is chosen, researchers are encouraged to identify computational needs and create data storage infrastructures appropriate to the project's scope. Following data collection, the focus shifts to data cleaning and post-processing. This phase emphasizes validation techniques to ensure data quality. Standard procedures include type normalization, imputing missing values, duplicate detection and removal, and noise reduction to produce datasets suitable for downstream analysis.

We outline a variety of analytical approaches ranging from descriptive and exploratory analysis to advanced machine learning and artificial intelligence methods capable of modeling sentiment, network structure, and spatiotemporal patterns. Throughout the process, documenting the research progress and tracking decisions are essential for reproducibility and future advancement. Finally, the chapter concludes by discussing limitations and recommendations for future research to support other scholars and communities examining related topics. By the end of this chapter, readers will gain a comprehensive understanding of how to manage the social media data pipeline, from project planning, data preparation, and cleaning to analysis and presentation.

Step 1. Research planning

Outlining research objectives is an important precursor to conducting social media data analysis. Researchers should begin by formulating clear research questions: what specific aspect of social media and health are you aiming to investigate using collected data? For example, are you interested in sentiments and public opinions around public health policies (Sukhwal and Kankanhalli 2022), impacts on mental health (Braghieri et al. 2022), or associations with birth outcomes (Nguyen et al. 2023)? Clearly defining

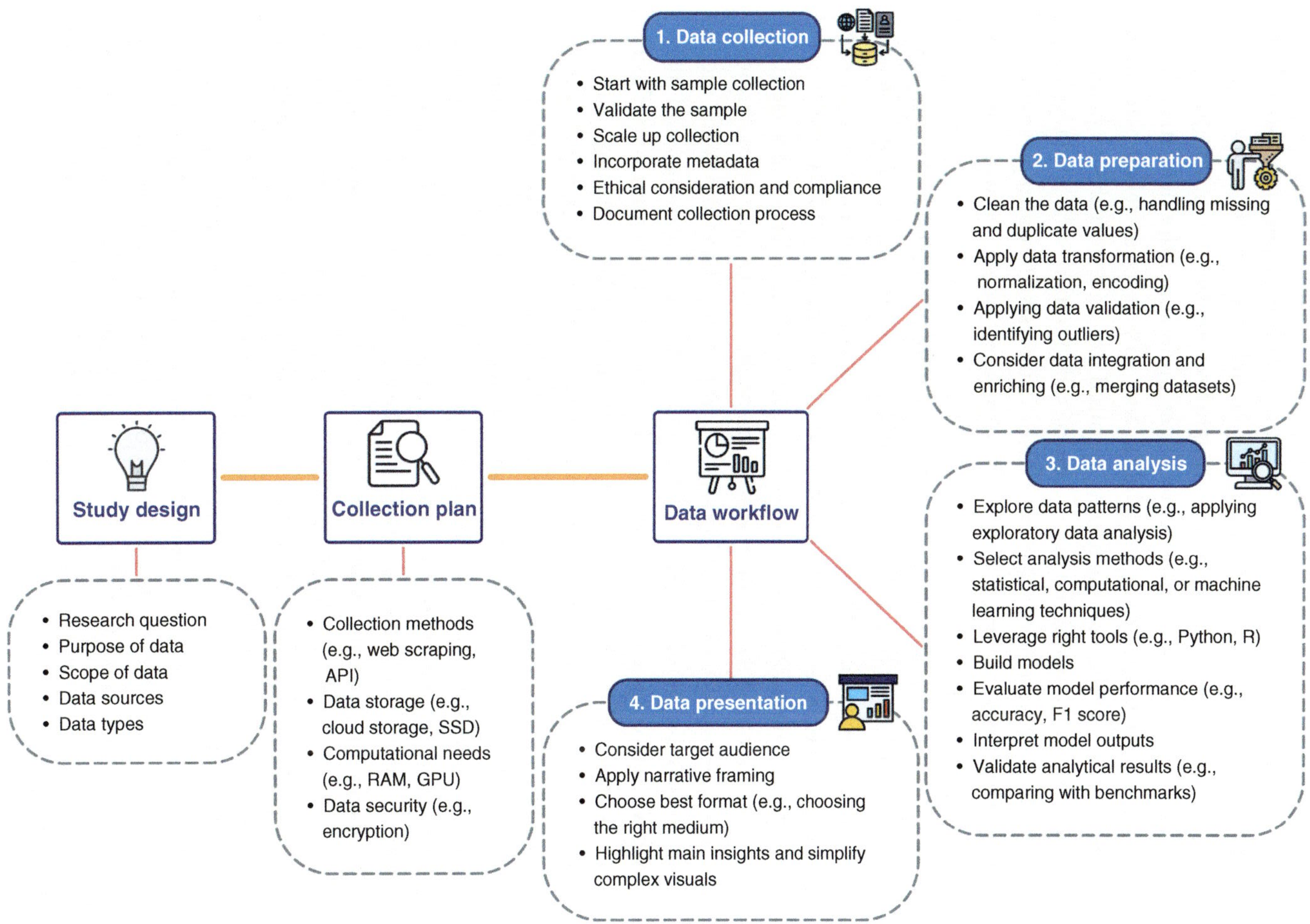

Figure 3.1 High-level guide to data collection, preparation, and presentation.

goals at the outset guides methodological choices and ensures that analytical strategies align with research needs. Evaluating potential data sources is critical, as social media platforms differ substantially in user demographics, content, accessibility, and metadata availability. For instance, X provides real-time textual data, whereas Instagram provides rich visual data. Determining the required data type will help identify the most suitable platforms. Researchers should thoroughly review the documentation provided by the various platforms to better understand the data structures, access policies, metadata availability, and API costs in relation to their research aims. The volume of data required should reflect the scope of the research question and the desired analytical granularity. While large datasets often provide advantages in statistical analysis, they also present challenges in access, storage, and post-processing, which we will explore in subsequent sections.

Moreover, researchers must consider potential biases, including data bias and method bias (Zhao et al. 2022). Platforms differ in user demographics, impacting the generalizability of the findings. For example, younger people tend to use TikTok more often (Bestvater 2024), while older adults are more active on Facebook (Gottfried 2024). Bias can arise from the design of the data collection process itself. For example, many projects rely on keyword-based filtering when downloading data from social media platforms. Keywords often carry multiple contextual meanings, and filtering without contextual validation may lead to misclassification or exclusion of relevant data. Similarly, decisions regarding data cleaning, such as removing perceived noise, may inadvertently exclude meaningful content. In addition, depending on platforms' restrictions, researchers may only be able to download small data samples, which may not fully represent the broader community or discussion under study. When applying preprocessing strategies such as removing stop words, emojis, or duplicates, careful consideration is necessary as these elements may encode subtle but valuable information. When applying post-processing, misclassifications from trained machine learning models may lead to biased conclusions as well. Recognizing and addressing these potential biases throughout the research design process enhances the reliability of the study findings.

Comprehensive documentation is also a critical component of planning. Researchers should record all their research-related decisions in a structured and accessible format so that team members or external collaborators can review and replicate them easily. This practice not only improves transparency and reproducibility but also facilitates future updates or extensions of the study.

Step 2. Collect Social Media Data

Creating a clear plan for data capture is essential to achieving research objectives in a timely and ethical manner. Such a plan should include well-defined data selection criteria, thoughtful consideration for data security, compliance, and a thorough assessment of potential ethical implications. Selecting appropriate data criteria involves defining filters (e.g., keywords, time range, geographic location, language, etc.) and identifying the types of data required: text, images, videos, or a combination. For multilingual or event-based studies, language, time, and location filters are critical in capturing relevant and context-rich information. Additionally, metadata such as user profiles, timestamps, and engagement metrics (e.g., follower and following counts, likes and shares counts, and comments) can help researchers better understand the broader context of social media users' behaviors.

Collecting data from social media platforms requires strict adherence to data security, compliance, and ethical guidelines. These platforms often maintain specific policies regarding how their data can be used, including restrictions on accessing users' information. Researchers must ensure full compliance with these guidelines. Researchers may implement protective multi-layered strategies that include secure data storage with controlled access, anonymization strategies such as masking or pseudonymization, and applying encryptions to alter data into a coded unreadable format. These safeguards help prevent unauthorized access and mitigate risks to privacy (Rubinstein and Hartzog 2016). It is also essential to prioritize informed consent and avoid collecting data that could harm individuals or communities (Varcoe et al. 2009). In addition, researchers should maintain transparency about the purpose and use of the data in the research process to gain trust and to uphold integrity. Institutional Review Board (IRB) approval or equivalent ethical clearance should be sought before any data collection. By carefully selecting data criteria, following security and ethical guidelines, researchers can build a solid foundation for responsible social media data collection.

Different social media platforms provide varying levels and methods of data access, ranging from user-friendly dashboards to API-based access. Figure 3.2 provides a visual illustration of the function of APIs. Meta provides approved users with multiple modes of data access through its Meta Content Library dashboard and its API, available via a restricted Meta enclave. In contrast, X requires approved users to programmatically download data through subscription-based API access. Table 3.1 provides an overview of platform-specific data access details.

The transition from Twitter to X marked a significant shift in how researchers and organizations collect data from the platform. Notably, this change involved the discontinuation of both the public API and the Academic Research API, which have been widely used by researchers for data collection. The Twitter Academic Research API was available for a set of services, including collecting historical tweets and daily streaming tweets at no cost to researchers and organizations (X Developer Platform 2020). Additionally, a public API allowed users to collect a random sample of tweets with a seven-day search index (tweets up to seven

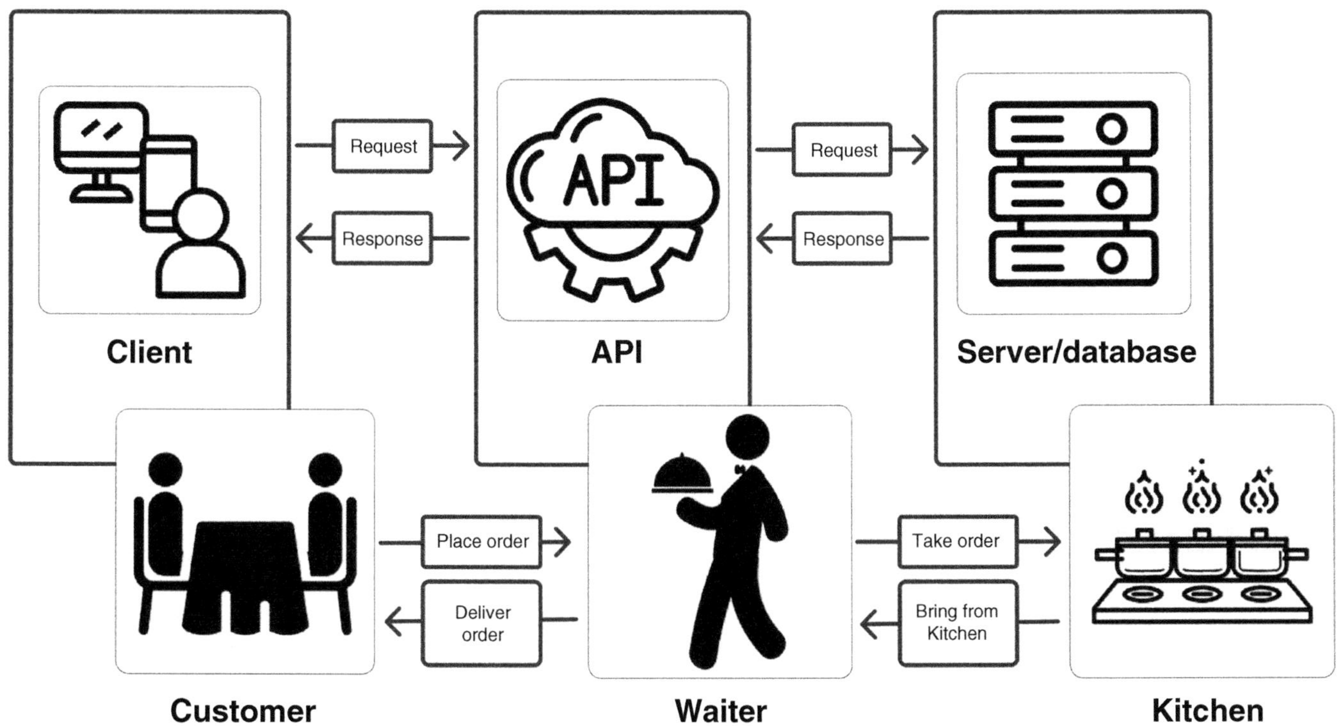

Figure 3.2 Visual illustration of the function of APIs.

Table 3.1 Social Media Data Collection by Platform

	X (Twitter)	Meta	Instagram	Reddit	Bluesky
Key features	Real-time data retrieval	Profile and page management, detailed user data	Images and videos content sharing	Full Reddit Data Analysis	Full Bluesky data available along with images (both historical and live data)
API type	X API v2	Content library API	Content library API	Reddit Data API	Bluesky XRPC Lexicon API
Rate limits	Tier-based: Free: 500 posts/month Basic: 10 K posts/month Pro: 1 M posts/month Enterprise: 50+ million posts/month	60 synchronous calls per minute. 1 asynchronous call per minute. 500,000 data records per 7-day	60 synchronous calls per minute. 1 asynchronous call per minute. 500,000 data records per 7-day	100 queries per minute per Auth client id. 10 queries per minute not using OAuth authentication	3,000 requests per 5 minutes per IP. One request can have a maximum of 100 posts
Cost	Access level-based: Free: free Basic: $200/month Pro: $5,000/month Enterprise: $42 K/month	Free	Free	Free	Free
Data access scope	Limited by tiers	Approved researcher accounts	Approved researcher accounts	Approved accounts	For public posts, no authentication required, open to the public

Citations for Social Media Platforms: X (X Developer Platform 2025c); Meta (Meta 2025b); Instagram (Meta 2025b); Reddit (Reddit 2025); and Bluesky (Bluesky 2025a)

X Data

days old; X Developer Platform 2025c). Under the current structure, X's v2 API free tier offers limited access, permitting up to 100 reads (data retrievals) and 500 posts per month.

While the free API access on X is now largely restricted in terms of data retrieval, researchers seeking access to larger amounts of data must evaluate the cost–benefit of subscription plans. The Basic plan ($200 per month, or $175/month with an annual membership) offers access to 10,000 posts per month. The Pro tier supports retrieval of up to 1,000,000 posts monthly for $5,000, with slight discounts for annual subscriptions ($4,500/month). The Enterprise tier, designed for commercial-scale use, is priced based on usage and begins at $42,000/month. Both the Pro and Enterprise tiers include two search endpoints: the Filtered Stream API, which provides real-time access to posts, and the Full-archive search, for historical data, respectively. Researchers can specify filtering parameters, such as keywords, geolocation, and language, to return root-level fields like "author_id," "id," "posts," and "created_at." This flexibility enables targeted data extraction that can be customized to research objectives.

Facebook and Instagram

Facebook and Instagram data were previously available through CrowdTangle, a public insights tool developed by Meta (Meta 2025a). However, CrowdTangle was officially discontinued in August 2024. Prior to its discontinuation, the tool granted access to over 7 million Facebook entities, including public pages with at least 50,000 likes, groups with over 95,000 members, all U.S.-based public groups with at least 2,000 members, and verified profiles. For Instagram, CrowdTangle provided access to 2 million accounts, including all verified profiles and those with at least 50,000 followers. Researchers using CrowdTangle were able to filter and refine by applying parameters such as time frame, pages, groups, keywords, or geographic region. Output data typically included post content, image URLs, post dates, and engagement metrics.

In November 2023, Meta introduced the Meta content library, a comprehensive multimedia database encompassing public data from Facebook, Instagram, and Threads, effectively replacing Crowdtangle. Researchers may access the Content Library through two interfaces: the Meta Content Library User Interface and a programmatic API accessed through a virtual enclave environment. An application process managed by the Inter-university Consortium for Political and Social Research (ICPSR) at the University of Michigan grants access to researchers who meet the requirements. Eligible researchers must be affiliated with an academic institution or a recognized not-for-profit research organization. The comprehensive application process requires information on the project personnel (e.g., principal investigator, collaborators, and team members), IRB documentation (approvals or exemptions), and signatures on a Restricted Data Use Agreement. Additionally, applicants must also submit detailed information on their intended research study, justification for data use, and a plan for maintaining data security in accordance with Meta's data governance policies (Meta 2025a).

The suitability of the user interface or the API depends on the user's specific requirements, as each offers distinct benefits and potential drawbacks. While the user Meta Content Library web-based tool is more intuitive, accessible, and easier to navigate, the data access can be more limited. The API enclave, on the other hand, provides the ability to extract larger volumes of through advanced querying capabilities, but requires technical expertise and secure enclave access. In the API enclave, users are provided free computational and data analysis resources. Researchers work within a secure version of JupyterHub, an open-source tool that enables users to access and share Jupyter notebooks through a web browser, providing a landscape that promotes collaborative work. The tool supports R, Python, SQL, and a range of standard statistical packages as well as CPU and GPU servers. Users can query up to eight different endpoints that can return up to 100,000 results per query. They are also able to analyze data while maintaining strict security guidelines. Removing, downloading, or copying the data in the enclave is strictly prohibited. Researchers must instead access and work with the data within the secure environment to conduct their research. Any analytical work and results derived from the data must undergo content review and receive approval prior to export.

Users approved for the Meta Content Library interface have access to advanced filtering options, such as date range, keyword, language, and branded content (paid content). The interface allows users to create dashboards based on these filters, providing an easy-to-navigate tool that can be viewed, edited, and shared. The Meta Content Library interface limits downloadable data to posts from Pages with 15,000 or more likes or followers, profiles with 25,000 or more followers, and verified profiles. However, for viewing and exploratory purposes, Pages, Groups, Events, and Profiles with 1,000 or more followers or a verified badge are accessible.

Beginning in November 2025, the Meta API is accessible to researchers through Meta's browser-based platform known as the Meta Secure Research Environment (SRE). The SRE system is a virtual data cleanroom accessible via an Amazon WorkSpaces Secure Browser instance running a modified Jupyter environment. This platform offers researchers access to standard statistical packages, including SQL, Python, and R, while safeguarding user data. Approved researchers can utilize this environment to analyze and, in some cases, integrate data under guidelines and restrictions designed to maintain data security.

Reddit

Reddit, launched in 2005, is a widely used U.S.-based social news and discussion platform. Registered users contribute multimedia content, which can be upvoted or downvoted by others, who may also leave threaded comments. Posts are organized into subject-based communities known as "subreddits," with highly upvoted content surfacing more prominently. In its early years, Reddit faced criticism for failing to curb the spread of hateful content. In 2015, the platform began instituting content moderation reforms, including the banning of explicitly racist forums such as "CoonTown" (Hern 2015). Reddit subsequently implemented "quarantining," measures to limit the visibility of certain subreddits, requiring users to acknowledge a content warning before access (Copland 2020). In 2020, the platform further expanded its policies to explicitly prohibit communities that promoted hate speech. Given Reddit's large and active user base, the platform serves as a valuable resource for studying hate speech and other issues relevant to population health.

Reddit provides a public API that allows researchers to collect Reddit posts, comments, and rating information and apply filters by keyword or date range. Retrieved metadata typically includes subreddit name, post title, post text, creation time, author name, and engagement metrics such as downvote/upvote count, downvote/upvote ratio, and media information such as posted images or videos. In our research, we have collected and analyzed Reddit data spanning from 2009 to 2024 using the Pushshift database, encompassing over 105 million users, over 15 billion comments and posts, and more than 4 million subreddits. The dataset is hierarchically structured across individual, subreddit, sentence, and post levels, facilitating fine-grained analyses of discourse, engagement, and sentiment patterns. This research builds upon foundational projects, particularly the Pushshift Reddit dataset and one of the first large-scale public health projects utilizing Pushshift data, conducted at George Washington University (Lama et al. 2019; Baumgartner et al. 2020).

Bluesky

Bluesky is a relatively new social media platform that gained attention as an alternative space for public discussions. Researchers can access Bluesky data through its publicly available API, which allows users to search and retrieve posts based on specific keywords or timeframes (Bluesky 2025a). As with other platforms, Bluesky's API offers filtering capabilities by date and keyword (Bluesky 2025b). However, individual API requests are limited to 100 posts per call (Bluesky 2025c), requiring multiple API calls to capture large data sets. Although this limitation demands more time and careful planning, the API remains a flexible and cost-free method for gathering data on a large-scale.

Despite the per-request limits, Bluesky's API is sufficiently robust for large-scale studies when paired with proper data collection planning. Common techniques to manage large data volumes are multi-threading and batching, which facilitate efficient data collection at scale. Multi-threading enables simultaneous retrieval of posts across multiple health-related keywords or timeframes, significantly reducing the time needed for data acquisition. Batching, on the other hand, divides data into manageable intervals, ensuring comprehensive coverage while minimizing data loss. In practice, exceeding Bluesky's rate limits may trigger an HTTP 429 (Too Many Requests) error, interrupting the data retrieval process (Bluesky 2025). To minimize such disruptions, sequential API calls are generally recommended for more reliable data retrieval. For example, instead of collecting posts for the keywords "Asian" and "Black" across several dates in parallel, researchers can process each (keyword, date) pair sequentially to reduce errors. In addition, batching—breaking large, continuous queries into smaller intervals—remains an effective way to keep requests within the API's limits. For instance, if a request fails for "Asian" on January 1st, only that batch needs to be retried, preserving the integrity of prior queries. By combining sequential calls with strategic batching, researchers can reduce data loss without triggering excessive rate-limit errors.

As with other platforms, researchers may encounter occasional technical issues such as timeouts or incomplete downloads. These challenges are often resolved with simple retry processes or automated scripts. Although Bluesky posts are predominantly text-based, image content is also available and can be incorporated into multimodal analysis when appropriate. Overall, Bluesky represents a promising resource for the study of emerging discourse. Effective use of its API calls, thoughtful batching, and retry logic enables researchers to build large, reliable datasets for analyzing social trends and public narratives.

Step 3. Process and Clean Social Media Data

Once data collection is complete, rigorous cleaning is required to enhance reliability. This includes removing duplicate or irrelevant data, handling missing data, standardizing data formats, and investigating automated accounts such as bots. Furthermore, based on project needs, processing steps, such as combining datasets from multiple sources, can be applied. This section outlines platform-specific considerations and preprocessing techniques, illustrated through examples from X, Facebook, Instagram, TikTok, and Reddit.

Data cleaning ensures analytical relevance and accuracy. For example, raw data collected from the former Twitter API was provided in JSON format, which often needs an extra step for format conversion. With natural language processing (NLP) analysis, researchers may need to remove noisy content such as stop words, special characters, and URLs from post texts to improve textual coherence. Ethical practice also mandates removing or anonymizing user identifiers (e.g., usernames or handles) to protect individual privacy. Common transformations include lowercasing text, correcting spelling errors, and filtering irrelevant posts. Keywords of interest can then be extracted and categorized to support thematic analysis or content classification. Cleaned textual datasets may then serve as input for sentiment analysis or topic modeling with machine learning models. Geolocation metadata often requires refinement. For example, while some X posts include exact geo coordinates, others use user-defined location fields, which may introduce noise through misspellings or inconsistent granularity (e.g., park name, city location). Standardizing and validating this information is critical for geographic analysis.

Building on these foundational preprocessing steps, further refinement may include deduplicating exact or near-duplicate posts from shared or cross-posted updates to avoid skewed results. However, researchers should carefully consider the study objectives, as retaining duplicates may be appropriate when examining the virality or amplification patterns of specific content. Language filtering can also be useful for multilingual datasets. By using language detection tools (Lui and Baldwin 2012), researchers can exclude irrelevant languages and narrow the focus to the target audience or analytical objectives.

Handling emojis and emoticons is another crucial aspect of cleaning social media data. Emojis often convey meaningful sentiment or contextual nuance (Novak et al. 2015), such as a "thumbs up" emoji signifying positivity. Depending on the project's goals, researchers may choose to remove, normalize, or convert emojis into textual representations (e.g., "thumbs_up") to retain their meaning. Hashtags, similarly, can provide valuable context for analysis. Depending on the research goal, these can be kept intact, stripped of their # symbol, or split into individual words (e.g., #ClimateChange becomes "Climate Change") to improve readability and align with analytical needs (Zappavigna 2015).

Timestamps require careful handling for temporal analysis. Social media data often contains timestamps in various formats and time zones. For example, X metadata is typically recorded in UTC (X Developer Platform 2025), so researchers may need to convert these timestamps to local time zones or retain UTC for consistency across global datasets.

Addressing incomplete or missing data is another important consideration. Empty text fields, missing geographic information, or other gaps in the dataset need to be managed appropriately. Strategies like imputing missing values or discarding incomplete records can help maintain the dataset's quality. Researchers should also normalize slang, abbreviations, and shortened terms frequently used on social media (e.g., "Y" for "Why") to enhance the performance of NLP models (Han et al. 2012).

Image Processing

Images constitute a valuable yet complex data source in social media research, requiring extensive preprocessing to ensure usability. Preprocessing typically begins with standardizing image formats and resolutions. Social media platforms such as Instagram, X, and Reddit host images in various file types (e.g., JPEG, PNG, GIF) and dimensions. Converting these to a consistent format and resizing them to a uniform resolution is essential for efficient processing with Python libraries such as Pillow or OpenCV (Pillow 2025; Open Source Computer Vision 2025). The next step involves filtering out irrelevant or low-quality images that can introduce noise into the dataset, reducing the accuracy of subsequent analyses. Techniques such as blur detection (Narvekar and Karam 2011) or resolution thresholding can be used to discard non-informative or degraded visual content.

Color space conversion is another critical preprocessing step in image analysis, involving the transformation of images between color spaces, such as RGB to grayscale or HSV (hue, saturation, value). For instance, converting an image to grayscale simplifies subsequent analysis by focusing on structural details rather than color information. This step is particularly useful for tasks like optical character recognition (OCR), where the primary goal is to extract textual content from images (Ye and Doermann 2015).

OCR becomes especially valuable when sentiment or context is embedded within images, such as in memes, which often combine visual and textual elements. By extracting textual content from these images, researchers can analyze sentiments, detect patterns, or classify content effectively. Finally, it's essential to filter out irrelevant content using keywords and ensure compliance with privacy and ethical standards by anonymizing personally identifiable information (Townsend and Wallace 2016). Thorough documentation of all steps not only ensures transparency and reproducibility but also reinforces the integrity of the research process.

As platforms continue to prioritize visual content, integrating computer vision techniques with public health research presents new opportunities for insight—but also demands careful methodological attention. For example, distinguishing between authentic health-related images and stylized or meme-based content requires tailored classification strategies. Pretrained convolutional neural networks (CNNs), such as VGG or ResNet, can be fine-tuned to detect relevant visual cues such as masks, pills, or clinical environments (Simonyan and Zisserman 2015; He et al. 2016). However, these models may struggle with noisy, satirical, or culturally nuanced imagery common on platforms like Instagram or Reddit. Researchers are encouraged to supplement automated pipelines with manual annotation strategies to improve labeling accuracy (AlSaad et al. 2024). As image data becomes more central in social discourse, leveraging such hybrid approaches ensures greater validity in visual analysis and enriches the multimodal understanding of health communication online.

The choice of preprocessing techniques should align with the research objective and the nature of the image data. Features relevant in one analytical context may be extraneous in another, and tool selection should reflect both theoretical goals and technical requirements.

Step 4. Data Analysis

After data collection and preprocessing, the next crucial step is data analysis to uncover patterns and insights. This phase can move beyond surface-level engagement metrics to deeper examinations of how different communities interact with public health content. Effective data analysis not only reveals disparities in outreach and engagement but also guides strategic decisions to address those inequities.

Descriptive Analytics: Understanding Trends and Patterns

Descriptive analytics serves as the foundation of social media data analysis, offering a structured approach to summarizing engagement metrics and identifying broad trends. These methods aggregate and visualize key indicators, enabling researchers to assess how users interact with health-related content across different platforms.

Primary aspects of descriptive analysis include:

- **Engagement Tracking**: Analyzing likes, shares, and comments using counts, percentages, and averages.
- **Data Visualization**:
  - Bar charts: Compare engagement across demographics.
  - Time-series plots: Reveal seasonal trends.
  - Heatmaps: Highlight geographic variations.

Beyond identifying overall trends, descriptive analytics can also detect disparities in engagement. By stratifying metrics by demographic categories such as age, gender, ethnicity, and location, researchers can uncover gaps in outreach efforts. As most social media platforms are inherently multimodal in nature, incorporating image-based data into descriptive analytics can enhance analytic depth. Posts that include images, memes, or infographics often receive higher engagement than text-only content, making it crucial to assess the impact of visual elements (Li and Xie 2019). By analyzing the frequency of image-based posts, engagement patterns for different media types, and correlations between text and visuals, researchers can better understand how different content formats influence user behavior.

Exploratory Data Analysis (EDA)

EDA involves an in-depth, systematic assessment of data characteristics prior to advanced modeling. This step ensures data quality and identifies potential sources of biases that might impact research findings.

- **Detecting Missing Data, Outliers, and Inconsistencies:**
  Prior to formal modeling, it's essential to understand the distribution and structure of key variables. Identifying and addressing issues such as missing values, duplicate records, and extreme outliers is critical for ensuring that the analysis is grounded in accurate, representative, and internally consistent data.
- **Examining Data Distributions:**
  Visualization and statistical summaries of data distributions can reveal trends and disparities. For example, plotting age-stratified engagement in a vaccine campaign may highlight underrepresented groups and inform targeted outreach strategies.
- **Using Statistical Techniques to Uncover Relationships:**
  Various statistical methods help uncover significant relationships between variables:
  - **Correlation Analysis:** Measures the strength of relationships between two variables (e.g., how misinformation spreads in relation to engagement rates).

- **Chi-Square Tests:** Assesses associations between categorical variables (e.g., differences in engagement levels by gender).
- **Clustering Techniques:** Group similar data points to discover patterns in audience behavior.

In addition to statistical methods, visual exploratory techniques play a critical role in identifying data patterns, detecting anomalies, and guiding modeling decisions. Tools such as pair plots, violin plots, and interactive dashboards allow researchers to visually assess the joint distributions of variables, helping to uncover nonlinear relationships and potential clusters in the data. For example, visualizing engagement metrics across different post types—text, image, video—can reveal skewed distributions that may affect predictive model performance. Similarly, plotting time-series heatmaps of keyword usage or engagement by hour can surface diurnal patterns or periodic spikes linked to external events. These visual cues not only enhance interpretability but also inform feature engineering and model selection, especially when dealing with high-dimensional or multimodal datasets. Incorporating visual EDA in the early stages of analysis ensures a deeper, more intuitive understanding of the data before proceeding to complex modeling tasks. Combining EDA with domain expertise can further help with distinguishing between true patterns and coincidental correlations.

Following Descriptive Analysis and EDA, the next steps depend on the research question and objectives, guiding whether the focus should be on Text Mining and NLP, Image and Video Analysis, and Geospatial & Temporal Mapping to uncover meaningful patterns and trends.

Text Mining and Natural Language Processing (NLP)

Social media produces an overwhelming volume of textual data, making text mining and NLP indispensable for understanding conversations, tracking emerging topics, and evaluating public sentiment. These techniques enable the extraction of relevant keywords, sentiment, and the identification of dominant discussion trends, providing valuable insights into online discourse.

Several key techniques help process and analyze textual data effectively. Keyword extraction identifies frequently mentioned terms, phrases, and hashtags that are central to discussions. Sentiment analysis classifies posts as positive, negative, or neutral using lexicon-based approaches like VADER (Hutto and Gilbert 2014) and TextBlob (TextBlob 2018), or more sophisticated transformer-based models such as BERT (Devlin et al. 2019) and RoBERTa (Liu et al. 2019). In our own research, we classified sentiment using a Support Vector Machine (SVM), a supervised machine learning model. The SVM model was trained using both publicly available data sources and manually annotated data from our research team (Nguyen et al. 2024). Topic modeling techniques, such as Latent Dirichlet Allocation

(LDA; Blei et al. 2003) and BERTopic (Grootendorst 2022), uncover hidden themes, making it easier to detect shifts in public opinion and trending subjects.

In the context of public health discussions, specific hashtags and terms can reveal key focus areas and user engagement patterns. For instance, discussions around the opioid crisis often include hashtags like #OpioidCrisis, #OverdoseAwareness, and #rehab, while mental health conversations frequently feature terms such as #MentalHealthAwareness, #Anxiety, and #DepressionHelp. By applying NLP and text mining, researchers can track these discussions, monitor engagement levels, and develop data-driven strategies to address critical issues.

Data Visualizations

Data visualization is the art of transforming complex and large-scale data into clear, coherent, and insightful visual representations that facilitate both comprehension and communication. At its core, data visualization is a form of evidence-based storytelling; it requires not only a deep understanding of the data and findings but also an awareness of the target audience. Effective visualizations extract practical and actionable insights from the data in ways that are easily understood even by individuals with varying levels of technical expertise. It is the art of condensing large amounts of data into digestible pieces of information that not only communicate findings effectively but also engage the audience and reinforce knowledge retention.

Beyond its communicative power, data visualization also benefits researchers, especially during the analysis process. It allows researchers to distill data into its most essential elements and helps uncover patterns and trends, gaps and clusters, correlations, and outliers, ultimately illuminating blind spots that statistical models and other methodologies may miss. This process deepens researchers' understanding of their dataset, strengthens the interpretability of findings, and can reveal new research directions previously unconsidered.

Selecting the Appropriate Visualization Strategy

Given the diversity of visualization types and the potential for multiple narrative framings, choosing the appropriate visualization should be guided by the specific analytic question and intended audience. Common objectives include comparative analysis, examining bivariate or multivariate relationships, and analyzing patterns across temporal and spatial dimensions. Selecting a visualization method that aligns with the analytical objective is critical to ensuring interpretability and insight clarity. Comparative visualizations (e.g., bar or column charts) are effective for highlighting differences across categorical groups. Relationship-oriented visualizations (e.g., scatter plots) are suited to exploring interactions or correlations between variables. Distribution plots (e.g., histograms and box plots) reveal how data points are spread or clustered. Geographical maps visualize data across regions, while line graphs and time-series bar charts track trends over time.

CASE STUDY 1. SOCIAL MEDIA SENTIMENT RELATED TO REFUGEES AND IMMIGRANTS

Dr. Nguyen and her team analyzed 6.3 million U.S.-based English-language posts from Twitter (2014–2023), Facebook (2014–2024), and Bluesky (2023–2024) to examine public narratives surrounding refugees and immigrants across platforms. Filtered posts contained one or more of 129 immigration-related keywords, grouped into 76 categories, and sentiment was classified using a supervised SVM model.

Figure 3.3 illustrates the evolution of social media sentiment related to refugees and immigrants on X over the period from 2014 to 2023. The figure depicts a yearly distribution of sentiment classification (positive, negative, and neutral) for posts containing refugee- and immigrant-related keywords. Neutral sentiment predominated throughout the timeframe, accounting for approximately 59.6–78.4% of posts in any given year. Negative sentiment followed in frequency, peaking at 37.9% in 2019. Positive sentiment was relatively minimal, with a lowest point at 2.4% in 2019. A marked increase in positive sentiment was observed in 2022 and 2023, nearly doubling in proportion, coinciding with a decline in negative sentiment.

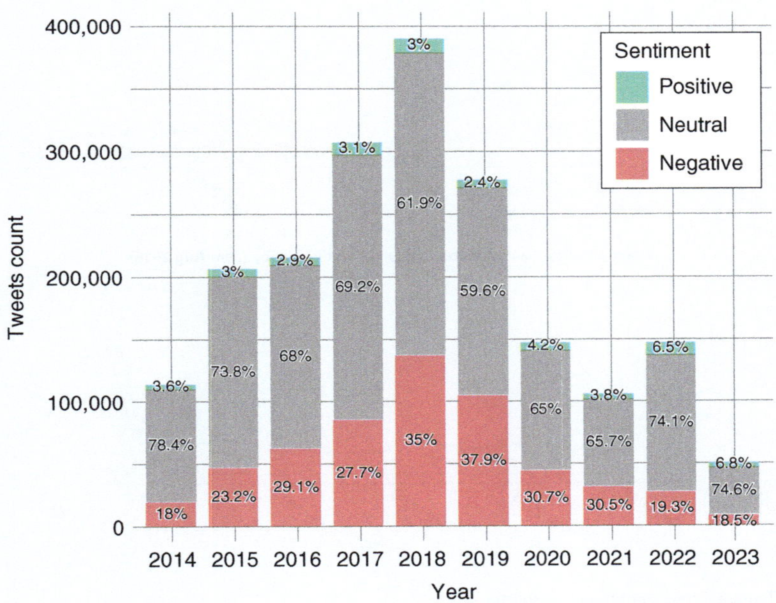

Figure 3.3 Yearly distribution of sentiment of posts containing refugee and immigrant keywords on Twitter (2014–2023).

Source: Nguyen et al. (2025) / Elsevier / CC BY 4.0.

To take a closer look at changes in sentiment for specific events, Figure 3.4 presents Twitter sentiment trends for three major immigration events: the Syrian refugee crisis (2014), the U.S. travel ban (2017), and the family separation policy (2018). In each case, neutral sentiment tweets were the most prevalent, followed by a substantial volume of negative sentiment. A notable spike in activity occurred in late November 2014, corresponding to the escalation of the Syrian refugee crisis, with Syrians becoming the largest refugee group globally (UNICEF 2020). Sentiment shifted dramatically in late January 2017, with a surge in negative tweets coinciding with the implementation of the U.S. travel ban. Another sharp increase in negative sentiment appeared in June 2018, aligning with the rollout of the family separation policy (Human Rights Watch 2018) aimed to deter illegal immigration but provoked widespread backlash due to

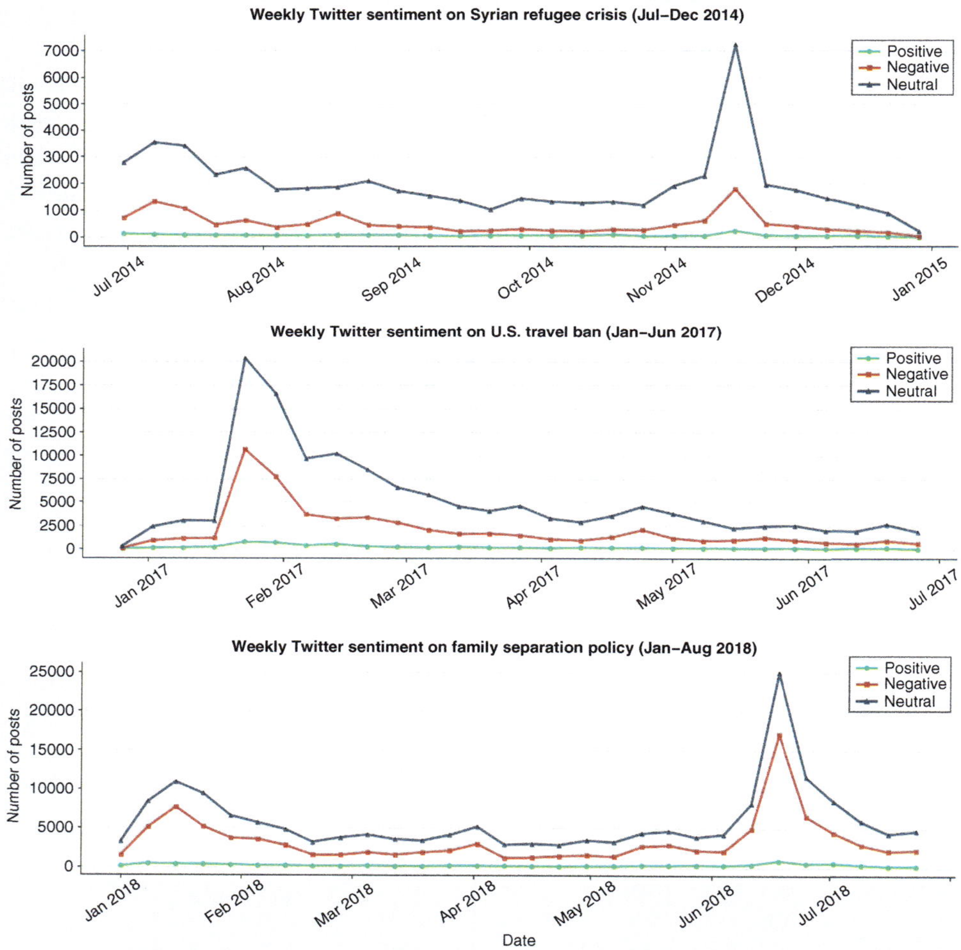

Figure 3.4 Temporal sentiment trends on Twitter.
Source: Nguyen et al. (2025) / Elsevier / CC BY 4.0.

its toll on families and lack of reunification infrastructure (Short 2022). These trends highlight the public's strong emotional response to immigration policies.

As data grows increasingly complex and multidimensional, so does the need for visualizations that convey multiple variables simultaneously. Scatter plots are particularly effective in this regard. In the context of social media, it is not merely the frequency of certain words that matters, but also the degree to which those words resonate with audiences. Figure 3.5 illustrates this concept by mapping keywords associated with refugee and immigration discourse on X between 2014 and 2023. Each point on the plot represents a keyword, positioned according to its frequency of use (x-axis, log scale) and engagement per use (y-axis, log scale). This dual-axis structure allows for the simultaneous examination of both popularity and audience reaction.

To aid interpretation, the chart is divided into four quadrants:

- **High Frequency, High Engagement (Top Right)**: Keywords like *Migrant Caravan*, *Travel Ban*, and *ICE* are widely used and also generate strong public interaction. These terms not only appeared frequently but also maintained consistently high engagement, often corresponding to major immigration events or policy debates.
- **Low Frequency, High Engagement (Top Left)**: Terms such as *Title 42* and *Migrant Protection Program* are less common but produce high engagement when they appear. These are labeled **overperformers**.
- **High Frequency, Low Engagement (Bottom Right)**: Keywords like *Illegal Alien* and *Border Control* appear frequently but provoke relatively low engagement per mention. These are considered **underperformers**, suggesting that audiences interacted less actively with these discussions.
- **Low Frequency, Low Engagement (Bottom Left)**: These terms *Norefugeeban* and *Rapefugee* are both rare and low in engagement, suggesting marginal resonance in broader discourse.

This visualization is particularly effective because it moves beyond word counts to evaluate qualitative impact through engagement metrics. By incorporating color coding and quadrant labeling, the graphic conveys meaning at a glance, enabling readers to quickly identify patterns and extract insights from complex social media discourse.

While Case Study 1 examined immigration-related discourse through a multidimensional lens encompassing temporal trends, emotional patterns, engagement dynamics, and geographic variation, Case Study 2 pivots toward a clinical application of social media analytics: pharmacovigilance. This case examines how user-generated posts can reveal real-time signals of adverse events associated with GLP-1 RA medications, underscoring the role of social media as a complementary surveillance tool in public health.

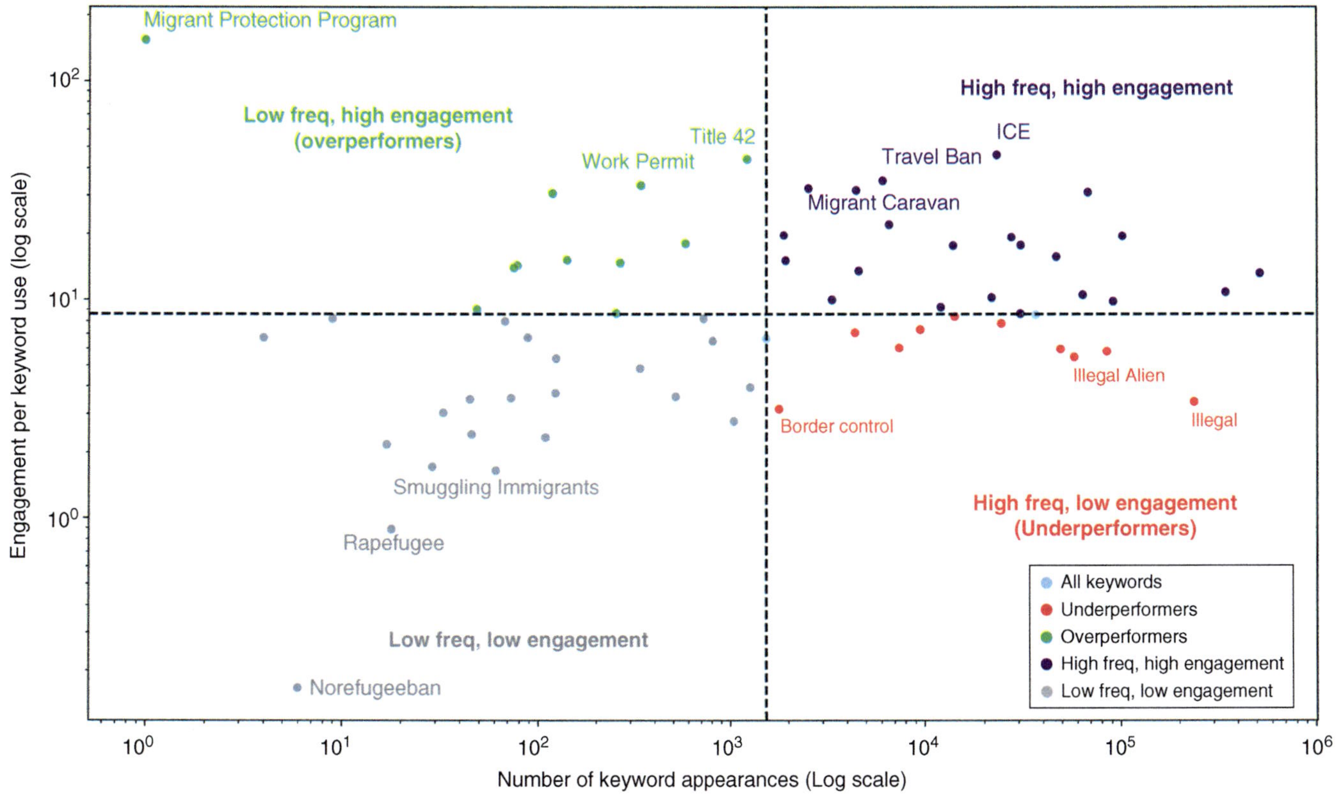

Figure 3.5 Keyword performance vs. engagement for refugee and immigration-related posts on Twitter (2014–2023).

Source: Nguyen et al. (2025) / Elsevier / CC BY 4.0.

CASE STUDY 2. SOCIAL MEDIA SURVEILLANCE OF ADVERSE EVENTS FROM GLP-1 RA WEIGHT LOSS MEDICATIONS (ALLIBILI ET AL. 2025 / JMIR PUBLICATIONS)

In recent years, Glucagon-Like Peptide-1 Receptor Agonists (GLP-1 RAs), such as Ozempic (semaglutide), Wegovy, and Mounjaro (tirzepatide), have garnered widespread public attention as effective weight loss medications (Singh et al. 2022). Originally developed for type 2 diabetes, these drugs have experienced a rapid surge in both off-label and FDA-approved use for obesity treatment, partly driven by increased media attention, celebrity endorsements, and the growing cultural acceptance of medicalized weight loss (Panic et al. 2020; Neumiller et al. 2025). The swift rise in usage has heightened concerns regarding the adverse events experienced by real-world users, particularly among populations excluded or underrepresented in clinical trials. Although clinical studies and regulatory reporting systems provide key insights into adverse events, they underrepresent the lived experiences of users (Muñoz et al. 2024). In contrast, social media offers an expansive, real-time, and unfiltered lens into how these medications are experienced and discussed by the public.

Allibilli and colleagues (2025) investigated how social media can inform early-stage pharmacovigilance for GLP-1 RAs by collecting and analyzing 59 293 publicly available Facebook posts (2022–2024). These posts encompassed discussions of semaglutide (Ozempic, Wegovy), tirzepatide (Mounjaro, Zepbound), and the broader class of GLP-1 RA medications. Using Meta's CrowdTangle platform, the study filtered for English-language U.S.-based posts to identify potential adverse events (AEs). The aim was to use social media content to identify frequently reported symptoms, identify co-occurrence patterns, assess temporal trends based on key events, and understand the broader themes shaping public narratives surrounding these weight loss medications.

To analyze the content, the investigators employed descriptive analytics, temporal trend analysis, and co-occurrence network analysis. The study found that gastrointestinal symptoms, especially nausea, vomiting, and pancreatitis, were the most common AEs mentioned across all GLP-1 RA medications, with Mounjaro and general GLP-1 RA posts showing the highest mention rates. Mental health-related adverse events, such as anxiety and depression, appeared more frequently in posts discussing semaglutide. Furthermore, temporal analysis revealed that social media discussion peaks corresponded to key public events, including the FDA's approval of Wegovy for adolescents in December 2022, Oprah Winfrey's public endorsement of weight loss medications in December 2023, and Medicare's expanded coverage of GLP-1 RAs in March 2024. Additionally, posts referenced broader topics such as cost, access, and effectiveness as public discourse increased.

Finally, the network analysis revealed three major clusters of co-mentioned side effects. Cluster 1 contained allergies, anxiety, depression, COPD, fatigue, fever, hypertension, indigestion, insomnia, GERD, hives, swelling, restlessness, and seizures. Cluster 2 contained constipation, dehydration, headache, diarrhea, dizziness, hypoglycemia, sweating, and jaundice. Cluster 3 contained gastrointestinal, nausea, pancreatitis, rash, and vomiting. The gastrointestinal symptoms, such as nausea, vomiting, pancreatitis, diarrhea, and indigestion, were strongly associated together ($\geq$100 co-occurrence mentions), while the mentioned neurological symptoms, such as anxiety, depression, and insomnia, were moderately correlated with each other

(50–100 co-occurrence mentions). These patterns highlight the complexity of patients' experiences and suggest possible interconnections among symptoms that warrant deeper clinical investigation.

This case study demonstrates the utility of social media as a complementary tool for pharmacovigilance. It can reveal real-time user concerns, detect rare or emerging adverse events, and expose patterns that may not yet be evident in clinical trial data. As GLP-1 RAs become more widely used, continued monitoring of social media platforms can assist clinicians, researchers, and policymakers in understanding how these medications are being experienced and perceived, ultimately contributing to more responsive and equitable healthcare practices.

CASE STUDY 3. USING TWITTER-DERIVED RACIAL SENTIMENT TO PREDICT BIRTH OUTCOMES IN THE UNITED STATES

Persistent racial disparities in birth outcomes, especially low birth weight (LBW) and preterm birth (PTB), continue to challenge public health systems in the U.S. While interpersonal and structural racism have been proposed as key drivers of these disparities, quantifying racial sentiment in a scalable way still remains as a challenge. Traditional approaches often rely on self-reported discrimination; however, this may not be a reliable indicator due to social desirability bias, internalized coping strategies, and limited geographic reach. To address this gap, Nguyen et al. (2020) used Twitter data to construct state-level indicators of racial sentiment. The study collected more than 26 million geotagged tweets within the U.S. between 2015 and 2017, which were collected using Twitter's Streaming API. First, 518 race-related keywords—sourced from census categories, racial slur databases, and prior literature—were used to filter relevant tweets. Tweets were aggregated by racial/ethnic groups and by U.S. states to generate composite measures of racial sentiment. The sentiment measures were then linked to over 9.9 million individual-level birth records from the National Center for Health Statistics over the same period. The analysis controlled for maternal age, education, smoking, BMI, prenatal care timing, and state-level demographics, including population density and economic disadvantage.

Findings indicated that mothers residing in states with the highest tertile of negative racial sentiment had an 8% higher incidence of both LBW and PTB compared to those in the lowest tertile. These associations were observed in the total population, among minoritized mothers, and White mothers. Subgroup analyses showed strong associations between tweets targeting Black and Middle Eastern individuals and adverse outcomes for corresponding minority populations. For example, Black mothers in states with the highest negativity toward Black individuals experienced a 13% higher risk of delivering LBW infants.

A follow-up study analyzed 56 million posts and 35 million births to investigate the association between Twitter-derived negative racial sentiment and birth outcomes for a longer time period, 2011–2021. It revealed similar findings, with negative racial sentiment associated with a higher incidence of PTB and LBW for the total population (Nguyen et al. 2023). In subgroup analyses, negative sentiment referencing Black people and birth outcomes among Black women showed the strongest and most consistent association.

Multimodal Models

Multimodal models represent a significant advancement in machine learning by enabling systems to process and integrate diverse types of data, such as text, images, audio, and video. Unlike traditional unimodal approaches that rely on a single data type, multimodal models capture complex, interdependent relationships across modalities. Early versions of these models used separate architectures for each input type and fused their outputs at the final stage. While this preserved modality-specific features, it often failed to capture deeper cross-modal interactions. In contrast, contemporary multimodal models are jointly trained on multiple data types from the outset, resulting in more cohesive and contextually rich representations. This paradigm shift mirrors how humans naturally interpret the world, synthesizing information from sight, sound, and language simultaneously to understand complex scenarios. In the same way, many AI systems today need to pull from different kinds of information at once to work effectively in real-world situations.

Figure 3.6 and Table 3.2 present a comparative overview of unimodal and multimodal AI models. Unimodal models process a single data type, such as text, image, or audio, through dedicated preprocessing and feature extraction steps, followed by a machine learning model for prediction. These models are typically simpler and faster to train but are limited in their ability to capture nuanced or contextual information, which may constrain model performance. Examples include BERT, ResNet, and VGG (Simonyan and Zisserman 2015; He et al. 2016). Unimodal models are well-suited for tasks like speech recognition or image classification, where one modality dominates.

Multimodal models, on the other hand, are designed to handle multiple data types (combining text with images or audio). Each data type is pre-processed separately, and their resulting features are combined in a *fusion* (see below) stage before prediction. This architecture enables richer, more integrated representations, enhancing their performance on complex tasks such as video captioning and meme detection. However, this complexity increases training time and computational demands. Prominent pre-trained multimodal models include CLIP and VisualBERT (Liu et al. 2019; Radford et al. 2021).

The strength of multimodal models lies in their ability to leverage complementary signals across different modalities, thereby resolving ambiguities and improving contextual understanding that unimodal approaches cannot address alone. For instance, visual context can disambiguate homonyms in text (e.g., "bat" as an animal vs. sports equipment), while textual descriptions can provide cues to interpret otherwise ambiguous or abstract visual scenes (Caglayan et al. 2019). These capabilities have proven particularly valuable in applications such as content moderation, where harmful content often relies on a subtle interplay of text and imagery; medical diagnostics, where patient data may include

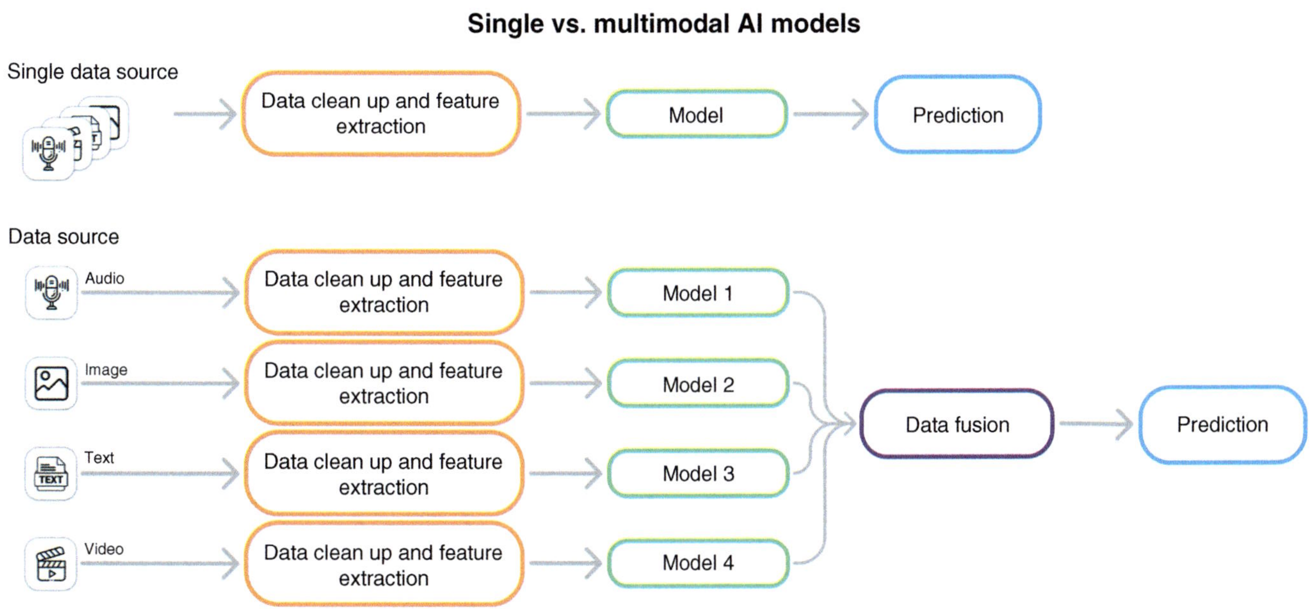

Figure 3.6 Comparison of unimodal and multimodal model pipelines.

Table 3.2 Unimodal vs. Multimodal Models: Key Differences

Criteria	Unimodal modals	Multimodal modals
Data input	Single modality such as text or images	Multiple modalities such as text and images, text and audio
Complexity	Simpler architecture	More complex
Performance	Single data input is processed which limits the learning depth and the accuracy	Richer information can be captured from multiple data inputs which can lead to a better understanding of the data and improved model accuracy
Training time	Usually faster	Usually slower due to model complexity
Model examples	BERT, ResNet, VGG	CLIP, VisualBERT, Flamingo
Applications	Best suited for single data type tasks such as speech recognition	Best suited for multiple data type tasks such as video captioning

both imaging scans and clinical notes; and multimedia analysis and assistive technologies for individuals with sensory impairments, such as systems that translate speech to text or describe images aloud. Multimodal model architectures can vary widely depending on the data types involved and the goals of the task. But in general, they follow three main steps: processing each type of input separately, combining the information, and then making a prediction.

Processing Each Input Type (Encoding): Each kind of input is first handled by a tool that's designed for that specific type of data. For example:

- Text may be processed by BERT, which converts words into contextual numerical representations.
- Images might be analyzed using VGGNet, which extracts key visual features.
- Audio can be processed by Wav2vec, which learns patterns directly from sound waves.

These tools turn raw inputs, such as sentences, images, or audio clips, into numerical summaries called embeddings, which serve as the foundation for multimodal integration.

Combining the Data (Fusion): Once each type of input is processed, the next step is to bring everything together. There are a few ways to do this:

- **Early fusion:** Combines inputs before learning begins. While it allows early intermodal learning, it can be challenging due to the differing nature of input data types, such as image and text data.
- **Late fusion:** Keeps each input separate until prediction combines results through averaging or voting. This approach retains the unique characteristics of each modality and offers modularity, allowing models to be trained or swapped separately. This is simpler but might miss deeper connections or interdependencies between the inputs.

- **Intermediate fusion:** Strikes a balance between early and late fusion by maintaining some independence while also enabling the model to learn nuanced intermodal relationships. Although computationally demanding, it often yields superior performance.

Prediction and Evaluation: After combining the inputs, the model makes its prediction, generating a description for an image or deciding if a post violates guidelines. Model performance depends on the task and is evaluated using specific metrics:

For classification tasks, standard metrics include:

Accuracy: the proportion of correctly predicted instances.

Precision: the ratio of correctly predicted positive instances to total predicted positives.

Recall: the ratio of correctly predicted positives to all actual positive instances.

F1-score: the harmonic mean of precision and recall, especially useful in imbalanced datasets.

AUROC (Area Under the Receiver Operating Characteristic Curve): measures the model's ability to distinguish between classes.

For generation tasks (e.g., text summarization, machine translation, or generative text), common evaluations are:

- **ROUGE** (Recall-Oriented Understudy for Gisting Evaluation): measures overlap between the model's output and a reference answer.
- **BLEU** (Bilingual Evaluation Understudy): often used in translation, measures a model's output similarity with human translation.

Account for Computational and Storage

Multimodal models, while powerful, often come with high computational and storage costs. Processing and storing multiple modalities often necessitate complex architectures and longer training times, especially when using complex fusion strategies that combine data at multiple stages. These limitations challenge real-time deployment models on devices with limited resources.

Despite these challenges, the benefits of multimodal models often outweigh the drawbacks, especially in tasks where combining information from different sources leads to a much better understanding or overall performance. For example, in medical diagnosis, integrating patient notes with scan images can improve accuracy. In content moderation or accessibility tools, capturing both visual and textual context is often necessary. In these cases, the added computation is justified by the value of the results. Still, it is important to evaluate the trade-offs for each application: in some situations, simpler unimodal models may be sufficient, while in others, the depth and flexibility of multimodal learning are well worth the investment.

CASE STUDY 4. HATE AND ANTI-HATE CONTENT DETECTION ON SOCIAL MEDIA USING MULTIMODAL MODELS

Traditional social media research has predominantly focused on text analysis to examine public attitudes and beliefs. However, memes and image-based content have evolved into a prominent feature of contemporary culture. Although memes were originally intended for humor, they are increasingly utilized to disseminate negative, disrespectful, or hostile attitudes toward marginalized groups. Their humor framing often obscures harmful intent, allowing them to evade content moderation and achieve widespread distribution.

To address this challenge, Nguyen et al. (2025) investigated the application of multimodal models for detecting hateful and anti-hateful content on social media. The study employed three complementary modeling approaches: CLIP, VisualBERT, and a custom intermediate fusion model. These architectures were selected for their ability to jointly process and reason over both text and images, a necessity in analyzing internet memes where harmful intent often arises from the interaction between modalities. VisualBERT employs a unified transformer-based architecture that directly integrates visual and textual embeddings, allowing it to model fine-grained relationships across modalities. It is particularly effective when textual cues are contextually harmful only in the presence of specific images. CLIP, through contrastive learning, aligns image-text pairs in a shared embedding space, enabling the detection of implicit or abstract semantic relationships. To complement these, the study implemented an intermediate fusion model, which combines features extracted separately from each modality and merges them at a later stage for joint representation learning. This fusion strategy strikes a balance between preserving data type-specific detail and enabling meaningful interactions across data types, particularly useful in cases where one modality carries a stronger signal than the other.

A significant challenge was high class imbalance, with a limited number of hate and anti-hate content compared to non-hate and non-anti-hate content. To address this, investigators employed a variety of strategies: weighted sampling to adjust for skewed class distributions during training, data augmentation (e.g., flipping or cropping images, paraphrasing captions) to diversify examples, and SMOTE (Synthetic Minority Oversampling Technique) to synthetically expand the underrepresented classes (Chawla et al. 2002). These methods were added to help reduce bias in model learning and improve generalization.

Additionally, the study incorporated topic distribution features from a topic model trained on the accompanying text. By including document-topic vectors as an additional input, investigators aimed to provide contextual cues that capture higher-level thematic patterns often associated with hate speech. For example, memes about race, religion, or gender may differ in tone depending on the underlying topic, and this signal can complement the semantic content of the text and image.

The evaluation revealed that while CLIP outperformed others in general accuracy, it showed overreliance on the textual component of memes. This limitation has prompted further work exploring enhanced visual attention mechanisms. In addition, the research team is extending their work to explore ensemble learning, combining the strengths of CLIP, VisualBERT, and our fusion model to improve classification robustness and overall performance.

This case study underscores the importance and challenges of using multimodal models for complex social media content analysis. Although multimodal models offer richer representations, their effectiveness is influenced by factors such as dataset imbalance, modality dominance, and the interaction between data types. Future work will focus on ensemble reasoning, detailed error analysis, and interpretability measures to enhance model transparency and guide design improvements. The overall aim is to build more reliable systems for understanding complex online discourse. These insights are not only relevant for hate speech detection but also extend to broader multimodal applications such as misinformation detection, content moderation, and cross-platform narrative tracking.

Opportunities and Pitfalls

Social media data provides real-time, large-scale insight into public sentiment, daily trends, and diverse user perspectives. The expansive reach of platforms like X, Facebook, Instagram, Reddit, and emerging sites such as Bluesky allows researchers to access near real-time snapshots of public discourse. This wealth of data supports studies across domains, including public health, misinformation, and cultural analysis, and facilitates longitudinal analyses of evolving trends. However, leveraging social media data also presents significant methodological and ethical challenges. APIs frequently change or are discontinued, affecting data accessibility. Bot activity and spam may distort datasets, while ethical and privacy considerations demand vigilance in handling user-generated content responsibly.

Researchers must also be prepared for platform-specific nuances like memes, slang, or ephemeral features that complicate data analysis, as well as for platform rebrandings, mergers, or shutdowns that can disrupt ongoing studies. Despite these hurdles, the sheer volume and diversity of social media data offer a unique window into real-world conversations and behaviors, making careful and methodical research well worth the effort. However, the abundance of data can also lead to overfitting if models are tuned too closely to platform-specific language or user behavior. Researchers should validate models across multiple datasets and consider domain adaptation or transfer learning strategies when possible. Careful documentation of training data composition, model assumptions, and temporal coverage is essential to ensure reproducibility and to avoid drawing conclusions that may not hold across platforms or populations. By applying rigorous cleaning procedures, ensuring ethical compliance, and maintaining transparent documentation, researchers can unlock powerful, actionable solutions from the dynamic ever-evolving realm of social media.

KEY POINTS AND TAKEAWAYS

- A robust social media research pipeline requires deliberate planning, structured preprocessing, and strategically designed analytical methods. This includes formulating clear research questions; selecting platforms, languages, and timeframes; establishing secure data storage; and implementing rigorous cleaning protocols. These foundational steps prepare the dataset for meaningful analyses such as sentiment classification, temporal trend detection, and co-occurrence pattern analysis, essential for extracting insights in public health contexts.

- Data acquisition from social media platforms requires navigating evolving access policies, platform-specific structures, and ethical constraints. Differences in API availability, data formats, scraping feasibility, and metadata granularity across platforms such as X, Facebook, Bluesky, and Reddit demand tailored strategies. A clear understanding of these constraints is essential to ensure data quality, compliance, and reproducibility in social media research.
- Applying multimodal models requires selecting appropriate architectures, modeling strategies, and preprocessing tools tailored to the data and task. Researchers can enhance performance by adopting architectures like CLIP, VisualBERT, or intermediate fusion models, addressing class imbalance using techniques such as SMOTE and data augmentation, and evaluating models with robust metrics. These strategies enable the construction of adaptable, task-specific pipelines for analyzing multimodal social media content in public health research.

Conclusion

Social media offers unprecedented opportunities to understand public health dynamics, user sentiment, and sociocultural trends in real time. However, transforming this vast, unstructured data into insight requires a systematic and ethically grounded approach. This chapter outlined the full data pipeline, from project planning and data acquisition to cleaning and modeling, emphasizing both technical workflows and ethical responsibilities. Across multiple case studies, we demonstrated how these methods advance public health research in practice: analyses of Facebook posts uncovered real-world adverse events associated with GLP-1 weight loss medications; temporal and co-occurrence analyses illuminated public responses to major health events and policy shifts; and multimodal models such as CLIP and VisualBERT enabled the detection of hate and anti-hate content in memes, supporting efforts to monitor harmful narratives and promote online safety. While these examples highlight the promise and versatility of social media data, they also underscore the challenges researchers face. Evolving access policies, class imbalances, and computational demands require researchers to approach these tools with transparency and methodological rigor. Yet, when applied thoughtfully, social media analytics and particularly multimodal approaches can offer a nuanced, real-time understanding that complements traditional public health data and informs more responsive and equitable interventions.

References

Alibilli, A. S., Jain, V., Mane, H., Yue, X., Ratzki-Leewing, A., Merchant, J. S., Criss, S., Nguyen, Q. C., McCoy, R. G., & Nguyen, T. T. (2025). Harnessing Facebook to investigate real-world mentions of adverse events of Glucagon-like peptide-1 receptor agonist (GLP-1 RA) medications: observational study of Facebook posts from 2022 to 2024. *JMIR Infodemiology, 5*, e73619. doi:10.2196/73619

AlSaad, R., Abd-Alrazaq, A., Boughorbel, S., Ahmed, A., Renault, M.-A., Damseh, R., & Sheikh, J. (2024). Multimodal large language models in health care: applications, challenges, and future outlook. *Journal of Medical Internet Research, 26*, e59505. doi:10.2196/59505

Baumgartner, J., Zannettou, S., Keegan, B., Squire, M., & Blackburn, J. (2020). The Pushshift reddit dataset. *Proceedings of the International AAAI Conference on Web and Social Media, 14*, 830–839. doi:10.1609/icwsm.v14i1.7347

Bestvater, S. (2024). How U.S. adults use TikTok. *Pew Research Center*. https://www.pewresearch.org/internet/2024/02/22/how-u-s-adults-use-tiktok/ (accessed 7 November 2025).

Blei, D., Ng, A., & Jordan, M. (2003). Latent Dirichlet allocation. *Journal of Machine Learning Research*, 993–1022. https://www.jmlr.org/papers/volume3/blei03a/blei03a.pdf (accessed 10 November 2025)

Bluesky (2025a). app.bsky.feed.searchPosts | Bluesky. https://docs.bsky.app/docs/api/app-bsky-feed-search-posts (accessed 2 December 2025).

Bluesky (2025b). Bluesky developer APIs. https://docs.bsky.app/ (accessed 2 December 2025).

Bluesky (2025c). Rate limits. https://docs.bsky.app/docs/advanced-guides/rate-limits (accessed 2 December 2025).

Braghieri, L., Levy, R., & Makarin, A. (2022). Social media and mental health. *American Economic Review, 112*(11), 3660–3693. doi:10.1257/aer.20211218

Caglayan, O., Madhyastha, P., Specia, L., & Barrault, L. (2019). Probing the need for visual context in multimodal machine translation. In J. Burstein, C. Doran, & T. Solorio (Eds.), *Proceedings of the 2019 Conference of the North American Chapter of the Association for Computational Linguistics: Human Language Technologies, Volume 1 (Long and Short Papers)* (pp. 4159–4170). Association for Computational Linguistics. doi:10.18653/v1/N19-1422

Chawla, N. V., Bowyer, K. W., Hall, L. O., & Kegelmeyer, W. P. (2002). SMOTE: synthetic minority over-sampling technique. *Journal of Artificial Intelligence, 16*, 321–357. https://www.jair.org/index.php/jair/article/view/10302

Copland, S. (2020). Reddit quarantined: can changing platform affordances reduce hateful material online? [Info:eu-repo/semantics/article]. 10.14763/2020.4.1516.

Devlin, J., Chang, M.-W., Lee, K., & Toutanova, K. (2019). BERT: pre-training of deep bidirectional transformers for language understanding. In J. Burstein, C. Doran, & T. Solorio (Eds.), *Proceedings of the 2019 Conference of the North American Chapter of the Association for Computational Linguistics: Human Language Technologies, Volume 1 (Long and Short Papers)* (pp. 4171–4186). Association for Computational Linguistics. doi:10.18653/v1/N19-1423

Gottfried, J. (2024). Americans' social media use. *Pew Research Center*. https://www.pewresearch.org/internet/2024/01/31/americans-social-media-use/ (accessed 2 February 2026).

Grootendorst, M. (2022). BERTopic: neural topic modeling with a class-based TF-IDF procedure (No. arXiv:2203.05794). *arXiv*. doi:10.48550/arXiv.2203.05794 (accessed 5 February 2026)

Han, B., Cook, P., & Baldwin, T. (2012). Automatically constructing a normalisation dictionary for microblogs. In J. Tsujii, J. Henderson, & M. Paşca (Eds.), *Proceedings of the 2012 Joint Conference on Empirical Methods in Natural Language Processing and Computational Natural Language Learning* (pp. 421–432). Association for Computational Linguistics. https://aclanthology.org/D12-1039/

He, K., Zhang, X., Ren, S., & Sun, J. (2016). Deep residual learning for image recognition. *2016 IEEE Conference on Computer Vision and Pattern Recognition (CVPR)*, 770–778. doi:10.1109/CVPR.2016.90

Hern, A. (2015). Reddit finally bans its white-supremacist subreddits. *The Guardian*. https://www.theguardian.com/technology/2015/aug/06/reddit-bans-white-supremacist-subreddits (accessed 10 February 2026).

Human Rights Watch (2018). Q&A: trump administration's "Zero-Tolerance" immigration policy | Human Rights Watch. https://www.hrw.org/news/2018/08/16/qa-trump-administrations-zero-tolerance-immigration-policy (accessed 11 February 2026).

Hutto, C., & Gilbert, E. (2014). VADER: a parsimonious rule-based model for sentiment analysis of social media text. *Proceedings of the International AAAI Conference on Web and Social Media, 8*(1), 216–225. doi:10.1609/icwsm.v8i1.14550

Lama, Y., Hu, D., Jamison, A., Quinn, S. C., & Broniatowski, D. A. (2019). Characterizing trends in human papillomavirus vaccine discourse on Reddit (2007–2015): an observational study. *JMIR Public Health and Surveillance, 5*(1), e12480. doi:10.2196/12480

Li, Y., & Xie, Y. (2019). Is a picture worth a thousand words? An empirical study of image content and social media engagement. *Sage Journals, 57*(1). https://journals.sagepub.com/doi/abs/10.1177/0022243719881113?casa_token=j9AZIIC8QNUAAAAA%3AgcOlAjlyOJczWMkIpnGYENnUORM1RhLepRODKOuc6b0C_O8yeDiLH5UFno6iv8lEU_LYA1BIwnmNUA

Liu, Y., Ott, M., Goyal, N., Du, J., Joshi, M., Chen, D., Levy, O., Lewis, M., Zettlemoyer, L., & Stoyanov, V. (2019). RoBERTa: a robustly optimized BERT pretraining approach (No. arXiv:1907.11692). *arXiv*. doi:10.48550/arXiv.1907.11692

Lui, M., & Baldwin, T. (2012). langid.py: an off-the-shelf language identification tool. In M. Zhang (Ed.), *Proceedings of the ACL 2012 System Demonstrations* (pp. 25–30). Association for Computational Linguistics. https://aclanthology.org/P12-3005/

Meta (2025a). Meta content library and API. https://developers.facebook.com/docs/content-library-and-api (accessed 9 November 2025).

Meta (2025b). Rate limiting and query budgeting. https://developers.facebook.com/docs/content-library-and-api/content-library-api/guides/rate-limiting/ (accessed 9 November 2025).

Meta (2025c). SOMAR application guide for meta content library and content library API. *Google Docs*. https://docs.google.com/document/d/1iN4KOvFaYGZro23cB4j1FveouXMBcZnKl-yTUyx6fCg/edit?tab=t.0&usp=embed_facebook (accessed 9 November 2025).

Muñoz, M. A., Dal Pan, G. J., Wei, Y. J., Xiao, H., Delcher, C., Giffin, A., Sadiq, N., & Winterstein, A. G. (2024). Sociodemographic characteristics of adverse event reporting in the USA: an ecologic study. *Drug Safety, 47*(4), 377–387. doi:10.1007/s40264-024-01397-6

Narvekar, N. D., & Karam, L. J. (2011). A no-reference image Blur metric based on the Cumulative Probability of Blur Detection (CPBD). *IEEE Transactions on Image Processing, 20*(9), 2678–2683. doi:10.1109/TIP.2011.2131660

Neumiller, J. J., Bajaj, M., Bannuru, R. R., et al. (2025). Compounded GLP-1 and dual GIP/GLP-1 receptor agonists: a statement from the American Diabetes Association. *Diabetes Care, 48*(2), 177–181.

Nguyen, T. T., Adams, N., Huang, D., Glymour, M. M., Allen, A. M., & Nguyen, Q. C. (2020). The association between state-level racial attitudes assessed from Twitter data and adverse birth outcomes: observational study. *JMIR Public Health and Surveillance, 6*(3), e17103. doi:10.2196/17103

Nguyen, T. T., Merchant, J. S., Criss, S., Makres, K., Gowda, K. N., Mane, H., Yue, X., Hswen, Y., Glymour, M. M., Nguyen, Q. C., & Allen, A. M. (2023). Examining twitter-derived negative racial sentiment as indicators of cultural racism: observational associations with preterm birth and low birth weight among a multiracial sample of mothers, 2011–2021. *Journal of Medical Internet Research, 25*(1), e44990. doi:10.2196/44990

Nguyen, T., Merchant, J., Yue, X., Mane, H., Wei, H., Huang, D., Gowda, K., Makres, K., Najib, C., Nghiem, H., Li, D., Drew, L., Hswen, Y., Criss, S., Allen, A., & Nguyen, C. (2024). A decade of tweets: visualizing racial sentiments towards minoritized groups in the United States between 2011 and 2021. *Epidemiology, 35*(1), 51–59. https://journals.lww.com/epidem/fulltext/2024/01000/a_decade_of_tweets__visualizing_racial_sentiments.7.aspx

Nguyen, T. T., Yue, X., Mane, H., Seelman, K., PSP, M., Dennard, E., Alibilli, A. S., Merchant, J. S., Criss, S., Hswen, Y., & Nguyen, Q. C. (2025). Decoding digital discourse through multimodal text and image machine learning models to classify sentiment and detect hate speech in race- and Lesbian, Gay, Bisexual, Transgender, Queer, Intersex, and Asexual Community–related posts on ****social media: quantitative study. *Journal of Medical Internet Research, 27*, e72822. PMID: 40354116; PMCID: PMC12107201. doi:10.2196/72822

Novak, P. K., Smailović, J., Sluban, B., & Mozetič, I. (2015). Sentiment of emojis. *PLOS ONE, 10*(12), e0144296. doi:10.1371/journal.pone.0144296

Open Source Computer Vision (2025). OpenCV: OpenCV modules. https://docs.opencv.org/4.x/index.html (accessed 11 November 2025).

Panic, G., Yao, X., Gregory, P., & Austin, Z. (2020). How do community pharmacies in Ontario manage drug shortage problems? Results of an exploratory qualitative study. *Canadian Pharmacists Journal (Ottawa), 153*(6), 371–377.

Pillow (2025). Pillow (PIL Fork) 11.3.0 documentation. *Pillow*. https://pillow.readthedocs.io/en/stable/index.html (accessed 11 November 2025).

Radford, A., Kim, J. W., Hallacy, C., Ramesh, A., Goh, G., Agarwal, S., Sastry, G., Askell, A., Mishkin, P., Clark, J., Krueger, G., & Sutskever, I. (2021). Learning transferable visual models from natural language supervision (No. arXiv:2103.00020). *arXiv*. doi:10.48550/arXiv.2103.00020

Reddit (2025). Developer platform & data API usage. https://support.reddithelp.com/hc/en-us/sections/14946321137172-Developer-Platform-Data-API-Usage (accessed 11 November 2025).

Rubinstein, I. S., & Hartzog, W. (2016). Anonymization and risk. *Washington Law Review, 91*, 703. https://heinonline.org/HOL/Page?handle=hein.journals/washlr91&id=719&div=&collection=

Short, K. (2022). Parents experience severe psychological trauma four years after family separation by the U.S. Government: *PHR report. PHR*. https://phr.org/news/parents-experience-severe-psychological-trauma-four-years-after-family-separation-by-the-u-s-government-phr-report/ (accessed 11 November 2025).

Simonyan, K., & Zisserman, A. (2015). Very deep convolutional networks for large-scale image recognition (No. arXiv:1409.1556). *arXiv*. doi:10.48550/arXiv.1409.1556

Singh, G., Krauthamer, M., & Bjalme-Evans, M. (2022). Wegovy (semaglutide): a new weight loss drug for chronic weight management. *Journal of Investigative Medicine, 70*(1), 5–13.

Sukhwal, P. C., & Kankanhalli, A. (2022). Determining containment policy impacts on public sentiment during the pandemic using social media data. *Proceedings of the National Academy of Sciences (PNAS), 119*(19). https://www.pnas.org/doi/full/10.1073/pnas.2117292119

TextBlob (2018). TextBlob: simplified text processing — TextBlob 0.15.2 documentation. *Readthedocs.io*. https://textblob.readthedocs.io/en/dev/.

Townsend, L., & Wallace, C. (2016). Social media research: a guide to ethics. https://www.gla.ac.uk/media/Media_487729_smxx.pdf.

UNICEF (2020). A timeline of the Syrian civil war and refugee crisis. *UNICEF Ireland*. https://www.unicef.ie/stories/timeline-syrian-war-refugee-crisis/ (accessed 3 December 2025).

Varcoe, C., Browne, A. J., Wong, S., & Smye, V. L. (2009). Harms and benefits: collecting ethnicity data in a clinical context. *Social Science & Medicine, 68*(9), 1659–1666. doi:10.1016/j.socscimed.2009.02.034

X Developer Platform (2020). Guide to the future of the X API. https://developer.x.com/en/products/x-api/early-access/guide (accessed 4 December 2025).

X Developer Platform (2025a). Data dictionary: standard v1.1. https://developer.x.com/en/docs/x-api/v1/data-dictionary/object-model/tweet (accessed 4 December 2025).

X Developer Platform (2025b). Standard search API. https://developer.x.com/en/docs/x-api/v1/tweets/search/api-reference/get-search-tweets (accessed 4 December 2025).

X Developer Platform (2025c). About the X API. *X*. https://docs.x.com/x-api/getting-started/about-x-api (accessed 4 December 2025).

Ye, Q., & Doermann, D. (2015). Text detection and recognition in imagery: a survey. *IEEE Transactions on Pattern Analysis and Machine Intelligence, 37*(7), 1480–1500. doi:10.1109/TPAMI.2014.2366765

Zappavigna, M. (2015). Searchable talk: the linguistic functions of hashtags. *Taylor & Francis, 25*, 274–291. https://www.tandfonline.com/doi/full/10.1080/10350330.2014.996948

Zhao, Y., He, X., Feng, Z., Bost, S., Prosperi, M., Wu, Y., Guo, Y., & Bian, J. (2022). Biases in using social media data for public health surveillance: a scoping review. *International Journal of Medical Informatics, 164*, 104804. doi:10.1016/j.ijmedinf.2022.104804

CHAPTER 4

ETHICAL CONSIDERATIONS FOR SOCIAL MEDIA RESEARCH

Yajie Xiong[1], Katrina Makres[2], Heran Mane[2], and Thu T. Nguyen[2]
[1]Department of Sociology, University of Maryland, College Park, MD, USA
[2]Department of Epidemiology and Biostatistics, School of Public Health, University of Maryland, College Park, MD, USA

LEARNING OBJECTIVES

1. Understand why ethical practices in social media research are critical, especially with health data impacting individuals and communities
2. Present an overview of the major ethical challenges in social media research; the roles and responsibilities of key stakeholders; current ethical guidelines; and future actions

Overview

Over the past two decades, social media has transformed the research enterprise, challenging traditional methodologies and long-standing ethical principles. A central question persists: has this shift fundamentally altered the foundations of research ethics? Scholars continue to debate whether social media research demands new ethical standards or whether existing principles—such as privacy, informed consent, and minimizing harm—remain relevant, albeit more complex in digital contexts. The blurred lines between public and private spaces online have made these longstanding concerns increasingly nuanced.

This chapter examines the ethical challenges unique to social media research. Many users lack a full understanding of how their data are collected, shared, or repurposed, particularly after content is deleted, posing difficulties for researchers committed to ethical integrity. Key concerns include anonymizing sensitive information, safeguarding user privacy, and obtaining informed consent in an environment where users may be unaware that their posts are being used for research, marketing, or other purposes (Figure 4.1). The chapter also considers the roles and responsibilities of platforms, researchers, and academic institutions in addressing these challenges. Although guidance from organizations such as the Association of Internet Researchers (AoIR) has expanded, gaps in oversight remain, particularly regarding varied data types and implications of post-deletion

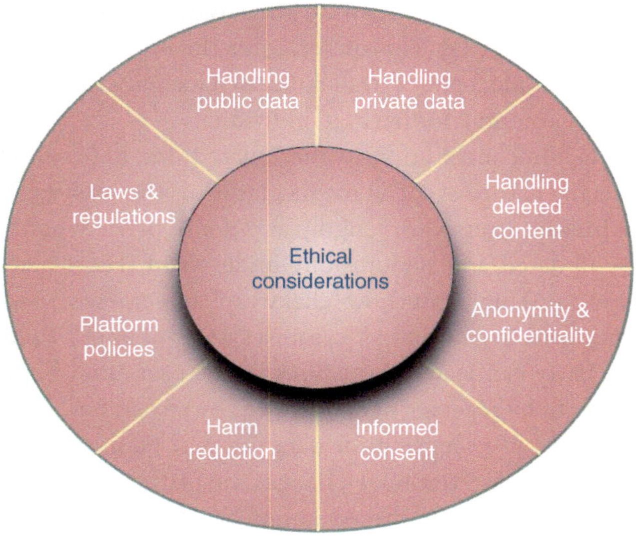

Figure 4.1 Key ethical considerations for social media use and research.

use. The chapter concludes with practical recommendations to strengthen ethical data management and enhance informed-consent practices in social media research.

Privacy Concerns in Social Media Research

Public vs. Private Data

Privacy concerns present a central ethical issue in social science research involving social media. As researchers increasingly turn to these platforms for data, they face a series of complex questions: What are users' expectations of data visibility? How can researchers balance privacy considerations with the need to ensure study validity? These questions are difficult to resolve, as the boundary between public and private data on social media is often ambiguous, given the fluid and dynamic nature of online sharing.

The complexity of this boundary partly stems from the contextual nature of privacy in digital spaces. Whether content is considered public or private often depends on the platform, the type of content shared, and the intended audience (Brown et al. 2016; Humphreys 2016). For instance, a tweet on X (formerly Twitter) designed for public engagement carries different privacy expectations than a Facebook post shared only with friends. The majority of X users have public accounts, furthering the ambiguity of posting privacy (Smith et al. 2021). While some content is technically public, users' intentions and expectations often differ based on context.

This mismatch between technical accessibility and perceived privacy is illustrated by Zimmer (2010), in his discussion of the "Tastes, Ties, and Time" study, which used publicly available data from a university-based social network. Although the data were publicly accessible, participants felt their privacy was breached. This underscores the importance of considering not just the technical public availability of data, but also the user intent, context, and the potential for harm to individuals.

Another factor contributing to the blurred line between public and private data is the nature of social media platforms themselves. These platforms often present users with lengthy and dense privacy policies, which are regularly updated and seldom fully understood (Hunter et al. 2018). Montgomery (2015) highlights how "clickwrap" agreements, in which users hastily accept terms to gain access, create a system of uninformed consent. This lack of clarity can lead to situations where users may be unaware of how their data can be accessed or repurposed by researchers and third parties. Consequently, user consent for data use may be more assumed than informed. In addition, continual changes in platform policies make it difficult for users to stay informed about how their data are governed (Obar and Oeldorf-Hirsch 2020).

The "right to be forgotten" (RTBF) introduces yet another layer of ethical complexity. The RTBF allows individuals to delete online content to protect privacy and reduce harm from outdated or sensitive posts (Stockmann and Tromble and 2017). This concept gained prominence through the European Court of Justice ruling in 2014 in the case of Google Spain SL, Google Inc. v AEPD, Mario Costeja González, which affirmed that individuals have the right to request the removal of personal data. However, the RTBF presents challenges for social science research, particularly for longitudinal studies that rely on data trends over time. Beyond methodological issues, the RTBF reflects a broader tension between privacy and the accessibility of information. Researchers must consider these difficult questions with sensitivity, ensuring that their work does not inadvertently harm individuals or communities, even as it seeks to contribute to broader societal understanding.

Anonymity and Confidentiality

Anonymity and confidentiality are often considered effective approaches to addressing privacy concerns in social media research. However, unlike traditional research data, social media posts are often accompanied by rich metadata and embedded within complex social networks, making it difficult to ensure true anonymity and confidentiality even when personally identifiable information is removed. This difficulty arises from several inherent features of online data environments, including the interconnectedness of platforms, sophisticated data aggregation techniques, and the evolving capability of re-identification technologies.

A core issue lies in the vulnerability of de-identified data to re-identification through advanced search engines and data analysis tools. Even when researchers follow standard protocols by removing identifiers such as names, email addresses, and phone numbers, de-identified social media data often remains traceable. Zimmer (2010) emphasizes that even after removing explicit identifiers, seemingly innocuous details, like timestamps, geolocations, and user interactions, can be leveraged to re-identify individuals. For example, Stefanidis et al. (2013) found that geotagged social media posts could be analyzed to infer personal information based on location patterns and user behavior. The sheer accessibility of online data, combined with sophisticated search capabilities, allows for the aggregation of disparate data points that can ultimately re-expose user identities. Consequently, removing explicit identifiers does not guarantee anonymity, raising ethical concerns about potential unintentional privacy breaches.

The networked nature of social media data further complicates efforts to maintain confidentiality. Social media data are relational, reflecting interactions and social connections that can reveal personal or sensitive attributes. Kosinski et al. (2013) showed that user interactions, such as likes, shares, and comments, could be analyzed to infer personal attributes, including political beliefs, sexual orientation, and personality traits. Advancements in artificial intelligence have further enhanced the ability to predict individual attributes from seemingly unrelated data. Companies and organizations using machine learning algorithms can infer users' preferences, relationships, and locations based on cross-platform behaviors. For instance, Facebook's advertising algorithms have been shown to infer and target users based on their online activities across multiple platforms (Andreou et al. 2018). While these tools are primarily used for commercial purposes, they show the potential for similar inference techniques to be employed in research contexts.

Another challenge is the re-identification of individuals through the combination of multiple anonymized datasets, also known as data linkage. Narayanan and Shmatikov (2009) showed that merging separately anonymized datasets can still lead to re-identification of individuals. In the context of social media research, this is particularly problematic due to the interconnected nature of social media profiles and interactions. Linking data across platforms—such as Facebook and X/Twitter profiles—or using third-party databases can undermine the effectiveness of traditional anonymization strategies. While the risk of re-identification due to data linkage is a known issue in traditional restricted data sources, it is now increasingly recognized as an important consideration for social media contexts (Rocher et al. 2019).

In conclusion, ensuring anonymity and confidentiality in social media research is far more complex than in traditional research settings due to the unique characteristics of social media data: its interconnected nature, the potential for data linkage, and the capabilities of advanced data analysis tools. Moving forward, it is important for researchers to consider the ethical implications of their methods, adopt new privacy-enhancing techniques, and balance data utility with participant privacy. As social media continues to evolve, ensuring the ethical handling of user data remains a critical issue and requires constant vigilance in research practice.

Risk of Harm to Participants and Communities

One of the primary ethical concerns in social media research is the potential for stigmatization of participants. Stigmatization occurs when individuals are publicly associated with socially or culturally sensitive issues, leading to labeling, discrimination, or social exclusion. This risk is amplified by the context-rich nature of social media data, which often includes user-generated content and metadata such as timestamps and locations. For instance, studies analyzing posts related to mental health disorders, substance abuse, or HIV/AIDS may inadvertently expose users' identities. Such identification can lead to negative outcomes, including job loss, social exclusion, online harassment, or increased marginalization within their communities. A notable example is discussed by Dawson (2014), in which a researcher disclosed usernames from an online community. This disclosure brought unwanted attention and scrutiny to one participant, leading them to feel pressured to leave the community they had been a part of for many years. This case illustrates how the risk of stigma can extend beyond individual harm, as it may deter people from discussing critical health or social issues due to fear of negative exposure. As such, researchers must exercise ethical vigilance to protect participant identities and prevent harm.

To mitigate these risks, researchers have proposed various protective measures and ethical strategies. One approach is integrating a "privacy-by-design" framework, which prioritizes privacy protections from the outset, including data anonymization and stringent controls on data access (Bender et al. 2017). Careful handling of data, including the use of content warnings and anonymized reporting, can help reduce the risk of emotional distress and limit re-identification. Ensuring that participants are fully informed about the risks, limitations, and purposes of the research fosters trust and minimizes potential harm. Complementing these efforts, researchers may choose to report only aggregated statistics derived from large datasets to protect the confidentiality of individual social media users.

Beyond technical safeguards, researchers should engage in continuous ethical reflection, considering the broader implications of social media research on communities and potential consequences for public perceptions and policy. Continued development of standardized ethical guidelines, policies, and best practices remains essential to ensure responsible conduct in social media research.

Informed Consent in Digital Space

Given the potential risks of harm discussed earlier, it is essential to consider whether social media users should provide consent for their posted content to be used in research. There is an ongoing debate among users and researchers on this issue, with arguments both for and against obtaining individual consent (Ford et al. 2021).

Many researchers adhere to the established view that consent is not required to collect information already in the public domain (Mikal et al. 2016; Azam 2018; Taylor and Pagliari 2018). This perspective is based on the notion that data mining constitutes a secondary data analysis of publicly available material. As long as data can be publicly accessed without login credentials, some argue that acquiring consent is unnecessary. Others further contend that anonymization sufficiently protects participant identities, thereby eliminating the need for a formal consent process (Bond et al. 2013; Monks et al. 2015).

However, other scholars caution that users should be asked for permission before their content is used. These concerns often relate to the original intent behind posts, questions of data ownership, and challenges associated with anonymizing direct quotes (Monks et al. 2015; Michaelidou et al. 2016; Valdez and Keim-Malpass 2019).

From a practical standpoint, the necessity of informed consent in social media research largely depends on the method of data collection: whether it involves large-scale data collection or the recruitment of specific participants. Mass data collection often involves the aggregation of publicly available data, which may qualify for a waiver of informed consent under ethical guidelines such as the Common Rule if no identifiable personal information is used (Zimmer 2010). In such contexts, obtaining consent from millions of users is often impractical. However, in studies involving focused, in-depth analyses of individual participants' social media data, informed consent becomes ethically necessary to respect participants' autonomy and expectations of privacy, even in a digital environment. Without such consent, researchers risk violating ethical norms and undermining public trust in research (Markham et al. 2012).

Even when guidelines are clear, real-world applications of informed consent in social media research remain challenging. Users may not fully grasp how their content is being used or may assume continued control over its dissemination. For instance, a tweet originally intended for a specific audience can be reshared or quoted in unintended contexts, complicating notions of ownership and consent (Roberts 2015). Moreover, privacy settings differ across platforms, meaning users operate under different assumptions about the visibility of their posts. These challenges are further compounded in longitudinal studies, where informed consent should be treated as a dynamic, ongoing process rather than a one-time agreement. As users change their behaviors, privacy settings, or consent preferences over time, researchers must remain responsive. For instance, when analyzing evolving online interactions, researchers may need to update consent protocols to address new data-sharing practices or emerging ethical concerns (Burkell et al. 2022). Viewing consent as dynamic helps ensure participants remain informed and reflects ethical standards that prioritize their rights and flexibility in research.

Responsibilities of Key Stakeholders

Social Media Platforms

Social media platforms hold significant responsibility for ensuring transparency in their data practices. They should clearly communicate how data are collected, stored, and shared, as ambiguous or overly complex policies can lead to misuse, particularly in research contexts. Prior studies emphasize the need for platforms to make privacy terms clear and accessible to both users and researchers (Smith et al. 2012). However, many platforms have been criticized for creating excessively long and difficult-to-understand terms and conditions, along with frequent and often confusing changes to their privacy policies (Hunter et al. 2018). To address these concerns, platforms should develop user-friendly policies that are straightforward and comprehensible. Simplifying terms and helping users understand how their data may be used are critical steps in this process (Milne and Culnan 2004). Platforms should also ensure that users are promptly notified of policy updates and prioritize transparency in communicating data-use practices.

Mitigating the risk of data breaches is another important responsibility. The growing privacy concerns surrounding the use of social media data in research have been extensively documented (Moreno et al. 2013). To minimize these risks, platforms may need to consider employing techniques such as differential privacy and anonymization tools, which can help ensure that data used for research purposes cannot be traced back to individual users. These measures align with ethical frameworks designed to safeguard user privacy and enhance data security (Bhatia-Lin et al. 2019).

Collaborating with researchers, academic institutions, and ethical review boards to establish clear and responsible guidelines for the use of social media data in research can help align research objectives with user privacy expectations and foster ethical practices in data utilization. Existing research underscores the importance of these partnerships in balancing the goals of academic inquiry with the need to protect user privacy (Di Minin et al. 2021).

Researchers

As the primary agents conducting social media research, researchers play a crucial role in ensuring the ethical use of social media data. Their responsibilities include adhering to foundational principles such as obtaining informed consent, protecting anonymity, and minimizing harm to participants. Given that social media data often include sensitive or personally identifiable information, researchers must prioritize user privacy and comply with relevant data protection laws (Golder et al. 2017). Ethical frameworks, such as those proposed by Pagoto and Nebeker (2019), emphasize the importance of ethical scrutiny throughout the research process from data collection to storage and publication. This includes careful consideration of data retention practices and the specific purpose for which data are used to ensure ethical accountability.

Transparency is another essential obligation. Researchers should clearly communicate their research goals, methods, and data sources, fostering trust and accountability. The dynamic nature of social media platforms requires researchers to continually adapt to changes in privacy settings, data-sharing mechanisms, and the ethical implications arising from platform updates (Lunnay et al. 2015).

Minimizing harm remains a cornerstone of ethical research. Researchers must carefully evaluate the potential risks associated with exposing sensitive information or inadvertently re-identifying individuals. This requires an understanding of the sociopolitical context in which data exists, as emphasized by Samuel et al. (2019). Effective mitigation strategies include data anonymization—removing usernames and other identifiable details—and ethical reporting of findings that avoids direct quotations from social media platform data (Moreno et al. 2013). Additionally, establishing strict access controls and conducting regular audits of data usage further enhances the protection of participant confidentiality.

Ethical responsibilities also extend beyond data collection and analysis to the sharing and publication of research findings. Researchers should avoid disseminating results that may harm or stigmatize individuals, either directly or indirectly (Bishop and Gray 2017). Rigorous data governance practices are essential, particularly when sharing datasets for secondary research. Datasets must be anonymized and managed to prevent misuse and protect participants' identities. Upholding these practices ensures that research remains ethically sound and respectful of the individuals whose data are studied.

Research Institutions

Research institutions play a pivotal role in fostering ethical practices in social media research by providing clear guidance, regulatory oversight, and institutional support.

One of their primary responsibilities is developing adaptable ethical guidelines tailored to the unique challenges of social media research. These guidelines should align with core ethical principles while addressing challenges unique to digital platforms, including issues around data collection, informed consent, privacy, and participant protection (Golder et al. 2017).

Another critical responsibility is providing institutional review and oversight. Institutional Review Boards (IRBs) play an essential role in evaluating the ethical implications of social media research proposals, ensuring a careful balance between the benefits of research and the potential risks to participants. Ideally, IRBs should adopt a risk-sensitive approach, with higher-risk studies requiring stricter scrutiny.

For example, analyzing the frequency of certain words in tweets may pose minimal risk, while observing sensitive discussions, such as those involving adolescent patients with HIV, requires significant oversight and stricter consent standards (Moreno et al. 2013). However, existing IRB frameworks often remain insufficient for social media studies, with many studies classified as exempt or "not human subjects research." This places significant ethical responsibility on researchers. To address these gaps, IRBs should expand their guidance, offering clearer policies on data anonymization, consent processes, and tailored risk mitigation strategies for online environments (Samuel et al. 2019).

Beyond oversight, research institutions must also invest in researcher training (Pagoto and Nebeker 2019). Targeted educational programs can equip researchers with the knowledge and skills needed to conduct ethical social media research. These programs should address digital privacy, the complexities of informed consent, and the ethical use of data. Workshops and resources can help researchers anticipate ethical dilemmas and develop appropriate responses, ensuring they are well-prepared to navigate the evolving ethical challenges of social media research.

Policymakers

The 1996 Telecommunications Act, particularly Section 230 of the Communications Decency Act, was a pivotal policy shaping the governance of social media platforms (GovInfo 1996). This provision granted immunity to online service providers from liability for user-generated content, enabling platforms to establish their own content moderation policies. However, this legal foundation has resulted in inconsistent policy enforcement across platforms.

Social media firms have historically resisted accountability for harmful or misleading content. In recent years, researchers and lawmakers have raised concerns over issues such as election interference, misinformation, and the adverse impact of social media on youth mental health. The COVID-19 pandemic further intensified these concerns as misinformation proliferated and political polarization deepened. These developments fueled debate over the boundaries between platform independence, freedom of speech, and government overreach in moderating content. Despite mounting public concern and proposed legislation, such as the Kids Online Safety Act (KOSA) and the Children and Teens' Online Privacy Protection Act (COPPA 2.0), Congress has yet to pass comprehensive federal legislation. In this vacuum, a patchwork of state-level regulations has emerged from states such as Utah (Utah Code Section 13–63-102) (Utah State Legislature, 2025), Arkansas (The Arkansas Social Media Safety Act, 2025 [SB611]), Louisiana (The Secure Online Child Interaction and Age Limitation Act [SB 162]) (Louisiana State Legislature, 2024), Georgia ("Protecting Georgia's Children on Social Media Act of 2024" [SB 351]),

Tennessee (The Protecting Children from Social Media Act [HB 1891]) (Tennessee General Assembly Legislation, 2024), and Texas (Securing Children Online through Parental Empowerment Act [HB 18]), which have enacted laws requiring age verification systems and parental consent for minors to access social media platforms. California has also implemented broader protections (Protecting Our Kids from Social Media Addiction Act (SB 976), Age-Appropriate Design Code Act (California Legislative Information AB-2273)) (California Legislative Information, 2022; California Legislative Information, 2023), while New York passed the SAFE Kids Act (SAFE for Kids Act [S7694/A8148]) (New York State Senate, 2023), which targets the exploitative use of algorithms on young users. However, many of these laws face legal challenges on First Amendment and federal preemption grounds. Contrary to the regulatory fragmentation in the United States, the EU has implemented more comprehensive regulations governing social media companies, such as the General Data Protection Regulation (GDPR) for data protection (GDPR 2025) and the Digital Services Act (DSA) for platform accountability and content moderation transparency (European Commission 2022).

Amid this complex governance landscape, policymakers play a fundamental role in fostering an environment conducive to ethical and impactful social media research. Promoting transparency and accountability is essential. Policymakers can require social media platforms and researchers to disclose data usage, practice regular audits, and conduct compliance checks to prevent data misuse (Samuel et al. 2019). Transparency initiatives such as those implemented in social media analytics demonstrate how open data practices can align research objectives with user trust (Taylor and Pagliari 2018).

Addressing the ethical challenges of social media research also necessitates collaboration among stakeholders, and policymakers are uniquely positioned to facilitate these partnerships. By establishing forums and fostering relationships among researchers, legal experts, and social media platforms, policymakers enable the co-development of ethical guidelines. UNESCO's efforts in promoting cross-sector partnerships around data governance exemplify the impact of shared responsibility in crafting ethical frameworks. These multi-stakeholder approaches help ensure that ethical guidelines are practical, inclusive, and responsive to evolving challenges (Hutchinson et al. 2017).

Another critical responsibility for policymakers is advancing education and public awareness about ethical considerations in social media research. Awareness campaigns that inform users of their data rights, alongside training programs for researchers and IRBs, encourage adherence to ethical data practices. Initiatives such as the Open Government Initiative highlight the importance of integrating educational components into data governance, cultivating a culture of ethical awareness and accountability (Mickoleit 2014).

Social Media Users

Social media users also have a role to play in protecting their privacy and supporting ethical research. First, users are encouraged to understand the implications of sharing personal data on public platforms. By familiarizing themselves with platform policies and how researchers use social media data, users can make more informed decisions about their participation and privacy preferences (Moreno et al. 2013).

Advocacy for privacy rights is another key responsibility. Users have the capacity to push for better privacy protections and demand greater transparency and accountability from both platforms and researchers, including calls for explicit consent mechanisms and clearer explanations of data usage. Researchers have noted the impact of user advocacy in influencing data governance practices, highlighting the potential for collective action to drive meaningful change (Golder et al. 2017).

Finally, responsible sharing practices are essential. Users should be mindful of the content they share online, avoiding oversharing sensitive information that could be exploited. By exercising digital caution and promoting ethical data practices, social media users contribute to a safer, more ethical and more accountable digital environment.

Research Data Sharing and Transparency in This Field

The benefits of data sharing in public health research are well established. It enhances the reproducibility of findings through independent validation, thereby strengthening the credibility of research outcomes. Data sharing also facilitates collaboration among researchers, enabling more comprehensive and innovative analyses that build upon prior work. In many instances, timely data sharing can accelerate responses to emerging health threats, improve disease surveillance, reduce duplication of efforts, and maximize the impact of publicly funded data collection efforts.

As social media becomes a vital source of data for public health research, there is a growing need to promote responsible and effective data-sharing practices. Major public health organizations, including the World Health Organization (2020) and the Centers for Disease Control and Prevention (2024), have published guidelines on data collection, storage, sharing, and use. Moreover, Wilkinson et al. (2016) proposed the FAIR principles, which stand for Findable, Accessible, Interoperable, and Reusable. According to these principles, metadata should be easy to find by both humans and machines; data should be accessible, interoperable with other resources, and well-documented for replication and reuse. The FAIR principles have been widely adopted by major funding organizations, including the National Institutes of Health (2025) and the European Research Council from the European Commission (2022). However, the FAIR principles do not make suggestions on any specific technology, standards, or implementation strategies. Achieving consensus remains challenging due to inconsistent platform policies, legal constraints, and ethical concerns related to user privacy and consent. Current scholarship highlights three key principles essential for fostering a sustainable and responsible data-sharing culture in this field (Walport and Brest 2011; Figueiredo 2017):

- **Standardization:** Data should be collected, preprocessed, and stored according to consistent rules (Kush and Goldman 2014). Standardization involves maintaining uniform formats, clear documentation of methods, and metadata that supports future data reuse.
- **Accessibility:** Shared datasets should be easy to access. This includes providing sufficient contextual information and clear instructions for replication to ensure usability by diverse research teams.
- **Research Ethics:** Data sharing must follow ethical principles that prioritize user privacy, platform policies, data use agreements, etc.

Despite this progress, substantial barriers to data sharing remain. Pisani and AbouZahr (2010) noted that academic structures often prioritize publications over data sharing, and the extensive labor involved in data curation and management is frequently undervalued. Researchers may also hesitate to share data due to concerns about authorship credit, competition, or the high cost and time investment required for data collection (Savage and Vickers 2009). A systematic review by Panhuis and his team (van Panhuis et al. 2014) identified twenty potential barriers to public health data sharing, including legal uncertainties, government restrictions, concerns about economic consequences, and a lack of clarity about responsibilities for data maintenance and access control. Disagreement over the appropriate use of sensitive health-related content further complicates sharing practices. Often, the burden of navigating these complexities falls disproportionately on individual researchers.

To address these challenges, the field must establish stronger collaborations among key stakeholders, including researchers, funders, government agencies, and platform providers. Investments in standardized repositories, privacy-preserving technologies, and transparent review mechanisms can help mitigate many of the technical and logistical barriers. Most importantly, these efforts must be accompanied by a cultural shift that recognizes data sharing as a valuable scholarly contribution, worthy of institutional and professional recognition.

Current Landscape of Ethical Guidelines

Ethical guidelines have increasingly been developed to help researchers address the complexities of social media studies. Notably, the AoIR offers a widely recognized framework featuring reflective questions for researchers to consider before starting their work (Markham et al. 2012). This adaptable, non-prescriptive approach has shaped ethical practices across disciplines and institutions within and beyond academia (Social Media Research Group 2016; Townsend and Wallace 2017; British Psychological Society 2017; British Sociological Association 2017; Williams et al. 2017; LSE Research Ethics Committee 2022; Government of Canada, Panel on Research Ethics 2022; Queen's University 2024).

These guidelines address core ethical issues specific to social media research. Key issues include determining when and how to obtain informed consent, the challenges of anonymizing content on platforms with long-term data storage and search functions, and strategies for modifying direct quotes to convey their meaning while reducing identifiability. Many also emphasize minimizing harm when working with sensitive data. For instance, the London School of Economics and Political Science Research Ethics Committee (2025) classifies data based on levels of public accessibility and specifies the corresponding consent requirements. Similarly, Williams and Burnap (2017) provide practical tools for risk assessment standards and ethical principles for social media research, while the Government of Canada (2022) clarifies when ethical review is necessary for studies involving social media platforms. Townsend and Wallace (2017) further use case studies to illustrate how researchers can ethically navigate diverse topics, data collection methods, and analytical strategies.

Despite their utility, these guidelines remain advisory rather than enforceable obligations. As Samuel et al. (2019) note, decisions about the ethical use of social media data often rely on individual researchers implementing a form of "personal ethics." Scholars argue that such flexibility is essential due to the limited empirical research on social media users' perceptions of research practices and the potential harms they might experience (Beninger et al. 2014; Taylor et al. 2014; Mikal et al. 2016; Williams et al. 2017). Nevertheless, critics contended that these voluntary frameworks may fall short in addressing all ethical concerns (Woodfield et al. 2013). Taylor and Pagliari (2018) highlight that researchers working with health-related social media data often overlook ethical issues. In many cases, discussions about ethics focus narrowly on meeting procedural requirements for IRB approval, such as acknowledging privacy risks and determining whether consent is needed, rather than critically examining the ethical and social implications of repurposing information originally shared for non-research purposes.

To address these shortcomings, we recommend that research institutions adopt clearer and more actionable ethical guidelines. Additionally, publications involving social media data can explicitly address the ethical considerations involved and specify the guidelines consulted. Such measures are essential to strengthening the ethical framework of social media research and safeguarding the rights and well-being of participants in an ever-changing digital environment.

KEY POINTS AND TAKEAWAYS

- **Understand why ethical practices in social media research are critical, especially with health data impacting individuals and communities.**
  In a dynamic social media landscape, health-related data may be sensitive with long-reaching implications for vulnerable populations. Therefore, upholding ethical principles is paramount to ensure confidentiality, maintain research integrity, and safeguard participant rights.
- **Present an overview of the major ethical challenges in social media research; the roles and responsibilities of key stakeholders; current ethical guidelines; and future actions.**
  As social media research continues to be harnessed as an innovative public health paradigm, major ethical challenges pose significant dilemmas: the blurred boundary between public and private social media data and the risk of participant stigmatization. These challenges heighten the responsibilities of key stakeholders to uphold anonymity, confidentiality, and informed digital consent. While ethical frameworks, such as the AoIR guidelines, have been developed, future advances are essential to provide explicit, actionable ethical social media research guidelines while safeguarding participant rights.

Conclusion

Ethical considerations are fundamental to social media research, particularly in health-related contexts where the potential risks to participants are significant. Protecting privacy, minimizing harm, and securing informed consent when appropriate are essential practices that safeguard both participants and the integrity of the research itself. The evolving nature of social media platforms and the ambiguity between public and private data make these issues especially challenging, requiring researchers to approach their work with sensitivity and responsibility. While existing ethical guidelines provide valuable frameworks, their non-prescriptive nature often relies on individual researchers' judgment. While this flexibility is beneficial in addressing diverse research contexts, it underscores the need for greater accountability to ensure consistent application of ethical standards.

The digital age has transformed how we study human behavior, and it has also tested the boundaries of traditional ethical principles such as privacy, consent, and harm reduction. The blurred boundary between public and private data, the potential for re-identification despite anonymization, and the risk of harm to individuals underscore the need for vigilance, adaptability, and collaboration across disciplines. Researchers must never lose sight of the fact that behind every data point is a real person, with lived realities and vulnerabilities.

Importantly, how we address these ethical challenges matters beyond just research. It sets a precedent for data governance in fields such as business, technology, and public policy. Ethical failures can erode public trust, not only in research but in the platforms that host this content. However, when conducted responsibly, social media research holds immense promise for advancing health and cultural understanding in ways that benefit individuals and communities alike.

References

Andreou, A., Venkatadri, G., Goga, O., et al. (2018). Investigating Ad transparency mechanisms in social media: a case study of Facebook's explanations. 10.14722/ndss.2018.23204, https://hal.science/hal-01955309/ (accessed 1 July 2025).

Arkansas State Legislature (2025). SB611 bill information. *State.ar.us*. https://arkleg.state.ar.us/Bills/Detail?id=sb611&ddBienniumSession=2025%2F2025R (accessed 1 July 2025).

Azam, R. (2018). Accessing social media information for pharmacovigilance: what are the ethical implications? *Therapeutic Advances in Drug Safety*, *9*(8), 385–387. doi:10.1177/2042098618778191

Bender, J. L., Cyr, A. B., Arbuckle, L., & Ferris, L. E. (2017). Ethics and privacy implications of using the internet and social media to recruit participants for health research: a privacy-by-design framework for online recruitment. *Journal of Medical Internet Research*, *19*(4), e7029. doi:10.2196/jmir.7029

Beninger, K., Fry, A., Jago, N., Lepps, H., & Silvester, H. (2014, February 20). Research using Social Media; Users' Views. https://www.researchgate.net/publication/261551701_Research_using_Social_Media_Users (accessed 1 July 2025)

Bhatia-Lin, A., Boon-Dooley, A., Roberts, M. K., Pronai, C., Fisher, D., Parker, L., Engstrom, A., Ingraham, L., & Darnell, D. (2019). Ethical and regulatory considerations for using social media platforms to locate and track research participants. *The American Journal of Bioethics: AJOB*, *19*(6), 47–61. doi:10.1080/15265161.2019.1602176

Bishop, L., & Gray, D. (2017). Ethical challenges of publishing and sharing social media research data. In *The Ethics of Online Research* (world; Vol. (Vol. 2, pp. 159–187). Emerald Publishing Limited. doi:10.1108/S2398-601820180000002007

Bond, C. S., Ahmed, O. H., Hind, M., Thomas, B., & Hewitt-Taylor, J. (2013). The conceptual and practical ethical dilemmas of using health discussion board posts as research data. *Journal of Medical Internet Research*, *15*(6), e2435. doi:10.2196/jmir.2435

British Psychological Society 2017. Ethics guidelines for Internet-mediated Research (2017). *Leicester*. https://www.bps.org.uk/news-and-policy/ethics-guidelines-internet-mediated-research-2017 (accessed 1 July 2025).

British Sociological Association 2017. Ethics guidelines and collated resources for digital research. https://www.britsoc.co.uk/media/24309/bsa_statement_of_ethical_practice_annexe.pdf (accessed 1 July 2025).

Brown, B., Weilenmann, A., McMillan, D., and Lampinen, A. (2016). Five provocations for ethical HCI research. In *Proceedings of the 2016 CHI Conference on Human Factors in Computing Systems*, pp. 852–863. 10.1145/2858036.2858313.

Burkell, J., Regan, P. M., & Steeves, V. (2022). Privacy, consent, and confidentiality in social media research. In A. Quan-Haase & L. Sloan (Eds.), *The SAGE handbook of social media research methods* (pp. 715–725). SAGE Publications.

California Legislative Information (2022). Bill text—AB-2273 The California age-appropriate design code act. Leginfo.legislature.ca.gov. https://leginfo.legislature.ca.gov/faces/billTextClient.xhtml?bill_id=202120220AB2273 (accessed 1 July 2025).

California Legislative Information (2023). Bill text—SB-976 protecting our kids from social media addiction act. *Ca.gov*. https://leginfo.legislature.ca.gov/faces/billTextClient.xhtml?bill_id=202320240SB976.

Centers for Disease Control and Prevention (2024). Data sharing and collection principles and standards. *Program Collaboration and Service Integration. CDC.* https://www.cdc.gov/program-collaboration-service-integration/php/data-security/principles.html (accessed 1 July 2025).

Dawson, P. (2014). Our anonymous online research participants are not always anonymous: is this a problem? *British Journal of Educational Technology, 45*(3), 428–437. doi:10.1111/bjet.12144

Di Minin, E., Fink, C., Hausmann, A., Kremer, J., & Kulkarni, R. (2021). How to address data privacy concerns when using social media data in conservation science. *Conservation Biology, 35*(2), 437–446. doi:10.1111/cobi.13708

European Commission. (2022). Digital services act. *In Europe Fit For the Digital Age: Priorities*, 2019–2024. https://commission.europa.eu/strategy-and-policy/priorities-2019-2024/europe-fit-digital-age/digital-services-act_en (accessed 1 July 2025)

European Commission European Research Council (2025). Open research data and data management plans. https://erc.europa.eu/sites/default/files/document/file/ERC_info_document-Open_Research_Data_and_Data_Management_Plans.pdf (accessed 1 July 2025).

Figueiredo, A. S. (2017). Data sharing: convert challenges into opportunities. *Frontiers in Public Health, 5*. doi:10.3389/fpubh.2017.00327

Ford, E., Shepherd, S., Jones, K., & Hassan, L. (2021). Toward an ethical framework for the text mining of social media for health research: a systematic review. *Frontiers in Digital Health, 2*. doi:10.3389/fdgth.2020.592237

GDPR (2025). General data protection regulation (GDPR). *GDPR*. https://gdpr-info.eu/ (accessed 1 July 2025).

Golder, S., Ahmed, S., Norman, G., & Booth, A. (2017). Attitudes toward the ethics of research using social media: a systematic review. *Journal of Medical Internet Research, 19*(6), e7082. doi:10.2196/jmir.7082

Government of Canada, Panel on Research Ethics (2022). Does research using social media platforms require Research Ethics Board review? Guidance in applying TCPS 2 (2022). https://ethics.gc.ca/eng/reb-cer_social-sociaux.html (accessed 1 July 2025).

GovInfo (1996). www.govinfo.gov. https://www.govinfo.gov/app/details/PLAW-104publ104 (accessed 1 July 2025).

Humphreys, A. (2016). *Social Media: Enduring Principles*. Oxford University Press.

Hunter, R. F., Gough, A., O'Kane, N., McKeown, G., Fitzpatrick, A., Walker, T., McKinley, M., Lee, M., & Kee, F. (2018). Ethical issues in social media research for public health. *American Journal of Public Health, 108*(3), 343–348. doi:10.2105/AJPH.2017.304249

Hutchinson, J., Martin, F., & Aim Sinpeng. (2017). Chasing ISIS: Network Power, Distributed Ethics and Responsible Social Media Research. https://www.researchgate.net/publication/330995106_Chasing_ISIS_Network_Power_Distributed_Ethics_and_Responsible_Social_Media_Research (accessed 1 July 2025)

Kosinski, M., Stillwell, D., & Graepel, T. (2013). Private traits and attributes are predictable from digital records of human behavior. *Proceedings of the National Academy of Sciences of the United States of America, 110*(15), 5802–5805. doi:10.1073/pnas.1218772110

Kush, R., & Goldman, M. (2014). Fostering responsible data sharing through standards. *New England Journal of Medicine, 370*(23), 2163–2165. doi:10.1056/NEJMp1401444

London School of Economics and Political Science (2025). Using data from the internet and social media in research: ethics & consent (Version 8) [PDF]. https://info.lse.ac.uk/staff/divisions/research-and-innovation/research/Assets/Documents/PDF/ethics-Using-internet-and-Social-media-data-v8.pdf (accessed 31 July 2025).

Louisiana State Legislature (2024). SB162. *La.gov*. https://www.legis.la.gov/Legis/BillInfo.aspx?s=23RS&b=SB162 (accessed 31 July 2025)

Lunnay, B., Borlagdan, J., McNaughton, D., & Ward, P. (2015). Ethical use of social media to facilitate qualitative research. *Qualitative Health Research, 25*(1), 99–109. doi:10.1177/1049732314549031

Markham, A., & Buchanan, E. (2012). Ethical Decision-Making and Internet Research Recommendations from the AoIR Ethics Working Committee (Version 2.0). ResearchGate. https://www.researchgate.net/publication/263564245_Ethical_Decision-Making_and_Internet_Research_Recommendations_from_the_AoIR_Ethics_Working_Committee_Version_20

Michaelidou, N., Moraes, C., & Micevski, M. (2016). A scale for measuring consumers' ethical perceptions of social media research. In M. W. Obal, N. Krey, & C. Bushardt (Eds.), *Let's Get Engaged! Crossing the Threshold of Marketing's Engagement Era* (pp. 97–100). Springer International Publishing. doi:10.1007/978-3-319-11815-4_33

Mickoleit, A. (2014). Social media use by governments: a policy primer to discuss trends, identify policy opportunities and guide decision makers. *OECD*. 10.1787/5jxrcmghmk0s-en, https://ideas.repec.org/p/oec/govaaa/26-en.html (accessed 31 July 2025).

Mikal, J., Hurst, S., & Conway, M. (2016). Ethical issues in using Twitter for population-level depression monitoring: a qualitative study. *BMC Medical Ethics, 17*(1), 22. doi:10.1186/s12910-016-0105-5

Milne, G. R., & Culnan, M. J. (2004). Strategies for reducing online privacy risks: why consumers read (or don't read) online privacy notices. *Journal of Interactive Marketing, 18*(3), 15–29. doi:10.1002/dir.20009

Monks, H., Cardoso, P., Papageorgiou, A., Carolan, C., & Thomas, L. (2015). Young people's views regarding participation in mental health and wellbeing research through social media. *International Journal of Emotional Education, 7*(1), 4–19.

Montgomery, K. C. (2015). Youth and surveillance in the Facebook era: policy interventions and social implications. *Telecommunications Policy, 39*(9), 771–786. doi:10.1016/j.telpol.2014.12.006

Moreno, M. A., Goniu, N., Moreno, P. S., & Diekema, D. (2013). Ethics of social media research: common concerns and practical considerations. *Cyberpsychology, Behavior, and Social Networking, 16*(9), 708–713. doi:10.1089/cyber.2012.0334

Narayanan, A. and Shmatikov, V. (2009). De-anonymizing social networks. In *2009 30th IEEE Symposium on Security and Privacy,* pp. 173–187. 10.1109/SP.2009.22.

New York State Senate (2023). NY state assembly bill 2023-A8148A. NYSenate.gov. https://www.nysenate.gov/legislation/bills/2023/A8148/amendment/A (accessed 31 July 2025).

Obar, J. A., & Oeldorf-Hirsch, A. (2020). The biggest lie on the internet: ignoring the privacy policies and terms of service policies of social networking services. *Information, Communication & Society, 23*(1), 128–147. doi:10.1080/1369118X.2018.1486870

Pagoto, S., & Nebeker, C. (2019). How scientists can take the lead in establishing ethical practices for social media research. *Journal of the American Medical Informatics Association, 26*(4), 311–313. doi:10.1093/jamia/ocy174

van Panhuis, W. G., Paul, P., Emerson, C., Grefenstette, J., Wilder, R., Herbst, A. J., Heymann, D., & Burke, D. S. (2014). A systematic review of barriers to data sharing in public health. *BMC Public Health, 14,* 1144. doi:10.1186/1471-2458-14-1144

Pisani, E., & AbouZahr, C. (2010). Sharing health data: good intentions are not enough. *Bulletin of the World Health Organization, 88,* 462–466.

Queen's University (2024). Guidelines on the use of social media in research [PDF]. https://www.queensu.ca/vpr/ethics/guidelines-policies/reb-social-media (accessed 1 August 2025).

Roberts, L. D. (2015). Ethical issues in conducting qualitative research in online communities. *Qualitative Research in Psychology, 12*(3), 314–325. doi:10.1080/14780887.2015.1008909

Rocher, L., Hendrickx, J. M., & de Montjoye, Y.-A. (2019). Estimating the success of re-identifications in incomplete datasets using generative models. *Nature Communications, 10,* 3069. doi:10.1038/s41467-019-10933-3

Samuel, G., Derrick, G. E., & van Leeuwen, T. (2019). The ethics ecosystem: personal ethics, network governance and regulating actors governing the use of social media research data. *Minerva, 57*(3), 317–343. doi:10.1007/s11024-019-09368-3

Savage, C. J., & Vickers, A. J. (2009). Empirical study of data sharing by authors publishing in PLoS journals. *PLOS ONE, 4*(9), e7078. doi:10.1371/journal.pone.0007078

Smith, M., Szongott, C., Henne, B., and von Voigt, G. (2012). Big data privacy issues in public social media. In *2012 6th IEEE International Conference on Digital Ecosystems and Technologies (DEST),* pp. 1–6. 10.1109/DEST.2012.6227909.

Smith, C. M., Widjaya, R., Rivero, G., and Aaron. (2021). The behaviors and attitudes of U.S. Adults on Twitter. *Pew Research Center.* https://www.pewresearch.org/internet/2021/11/15/the-behaviors-and-attitudes-of-u-s-adults-on-twitter/ (accessed 1 August 2025).

Social Media Research Group 2016. Using social media for social research: an introduction. https://www.gov.uk/government/uploads/system/uploads/attachment_data/file/524750/GSR_Social_Media *Research_Guidance-*_Using_social_media_for_social_research.pdf (accessed 1 August 2025).

Stefanidis, A., Crooks, A., & Radzikowski, J. (2013). Harvesting ambient geospatial information from social media feeds. *GeoJournal, 78*(2), 319–338. doi:10.1007/s10708-011-9438-2

Stockmann, D., & Tromble, R. (2017). Lost Umbrellas: Bias and the Right to be Forgotten in Social Media Research. In M. Zimmer & K. Kinder-Kurlanda (Eds.), *New Challenges, Cases, and Contexts* (pp. 75–90).

Taylor, J., & Pagliari, C. (2018). Mining social media data: how are research sponsors and researchers addressing the ethical challenges? *Research Ethics, 14*(2), 1–39. doi:10.1177/1747016117738559

Taylor, H. A., Kuwana, E., & Wilfond, B. S. (2014). Ethical implications of social media in health care research. *The American Journal of Bioethics, 14*(10), 58–59. doi:10.1080/15265161.2014.947820

Tennessee General Assembly Legislation (2024). *Tn.gov.* https://wapp.capitol.tn.gov/apps/BillInfo/default.aspx?BillNumber=HB1891&GA=113 (accessed 1 August 2025).

Townsend, L., & Wallace, C. (2017). The ethics of using social media data in research: a new framework. In K. Woodfield (Ed.), *The Ethics of Online Research* (Vol. 2, pp. 189–207). Emerald Publishing Limited. doi:10.1108/S2398-601820180000002008

Utah State Legislature (2025). *Utah.gov.* https://le.utah.gov/xcode/historical.html?date=1/16/2024&oc=/xcode/Title13/Chapter63/C13-63-S102_2023050320230503.html (accessed 1 September 2025)

Valdez, R., & Keim-Malpass, J. (2019). Ethics in health research using social media. In J. Bian, Y. Guo, Z. He, & X. Hu (Eds.), *Social Web and Health Research: Benefits, Limitations, and Best Practices* (pp. 259–269). Springer International Publishing. doi:10.1007/978-3-030-14714-3_13

Walport, M., & Brest, P. (2011). Sharing research data to improve public health. *The Lancet, 377*(9765), 537–539.

Wilkinson, M. D., Dumontier, M., Aalbersberg, I. J., Appleton, G., Axton, M., Baak, A., Blomberg, N., Boiten, J.-W., da Silva Santos, L. B., Bourne, P. E., Bouwman, J., Brookes, A. J., Clark, T., Crosas, M., Dillo, I., Dumon, O., Edmunds, S., Evelo, C. T., Finkers, R., & Gonzalez-Beltran, A. (2016). The FAIR guiding principles for scientific data management and stewardship. *Scientific Data, 3*(1). https://www.nature.com/articles/sdata201618

Williams, M. L., Burnap, P., & Sloan, L. (2017). Towards an ethical framework for publishing Twitter data in social research: taking into account users' views, online context and algorithmic estimation. *Sociology, 51*(6), 1149–1168. doi:10.1177/0038038517708140

Woodfield, K., Morrell, G., Metzler, K., et al. (2013). Blurring the boundaries? New social media, new social research: developing a network to explore the issues faced by researchers negotiating the new research landscape of online social media platforms [Working Paper]. *NCRM.* https://eprints.ncrm.ac.uk/id/eprint/3168/.

World Health Organization (2020). WHO data principles. *World Health Organization.* https://data.who.int/about/data.who-data-principles (accessed 1 September 2025).

Zimmer, M. (2010). "But the data is already public": on the ethics of research in Facebook. *Ethics and Information Technology, 12*(4), 313–325. doi:10.1007/s10676-010-9227-5

CHAPTER 5

QUANTITATIVE AND MACHINE LEARNING METHODS FOR SURVEILLANCE AND EXPLORING TEMPORAL AND GEOGRAPHIC TRENDS

Thu T. Nguyen[1], Amrutha S. Alibilli[1], Xiaohe Yue[1], Vidur Jain[1], and Yulin Hswen[2]

[1]Department of Epidemiology and Biostatistics, School of Public Health, University of Maryland, College Park, MD, USA

[2]The Artificial Intelligence Interdisciplinary Institute at Maryland (AIM), College of Computer, Mathematical, and Natural Sciences (CMNS), Department of Epidemiology and Biostatistics, School of Public Health, University of Maryland, College Park, MD, USA

Overview

The turn of the 21st century has catalyzed seismic societal shifts and propelled rapid advancements in social media and artificial intelligence (AI) technologies, reshaping communities, industries, information, and communication. Social media represents a form of Big Data due to its vast scale, high density of information, and complexity. Data samples can be in the millions or billions of posts, containing mixed types of text, images, and videos. These data are visualized and analyzed to uncover patterns, test hypotheses, track trends, and identify emerging symptoms, diseases, or behaviors. Key data attributes of interest to researchers include timestamp data and geographic markers, which help analyze temporal and geographic trends. Time and geographic information also allow for the integration of social media data with other datasets, such as health or hate crimes data. Engagement metrics such as reactions, likes, shares, followers, and following counts can offer valuable insights into the reach and influence of posts. This chapter explores quantitative analyses leveraging AI and machine learning to process and analyze social media data. Case studies include the use of social media for

LEARNING OBJECTIVES

1. Provide a broad overview of disease surveillance
2. Discuss limitations of official counts or reports for disease surveillance
3. Discuss potential ways social media can address some of these limitations to provide complementary data that can supplement but not replace traditional surveillance, using examples of Zika and COVID-19
4. Discuss some of the strengths and limitations of social media data for disease surveillance
5. Offer applied examples of using social media data to track trends in online discussions of marginalized populations

outbreak surveillance, demonstrating how social media can act as a forecasting system and provide real-time data on public behaviors and beliefs about diseases. Additional examples explore key social movements, including the Black Lives Matter Movement, the rise and recognition of anti-Asian racism during the COVID-19 pandemic, and national conversations about LGBTQ+ and transgender rights and protections.

Disease Surveillance—Key Concepts

Indicator-based surveillance (IBS) is a traditional surveillance approach where data from health facilities are routinely collected using standard case definitions to track trends and identify outbreaks. It is primarily used for well-established diseases and conditions with predefined standard case definitions (World Health Organization 2017).

Event-based surveillance (EBS) is a less traditional approach that collects data on health-related events or risks from diverse sources, including social media, news media, and non-governmental organizations. EBS can complement IBS systems, as there is often a delay for official counts and reports (Velasco et al. 2014).

Social Media and Health Surveillance

The COVID-19 pandemic has demonstrated the pressing need for digital health surveillance through nontraditional sources to support more efficient diagnosis and treatment. Public health professionals have historically relied on established indicator-based health databases to monitor infectious diseases, but these platforms depend on timely updates from physicians and health officials (Velasco et al. 2014). Indicator-based health reporting is constrained by time delays and the inability to detect novel, unexpected disease occurrences due to the need for predefined case definitions (Velasco et al. 2014). Social media provides unique advantages for monitoring the following types of health events:

1. Rare or unexpected health events that fall outside standard indicator-based reporting
2. Real-time health events that have not been detected in indicator-based reporting due to time delays
3. Health events affecting marginalized populations with limited access to formal indicator-based reporting systems

With the advent of the Internet, social media has emerged as a predominant platform for public discourse. In particular, geotagged social media data with precise timestamps and geographic coordinates enable temporal and geographic analyses. For instance, the Social Media and Research Testbed (SMART) database processed and sorted tweet data according to public health relevance (Tsou et al. 2016). Compared with relying on a single source alone, diverse social media platforms offer invaluable public data that can assist in disease prediction and surveillance, providing epidemiologists with timely information to develop effective public health interventions.

Leveraging Artificial Intelligence and Machine Learning Techniques in Analyzing Social Media Discourse During the COVID-19 Pandemic

Several studies have explored the use of social media data to enhance public health surveillance during the COVID-19 pandemic, demonstrating the potential of natural language processing (NLP) and machine learning (ML) techniques to detect disease-related signals in real time for accurate results.

A study using X (formerly Twitter) data found a high correlation between tweets and real-time COVID-19 data, demonstrating X as a valuable tool for epidemiological monitoring (Comito 2021). Hasan et al. (2022) developed a novel end-to-end NLP pipeline to automatically triage and diagnose COVID-19 from patient-authored social media posts. Their study focused on individual-level posts, particularly from UK users during the early pandemic phase, and demonstrated how symptom concepts (such as "breathing hurts") and relations (e.g., linking symptoms to body parts) could be annotated and used to train ML classifiers. The researchers engaged frontline clinicians to validate the triage and diagnosis decisions, revealing that support vector machine (SVM) models trained on either ground-truth or predicted annotations could inform clinical decision-making (Hasan et al. 2022). While the individual-level diagnosis was limited by the noisy nature of social media data, the aggregate patterns were found to be valuable for public health surveillance.

Kellner et al. (2023) expanded this approach to a broader population-level application, addressing the limitations of official case reporting systems that are often delayed and inconsistent. They demonstrated that integrating heterogeneous user-generated content (UGC) from platforms like Reddit and X can improve the prediction of real-world metrics such as COVID-19 incidence and hospitalization rates up to 14 days in advance. Unlike earlier studies that relied on a single platform or static models, Kellner et al. (2023) employed adaptable models that accounted for temporal shifts in information relevance. Their findings emphasized the importance of data fusion across platforms to improve model robustness and timeliness in disaster response contexts. The ability to use early symptom self-reporting from users, often occurring before formal testing, proved to be a powerful predictor for healthcare system strain.

Together, these studies underscore the utility of NLP-driven methods for extracting actionable insights from real-time data sources during health crises. Additionally, they reveal a key research opportunity: while Hasan et al. (2022) illustrated the technical feasibility of extracting structured clinical information from free-text social media posts, Kellner et al. (2023) highlighted the epidemiological value of combining this information across diverse platforms. Building upon these foundations, future research can further investigate geospatial and temporal trends in self-reported symptoms using clustering algorithms and visualizations to inform health promotion strategies.

Zika Surveillance and Management

Transmitted by mosquitoes, the Zika virus was first identified in 1947 in a Rhesus macaque in Uganda. By the 1950s, infections were reported in other African countries. Initially, Zika infections were characterized by mild symptoms of fever and rash lasting for several days (Macnamara 1954). In 2015, the Zika virus emerged in the Americas and Brazil. Concerns about the Zika virus grew as it became increasingly associated with Guillain–Barré syndrome, an autoimmune disorder, and microcephaly, a birth defect resulting in an abnormally small head. In February 2016, the World Health Organization (WHO) declared Zika as a public health emergency of international concern (World Health Organization 2016).

Using Event-Based Surveillance with Zika

Officially reported Zika case counts are generally delayed by several weeks. To complement government tracking and reporting of Zika cases, a study examined Google searches, Twitter microblogs, and the HealthMap digital surveillance system, which monitors, compiles, and visualizes reports of nongovernmental alerts of infections, along with official historical suspected Zika case counts, to evaluate the combination of data sources that best predicted suspected Zika cases for five countries: Colombia, El Salvador, Honduras, Venezuela, and Martinique. For Google Correlate and Google Trends data, researchers analyzed country-specific Zika-related search terms. For Twitter data, the researchers collected a random sample of tweets with "Zika," "microcephaly," and "microcefalia" and calculated the percentage of Zika-related tweets to the total number of tweets as the predictor variable. The study found that Google and Twitter data, coupled with historical data, best predicted case counts one week ahead. Without historical data, Google and Twitter data most accurately predicted case counts two to three weeks ahead, suggesting that official case count information two to three weeks out was less useful for longer-term forecasting. This study illustrates the potential value of Google and Twitter data in tracking Zika trends and can be adapted to monitor other new and emerging diseases (McGough et al. 2017).

CASE STUDY 1. MISINFORMATION AND VACCINE HESITANCY

Beyond disease surveillance, social media can be used to understand the public's beliefs regarding important public health issues, including vaccinations. This section explores vaccine hesitancy and misinformation surrounding the Zika and COVID-19 vaccines.

Misinformation is defined as information that is inadvertently false and is shared without the intent to cause harm. In contrast, **disinformation** is false information that is deliberately developed and shared with the intent to cause harm (Wang et al. 2019).

Even before the Zika virus vaccine was fully developed and approved, there was a rise in skepticism and misinformation surrounding the Zika virus and the vaccine. Studies examining misinformation on the Zika virus found the following themes: attributing microcephaly to a mosquito larvicide; microcephaly as an adverse side effect of existing vaccines such as the Measles, Mumps, and Rubella (MMR) or Tdap (Dredze et al. 2016); conspiracy theories around the creation of the Zika virus as a bioweapon; and the development of the Zika virus with the purpose of decreasing the world population (Sommariva et al. 2018).

Similar themes reappeared in an analysis of COVID-19 vaccine hesitancy using social media data. Vaccine hesitancy is impacted by the broader societal and historical context. In the United States, historical medical injustices, such as the Tuskegee Study of Untreated Syphilis, in which African American men were enrolled to document the natural progression of syphilis without treatment, have contributed to medical mistrust that can impact engagement with the health care system. Additionally, contemporary experiences of discrimination in health care settings further perpetuate medical mistrust (Armstrong et al. 2013). For instance, Black Americans report higher rates of racial discrimination in the health care setting than other racial groups. Against this backdrop, Criss et al. (2021) conducted a qualitative content analysis of Twitter posts from October 2020 to January 2021. Tweets were collected using Twitter's Streaming application programming interface (API)and filtered for race-related, vaccine-related, and COVID-19 keywords. Using a thematic content analysis, the researchers identified six major categories: vaccine support, opposition, misinformation, disparities, representation, and politics.

For vaccine hesitancy, various tweets expressed opposition to the COVID-19 vaccine or concerns over potential adverse reactions. There were frequent mentions of conspiracy theories and misinformation; for instance, misinformation included the beliefs that the vaccine was a tool for extermination and that mere protective behaviors were sufficient in protecting oneself from COVID-19 without the vaccine. For vaccine support, there were expressions of excitement and positivity related to the development of the vaccine and people receiving their COVID-19 shots. Some tweets emphasized the importance of vaccination for people of color, while others criticized vaccine hesitancy and opposition. Vaccine support tweets emphasized pride in vaccine development, especially highlighting prominent Black scientists like Dr. Kizzmekia Corbett (Criss et al. 2021). Emergent themes also included the persistence of health disparities, the history of medical racism, and the importance of reducing barriers to vaccine access. Additionally, there were debates about the role of politics in vaccination efforts (Criss et al. 2021). These studies highlight the value of using social media to gain greater understanding and insight into the public's fears, beliefs, and attitudes related to public health issues. Such information can be used to develop targeted communication strategies to promote vaccine uptake, decrease medical mistrust, and address barriers to vaccine access.

CASE STUDY 2. SOCIAL MEDIA DATA FOR UNDERSTANDING DISCUSSIONS RELATED TO HISTORIC MOMENTS AND MOVEMENTS

The COVID-19 pandemic was marked by an extended period of uncertainty and fear, especially in the early phases of the pandemic when there was limited information about the virus' origin and transmission. Additionally, there was widespread misinformation related to COVID-19's source in China (Leng et al. 2021). Although news reports, first-hand accounts, and second-hand sources regarding anti-Asian racism emerged across the globe, there were few empirical investigations. This study aimed to address the dearth of literature on changes in anti-Asian sentiment at the beginning of the COVID-19 pandemic.

For this study, Nguyen et al. (2020) collected U.S. tweets referencing Asians from November 2019 to June 2020. In total, 3,377,295 tweets from 521,161 Twitter users were analyzed. Sentiment analysis was conducted using SVMs to examine temporal trends in negative racial sentiment before and after the emergence of COVID-19 (Nguyen et al. 2020). SVMs are flexible and robust supervised ML models that require training data (e.g., human-labeled data) to understand how individuals perceive posts as positive or negative in sentiment (Joachims 1998). Training data were obtained from Sentiment140 (n = 498; VanderWeele and Vansteelandt 2009), Kaggle (n = 7086; Kaggle: University of Michigan; 2018), and Sanders (n = 5113; Sanders Analytics: GitHub; 2011), with an additional 6471 tweets labeled by our research group. Sentiment140, Sanders, and Kaggle datasets are all publicly available training datasets specifically labeled for sentiment analysis. Tweets were labeled 1 if negative (0 for positive or neutral tweets). Fivefold cross-validation was used to assess model performance, and the final models had an accuracy of 91% for negative sentiment classification and an F1 score of 84%. Accuracy for positive sentiment classification was 89% with an F1 score of 81%. Once trained and tested, this model was used to label collected tweets from 2019 to 2020.

The study found that the percentage of tweets referencing Asians that were negative rose from 9.8% in early November 2019 to 16.5% by the end of March 2020, representing a 68% increase. By April 2020, the proportion of negative sentiment tweets referencing Asians declined to 13.2%. In June 2020, negative sentiment toward Asians declined further but remained higher compared to levels observed prior to the COVID-19 pandemic (Figure 5.1).

Investigators examined whether this trend was specific to tweets referencing Chinese individuals in particular or broadly to Asians. A sensitivity analysis was conducted to examine the sentiment of tweets using the terms: "Chinese," "chinaman," "ching chong," and "chink." The results closely mirrored the trends observed for Asian tweets overall, indicating spillover effects regarding discussions of COVID-19 toward Chinese people and Asians in general.

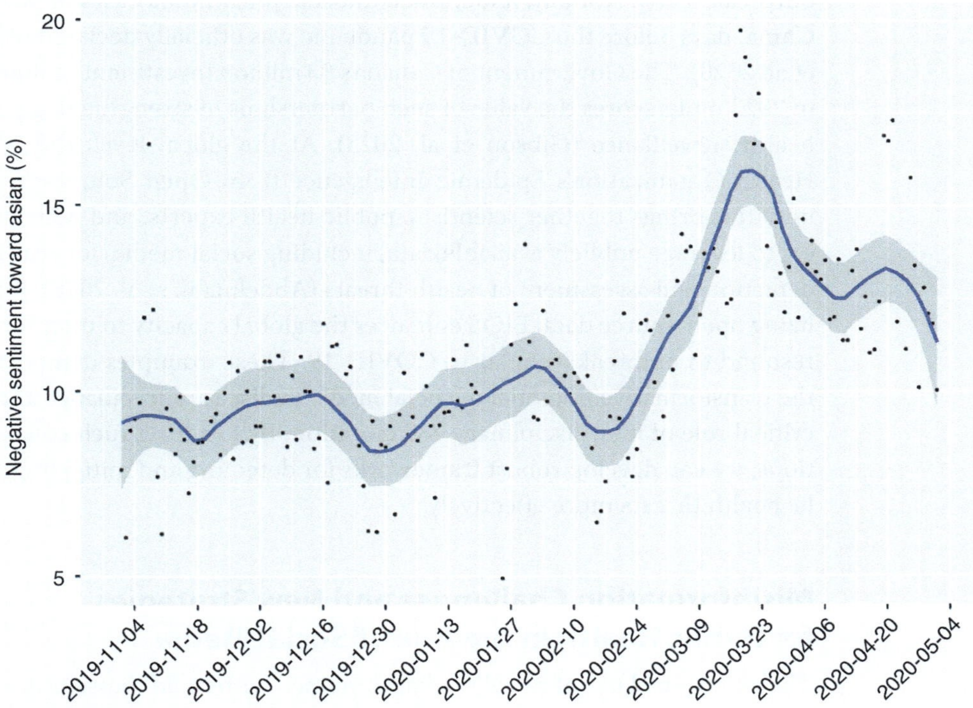

Figure 5.1 Temporal changes in negative Asian sentiment, November 2019–April 2020. $N = 235{,}263$ tweets. LOESS (locally estimated scatterplot smoothing) was performed to fit smooth curves to the daily prevalence of negative sentiment. The shaded area represents 95% confidence bands around the smoothed trend line.

Source: Nguyen et al., 2020 / MDPI / CC BY 4.0.

Future Directions for Social Media Research

Interdisciplinary and Cross-Sector Collaborations

To fully unlock the potential of social media in disease surveillance, interdisciplinary collaboration among scientists, public health professionals, and policymakers is essential. Interdisciplinary partnerships have led to innovative platforms and strategies that leverage social media and other digital data sources to enhance public health responses. For instance, the HealthMap platform, developed through a partnership among researchers, epidemiologists, and software developers, integrates data from online news, social media, and user submissions to provide real-time surveillance of emerging public health threats. This platform played a pivotal role in detecting the 2014 Ebola outbreak in Guinea by analyzing informal data sources and threats before official alerts were issued (Milinovich et al. 2015).

Similarly, BlueDot, a Canadian health intelligence company, exemplifies collaboration between public health authorities and data scientists. In partnership with the Government of Canada, BlueDot processes data from social media, flight patterns, and medical reports to identify disease outbreaks early. Notably, it identified unusual pneumonia cases in Wuhan, China, days before the COVID-19 pandemic was officially declared (Allam et al. 2020). The Government of Canada's $3 million investment in BlueDot in 2023 underscores the value of such partnerships in strengthening public health surveillance (Gibson et al. 2023). At the global level, the World Health Organization's Epidemic Intelligence from Open Sources (EIOS) initiative brings together scientists, public health experts, and policymakers to leverage publicly available data, including social media, for real-time detection and assessment of health threats (Abdelmalik et al. 2018). By utilizing open-source data, EIOS enhances the global capacity to monitor and respond to outbreaks similar to COVID-19. These examples demonstrate the transformative potential of social media in disease surveillance and the critical role of interdisciplinary collaboration. By fostering such collaborations, we can develop robust frameworks for detecting and mitigating public health threats more effectively.

Misinformation Challenges and New Strategies for Public Health in the Age of Social Media

The widespread use of social media, combined with rapid message dissemination and minimal entry barriers, has transformed these platforms into a primary channel for the spread of health-related misinformation. As platforms expand and diversify, the strategies used to disseminate misleading content do as well. False text, manipulated images, and increasingly sophisticated AI-generated videos complicate efforts to distinguish between credible and deceptive information. The use of bots, fake accounts, and paid users further amplifies the reach of misinformation. These messages are often emotionally charged, encouraging engagement and resharing without critical evaluation. Compounding this challenge is the blending of factual and false information within the same message, further complicating discernment between accurate and misleading content. The implications of such misinformation are profound: it can erode trust, promote harmful behaviors, and hinder timely responses to health emergencies.

However, traditional methods of detecting and addressing misinformation are often insufficient in this rapidly changing environment. Older methods, such as keyword flagging or basic content analysis, are increasingly inadequate in capturing the complexity and multimodal nature of these evolving tactics. To address these challenges, future social media public health research must adopt more advanced methods. One promising approach involves tracking misinformation alongside corrective responses. Prior studies, such as research by Vraga and Bode (2017), found that when organizations like the Centers for Disease Control and Prevention (CDC) issue corrective information, it does not harm the organization's credibility, and public misperceptions are reduced. This evidence supports immediate and authoritative rebuttals of health misinformation as an effective intervention. Another critical strategy is improving public health literacy. Empowering users to evaluate health information critically can help individuals identify questionable content and make informed decisions.

Beyond the organic spread of misinformation by individual users, social media platforms themselves can actively shape what content gains visibility by algorithmic amplification. These algorithms are designed to maximize user engagement, often by prioritizing content that provokes strong emotional reactions such as anger, fear, or outrage. As a result, misleading or sensationalist health information is more likely to be promoted over balanced, evidence-based messaging. Prior research has indicated that false health claims, such as "miracle" cures or vaccine conspiracies, often outperform factual posts in terms of likes, shares, and reach due to their emotional value (Bandy and Diakopoulos 2021). Furthermore, recommendation systems on platforms like YouTube and Facebook can trap users in "filter bubbles," where they are continuously shown similar content; this reinforces existing beliefs and increases exposure to misinformation. These algorithmic patterns can disproportionately affect vulnerable populations and communities with limited health literacy, thereby reinforcing preexisting disparities and reducing access to correct or authoritative health information. Understanding and mitigating algorithmic bias is crucial for reducing the spread of harmful narratives and promoting equitable information environments.

The landscape of online misinformation is further complicated by the presence of bots and coordinated disinformation campaigns. Unlike human users, bots can rapidly disseminate content across platforms, interact with other users, and generate artificial popularity for posts through user-engagement metrics. During the early stages of COVID-19, researchers found that these bots were responsible for amplifying hashtags that falsely alleged that hospitals were empty and the pandemic was overblown (Ahmed et al. 2020). In some cases, they were part of coordinated operations backed by domestic and foreign individuals hoping to stir confusion or distrust in health authorities. Moreover, bots often target health topics that are emotionally charged and powerful to maximize potential disruption. This activity can overwhelm public discourse, skew perception of public sentiment, and reduce the reach of trustworthy and valid content.

Efforts by platforms to moderate content, such as removing false claims or banning accounts, are critical but complex. While content removal can prevent further spread of harmful misinformation, it often triggers backlash and deepens mistrust. This is particularly seen among users who perceive such actions as censorship. A notable example occurred during the COVID-19 pandemic with the removal of the viral "Plandemic" video. Despite its quick takedown for promoting incorrect information about the virus and vaccines, the video continued to spread across lesser-known platforms and became prominent for conspiracy theorists who claimed that "truth" was being suppressed. In some cases, attempts at moderation have had the adverse effect of lending perceived credibility to false claims and fueling antiestablishment narratives. Furthermore, takedown policies are often inconsistently applied across languages and countries (Simpson and Conner 2020; Saumya et al. 2024). This allows some misinformation to persist in under-moderated languages or regions, such as posts in Spanish and Arabic, while other content, such as English-language posts, may be erroneously removed due to strict filters. These inconsistencies highlight the need for more transparent, consistent, and culturally competent moderation policies that account for both the harms of misinformation and the risks of perceived silencing, especially within historically marginalized communities.

Despite the growing number of strategies, there is limited comparative evidence about their effectiveness across different contexts. Variables, such as culture and religion, can affect the feasibility of the strategies. To address the complex issue of misinformation, researchers are increasingly turning to multimodal models to detect misinformation. As introduced in Chapter 3 in the context of hate speech detection, these models combine multiple data types, such as text and images, to improve classification accuracy. Similar models can be applied to address misinformation issues on social media as well. Given the differences in platform design and policy, researchers are encouraged to design platform-specific multimodal detectors. Finally, more studies are needed to investigate the underlying drivers of misinformation. This includes examining platform-level priorities and characteristics of viral misinformation. These insights can inform more effective, context-specific intervention designs. It would be valuable for future research to measure both short-term user responses and long-term behavioral impacts. Additionally, assessments of unintended consequences, such as user resistance to correction or increased mistrust, are needed. While major platforms often prioritize misinformation filtering around high-profile events such as elections or pandemics, more routine health misinformation receives less attention. Closer collaboration between researchers and platform providers is essential to broaden the scope and effectiveness of intervention strategies.

Opportunities and Pitfalls

There are important limitations to using social media data. The number of social media posts is not necessarily related to the importance of issues. Similarly, we often observe temporary spikes and then declines related to important events or issues, but this does not mean the issue is now resolved. It can reflect post activity, public attention, and discourse. Social media has the capacity to spread both factual information and misinformation. As a result, information on social media needs to be evaluated and verified against validated information.

Despite these limitations, social media and online data can be valuable data sources to complement existing traditional methods that are routinely collected by health facilities to provide timely data for intervention and to investigate new and emerging conditions where little information is known or there is a delay in data collection. Because social media data are continually being created across the globe, these data can be used to examine important national and international moments in real-time. Researchers can use social media data to examine how the public, political leaders, and health officials are discussing and responding to these events and to track sentiment, behaviors, and outcomes. Even when information is misleading on social media, it provides an important opportunity to monitor the public's understanding, attitudes, and beliefs about crucial issues.

KEY POINTS AND TAKEAWAYS

- **Provide a broad overview of disease surveillance.**
  There are two primary types of disease surveillance: indicator-based and event-based. While traditional indicator-based surveillance relies on routinely reported public health data to monitor known diseases, event-based surveillance uses nontraditional public health sources, such as social media, to respond to novel disease outbreaks.
- **Discuss limitations of official counts or reports for disease surveillance.**
  Official indicator-based reports may be delayed or incomplete. There is under-reporting, especially in areas where there is limited healthcare or public health infrastructure. Furthermore, indicator-based reporting has limited ability to detect novel diseases because this type of surveillance depends on standard case definitions.
- **Discuss the strengths and limitations of social media data for disease surveillance.**
  As depicted by the Zika and COVID-19 case studies, social media serves as a complementary tool for disease surveillance, providing real-time, wide-reaching data to help predict early outbreaks and monitor disease trends. While social media may be susceptible to misinformation and privacy concerns, it can offer timely insights into broader public sentiment, aiding public health professionals and policymakers to engage in effective, targeted interventions.
- **Offer applied examples of using social media data to track trends in online discussions of marginalized populations.**
  Applied examples, such as temporal sentiment analysis and geographic mapping, can highlight how social media image and text data can be merged with complementary data sources to reveal deeper insights into health trends. In addition, social media provides a unique platform to analyze the experiences of marginalized populations during public health crises, revealing insights

that may be otherwise inaccessible through other traditional methods. Overall, social media analysis helps monitor misinformation, assess vaccine hesitancy, and develop targeted communication strategies to improve public trust.

- **Highlight** the Importance of Key Stakeholder Collaboration
  Interdisciplinary collaboration is key. Effective surveillance requires collaboration among data scientists, epidemiologists, and policymakers, as seen in platforms like HealthMap and BlueDot that integrate digital and traditional data sources.

Conclusion

Social media data provides real-time access to experiences and information from across the globe. It can be harnessed to track new and emerging threats, whether real, perceived, or misinformed. By offering insights and understanding of these threats, researchers, policymakers, and the public are better equipped to respond and identify opportunities for intervention. To unlock the full potential of social media in disease surveillance, sustained collaboration among data scientists, public health professionals, and policymakers is essential. These interdisciplinary partnerships play a pivotal role in developing robust analytical frameworks, safeguarding data privacy, ensuring ethical use, and translating insights into actionable public health strategies.

References

Abdelmalik, P., Peron, E., Schnitzler, J., Fontaine, J., Elfenkamper, E., & Barboza, P. (2018). *The Epidemic Intelligence from Open Sources initiative: A collaboration to harmonize and standardize early detection and epidemic intelligence among public health organizations* [L'initiative «Epidemic Intelligence from Open Sources»: une collaboration visant à harmoniser et à standardiser les procédures de détection précoce et de renseignement épidémiologique entre les organisations de santé publique]. *Weekly Epidemiological Record, 93*(20), 267–270.

Ahmed, W., Vidal-Alaball, J., Downing, J., & López Seguí, F. (2020). COVID-19 and the 5G conspiracy theory: social network analysis of Twitter data. *Journal of medical Internet research, 22*(5), e19458. doi:10.2196/19458

Allam, Z., Dey, G., & Jones, D. S. (2020). Artificial intelligence (AI) provided early detection of the coronavirus (COVID-19) in China and will influence future urban health policy internationally. *AI, 1*(2), 156–165.

Armstrong, K., Putt, M., Halbert, C. H., Grande, D., Schwartz, J. S., Liao, K., Marcus, N., Demeter, M. B., & Shea, J. A. (2013). Prior experiences of racial discrimination and racial differences in health care system distrust. *Medical Care, 51*(2), 144–150.

Bandy, J., & Diakopoulos, N. (2021). More accounts, fewer links: how algorithmic curation impacts media exposure in Twitter timelines. *Proceedings of the ACM on Human-Computer Interaction, 5*(CSCW1) Article 78, 1–28. doi:10.1145/3449152

Comito, C. (2021). How COVID-19 information spread in US? The role of Twitter as early indicator of epidemics. *IEEE Transactions on Services Computing, 15*(3), 1193–1205.

Criss, S., Nguyen, T. T., Norton, S., Virani, I., Titherington, E., Tillmanns, E. L., Kinnane, C., Maiolo, G., Kirby, A. B., & Gee, G. C. (2021). Advocacy, hesitancy, and equity: exploring US race-related discussions of the COVID-19 vaccine on Twitter. *International Journal of Environmental Research and Public Health, 18*(11), 5693.

Dredze, M., Broniatowski, D. A., & Hilyard, K. M. (2016). Zika vaccine misconceptions: a social media analysis. *Vaccine, 34*(30), 3441–3442.

Gibson, E., DeWolfe, C., & Luther, I. (2023). Digital surveillance of COVID-19: privacy and equity considerations. *Canadian Journal of Law and Technology, 19*(1), 37.

Hasan, A., Levene, M., Weston, D., Fromson, R., Koslover, N., & Levene, T. (2022). Monitoring COVID-19 on social media: development of an end-to-end natural language processing pipeline using a novel triage and diagnosis approach. *Journal of Medical Internet Research, 24*(2), e30397.

Joachims, T. (1998l). Text categorization with Support Vector Machines: learning with many relevant features. In *Proceedings of the 10th European Conference on Machine Learning* (pp. 137–142).

Kaggle.: University of Michigan; 2018 (n.d.). UMICH SI650—sentiment classification. https://www.kaggle.com/c/si650winter11 https://www.zotero.org/google-docs/?8z9P9c (accessed 9 June 2025).

Kellner, D., Lowin, M., & Hinz, O. (2023). Improved healthcare disaster decision-making utilizing information extraction from complementary social media data during the COVID-19 pandemic. *Decision Support Systems, 172,* 113983.

Leng, Y., Zhai, Y., Sun, S., Wu, Y., Selzer, J., Strover, S., Zhang, H., Chen, A., & Ding, Y. (2021). Misinformation during the COVID-19 outbreak in China: cultural, social and political entanglements. *IEEE Transactions on Big Data, 7*(1), 69–80.

Macnamara, F. (1954). Zika virus: a report on three cases of human infection during an epidemic of jaundice in Nigeria. *Transactions of the Royal Society of Tropical Medicine and Hygiene, 48*(2), 139–145.

McGough, S. F., Brownstein, J. S., Hawkins, J. B., & Santillana, M. (2017). Forecasting Zika incidence in the 2016 Latin America outbreak combining traditional disease surveillance with search, social media, and news report data. *PLoS Neglected Tropical Diseases, 11*(1), e0005295.

Milinovich, G. J., Magalhães, R. J. S., & Hu, W. (2015). Role of big data in the early detection of Ebola and other emerging infectious diseases. *The Lancet Global Health, 3*(1), e20–e21.

Nguyen, T. T., Criss, S., Dwivedi, P., Huang, D., Keralis, J., Hsu, E., Phan, L., Nguyen, L. H., Yardi, I., & Glymour, M. M. (2020). Exploring US shifts in anti-Asian sentiment with the emergence of COVID-19. *International Journal of Environmental Research and Public Health, 17*(19), 7032.

Sanders Analytics (2011). *Twitter Sentiment Corpus. GitHub.* https://github.com/zfz/twitter_corpus[accessed2020-05-07https://www.zotero.org/google-docs/?8z9P9c (accessed 9 June 2025).

Saumya, S., Kumar, A., & Singh, J. P. (2024). Filtering offensive language from multilingual social media contents: a deep learning approach. *Engineering Applications of Artificial Intelligence, 133*(Part B), 108159. doi:10.1016/j.engappai.2024.108159

Simpson, E., & Conner, A. (2020). *Fighting Coronavirus Misinformation and Disinformation: Preventive Product Recommendations for Social Media Platforms*. Center for American Progress. https://www.americanprogress.org/article/fighting-coronavirus-misinformation-disinformation/

Sommariva, S., Vamos, C., Mantzarlis, A., Đào, L. U.-L., & Martinez Tyson, D. (2018). Spreading the (fake) news: exploring health messages on social media and the implications for health professionals using a case study. *American Journal of Health Education, 49*(4), 246–255.

Tsou, M.-H., Jung, C.-T., & Peddecord, M. (2016). Situational awareness of health events using social media and the SMART dashboard. *Online Journal of Public Health Informatics, 8*(1), e61882.

VanderWeele, T., & Vansteelandt, S. (2009). Conceptual issues concerning mediation, interventions and composition. *Statistics and Its Interface, 2*, 457–468.

Velasco, E., Agheneza, T., Denecke, K., Kirchner, G., & Eckmanns, T. (2014). Social media and internet-based data in global systems for public health surveillance: a systematic review. *The Milbank Quarterly, 92*(1), 7–33.

Vraga, E. K., & Bode, L. (2017). Using expert sources to correct health misinformation in social media. *Science Communication, 39*(5), 621–645. doi:10.1177/1075547017731776 (Original work published 2017)

Wang, Y., McKee, M., Torbica, A., & Stuckler, D. (2019). Systematic literature review on the spread of health-related misinformation on social media. *Social Science & Medicine, 240*, 112552.

World Health Organization (2016). Zika situation report: Zika virus, microcephaly and Guillain-Barré syndrome. https://www.zotero.org/google-docs/?8z9P9c (accessed 3 July 2025).

World Health Organization. (2017). *Strengthening Surveillance of and Response to Foodborne Diseases: A Practical Manual. Stage 1: Using Indicator-and Event-Based Surveillance to Detect Foodborne Events*. World Health Organization.

CHAPTER 6

QUALITATIVE AND MIXED METHODS FOR ANALYZING SOCIAL MEDIA DATA

Thu T. Nguyen[1], Amrutha S. Alibilli[1], Elizabeth Dennard[1], and Shaniece Criss[2]

[1]Department of Epidemiology and Biostatistics, School of Public Health, University of Maryland, College Park, MD, USA

[2]Department of Health Sciences, Furman University, Greenville, SC, USA

Overview

Qualitative research methods are designed to capture rich, detailed insights into individuals' experiences, perceptions, and social contexts. Specifically, qualitative content analysis can be used to gain a deeper understanding of social media discussions. This chapter provides practical guidance for conducting a qualitative content analysis, outlining key steps such as developing and refining a codebook, coding the data sample using the codebook, resolving any coding disagreements, conducting thematic analysis, and interpreting the findings. Attention is also given to considerations unique to analyzing social media data qualitatively.

While both qualitative and quantitative research methods are powerful independently, combining them through a mixed-methods approach enables researchers to leverage the strengths of each approach. Mixed-methods research offers a holistic perspective, allows for diverse ways to evaluate data, and enhances the strength of findings through cross-validation and triangulation. Quantitative approaches support generalization of larger populations, while qualitative methods provide a nuanced perspective, offering depth and context. The latter half of this chapter explores how qualitative and quantitative research methods complement each other for social media studies. The decision on when and how to incorporate

LEARNING OBJECTIVES

1. Define qualitative, quantitative, and mixed methods
2. Discuss the strengths and limitations of qualitative and quantitative methods
3. Highlight the strengths of mixed-methods research
4. Discuss applied examples of qualitative and mixed methods research

each approach is vital, so we will discuss the implications of sequential and concurrent designs. Finally, we illustrate the application of mixed-methods research in the context of online discourse involving minoritized communities. This includes case studies on neighborhood dynamics affecting Mexican American women and social media responses to the killings of Ahmaud Arbery, Breonna Taylor, George Floyd, and the Atlanta spa shootings. These examples demonstrate how mixed methods can be employed to examine themes of hostility, bias, resilience, solidarity, and support within digital environments.

Qualitative Methods

Qualitative methods aim to understand experiences, uncover contextual meaning, and develop theories (Scharrer and Ramasubramanian 2021). This methodology is marked by its iterative and interpretive approach, emphasizing both observation and the subjective meanings that shape experiences, behaviors, and phenomena (Aspers and Corte 2019). Characterized by adaptability, qualitative research is especially vital to investigating exploratory research questions with no predefined variables. For instance, an Australian Aboriginal research study strived to investigate the underlying reasons for patient self-discharges from hospitals (Askew et al. 2021). Due to the lack of predetermined variables, researchers conducted qualitative semi-structured interviews and learned key unmet patient needs: respect, peace of mind, basic comforts, informational awareness, and confidence in healthcare quality. Thus, the qualitative research revealed novel insights that might not have emerged through quantitative methods alone. Beyond interviews, qualitative research encompasses a wide range of techniques such as focus groups, thematic content analysis, photovoice, observational studies, case studies, and ethnography (Busetto et al. 2020).

Steps for Qualitative Research Analysis

Although qualitative research can be conducted through various approaches, this section outlines commonly used steps in the analysis process to provide a foundational overview.

Developing and Refining the Codebook: First, review the literature to identify potential codes relevant to the study. Each researcher independently examines a subsample of the data to generate preliminary themes, which are then collaboratively reviewed and refined during team discussions. This iterative refinement often includes piloting the codebook on a subset of the data and adjusting code definitions for clarity and consistency.

Coding the Data Sample: For the first round of coding, at least two researchers typically code a section of data together to build consensus and discuss any ambiguities in code interpretation. Following this calibration, they independently apply the codebook to a broader data sample. A common benchmark for inter-coder reliability is achieving 80% agreement or greater, ensuring consistency in code application.

Resolving any Coding Disagreements: When coding disagreements occur, at least two researchers review and discuss the inconsistencies until consensus is reached. The agreed-upon coding decisions are used to update and refine the codebook.

Thematic Analysis: Following the coding process, the team conducts a deeper thematic analysis for each code. This step involves identifying recurring themes and subthemes that reflect broader patterns in the data. Each code can comprise multiple themes and subthemes. Themes can also appear across multiple codes.

Writing of the findings: In the final stage, the research team synthesizes the identified themes to craft a coherent narrative that effectively communicates the findings to the target audience.

Evaluation of Qualitative Research

Evaluating qualitative research is essential to ensure transparency, credibility, and reproducibility. According to a scoping review of qualitative methods, the following criteria are among the most prevalent for evaluating qualitative research (Busetto et al. 2020):

- **Standards for Reporting Qualitative Research (SRQR):** While quantitative research benefits from standardized reporting guidelines, qualitative research has historically lacked such uniformity. The SRQR checklist provides a widely adopted framework for transparent research reporting, enabling consistent evaluation of qualitative studies (O'Brien et al. 2014).
- **Reflexivity:** The investigator is not isolated from the research process. Transparent reporting of information, such as recruitment strategies, researcher backgrounds, and experience, offers an opportunity for the researchers and the readers to be aware of potential biases that may influence the qualitative findings.
- **Iterative and Information-Rich Sampling:** Iterative data collection enables researchers to explore complex phenomena dynamically by adapting their research methodology. For instance, as qualitative themes emerge in the initial dataset, they may pave the way for novel themes to be explored in the subsequent data collection iterations. This iteration allows for more holistic, diverse sampling (Busetto et al. 2020). The iterative sampling continues until the saturation point (no new relevant information) is reached (Busetto et al. 2020). Purposive sampling is recommended to identify the cases and participants needed to ensure the research question is addressed from all possible relevant perspectives.

- **Respondent Validation of Findings:** This technique involves soliciting feedback from participants on the study's interpretations. Their feedback can be considered as part of the data collection and analysis (Busetto et al. 2020).
- **Stakeholder Involvement:** Beyond participants and depending on the research question, stakeholders can be consulted in order to incorporate their perspectives as well, broadening the holistic scope of the research (Busetto et al. 2020).

Quantitative Methods

Quantitative methods are employed to test hypotheses, examine relationships between variables, and make generalizations from a sample to a wider population (Scharrer and Ramasubramanian 2021). These approaches rely on numerical data and statistical analysis to identify measurable patterns and associations. While quantitative methods are powerful for identifying trends across large datasets, they are often limited in capturing individual social media users' emotions, behaviors, and lived experiences. The lack of understanding of the context surrounding numerical data may lead to inaccurate conclusions or oversimplifications. In addition, quantitative analyses necessitate known predefined variables, limiting their applicability to understudied research questions.

Social Media Research

Social media data represent an example of "big data" characterized by high volume, velocity, and variety. To fully understand such data, both qualitative and quantitative methods are essential. Qualitative methods illuminate human experiences and narratives underlying social media discourse, while quantitative methods, including machine learning, enable large-scale analyses that uncover temporal and geographic trends. These combined strategies facilitate hypothesis testing, trend detection, and the identification of emerging topics across vast, dynamic digital landscapes.

Mixed Methods

Mixed-methods research combines the strengths of both quantitative and qualitative approaches to investigate social media trends more comprehensively. While quantitative analysis offers a broad overview of patterns and correlations, qualitative inquiry provides contextual depth and the underlying reasons behind observed phenomena. Together, they help corroborate findings and offer richer contextualization of complex trends and user sentiment.

Key advantages of mixed methods include triangulation for validation, complementary for depth, expansion to a broader inquiry, and explanation of any unexpected results, and the ability to compensate for the limitations of one method with the strengths of the other (Busetto et al. 2020). For instance, quantitative analysis may highlight patterns of discourse, while qualitative research may reveal specific contextual or emotional nuances driving those patterns.

Among the most common mixed-methods approaches are convergent parallel, explanatory sequential, and exploratory sequential (Snelson 2016). Convergent parallel design leverages triangulation to simultaneously conduct quantitative and qualitative analyses, integrating the parallel results in the final interpretation. Explanatory sequential design begins with quantitative analysis, followed by qualitative methods to explain or elaborate on the quantitative findings. An exploratory sequential design starts with qualitative research, and the findings are then used to inform or generalize subsequent quantitative analysis.

Mixed-methods designs have unique strengths, but they also present challenges. Large, complex datasets from various sources may be challenging to synthesize, requiring specialized skills and a well-designed experimental protocol to ensure replicability. The sequential designs (explanatory and exploratory) offer flexibility but require careful consideration of how early results influence later phases. Mixed-methods research, when applied strategically, offers a powerful framework for capturing both the measurable patterns and the rich contextual meaning embedded in social media discourse.

CASE STUDY 1. NEIGHBORHOOD CONTEXTS EXPERIENCED BY MEXICAN AMERICAN WOMEN: A MIXED-METHODS STUDY

This study employed a qualitative descriptive design to elucidate the impact of neighborhood contexts on young Mexican American women (Richardson & Nuru-Jeter 2012). It integrated two complementary qualitative methods: (1) participatory photography and photo-elicitation and (2) focus groups to capture how participants defined and experienced their neighborhoods. These methods offered insights into broader environmental influences on adolescent reproductive health while fostering active participant engagement and enhancing participants' control of data, thereby improving data validity. Triangulating photography and focus group data allowed for a vivid, descriptive, in-depth understanding of the impact of specific contexts on health.

This mixed-methods study had notable strengths. The combination of participant-generated photography in conjunction with focus groups developed an understanding of neighborhood contexts experienced by participants. For instance, while "gangs" were broadly discussed during focus groups, photovoice allowed participants to depict and discuss their specific, everyday encounters, sharing both negative experiences (e.g., violence) and positive aspects (e.g., family and community connections). However, the study's small sample size of 10 young Mexican American women limits its generalizability. Nonetheless, this novel study underscored the importance of neighborhood contexts, facilitating research queries and future public health research.

CASE STUDY 2. KILLINGS OF AHMAUD ARBERY, BREONNA TAYLOR, AND GEORGE FLOYD

Social media has been harnessed to examine important historical moments and movements in the United States and globally. Social media data can provide meaningful insights into the discussions, reflections, and activities of individuals navigating both everyday experiences and pivotal historic moments. The killings of Ahmaud Arbery, Breonna Taylor, and George Floyd in 2020 sparked national discussions on the fundamental rights and protections of Black Americans against police violence. To examine these discussions, Nguyen et al. (2021) collected a 1% random sample of U.S. race-related tweets from November 2019 to September 2020 using X's (formerly Twitter's) application programming interface (API). Based on keywords used, the tweets were classified into four racial or ethnic categories: Asian, Black, Latinx, and White. The study focused on 3,380,616 tweets referencing Black people from 430,189 unique users. Sentiment analysis was conducted using a support vector machine, a supervised machine learning model trained to classify tweets as positive, negative, or neutral based on linguistic features. This computational approach enabled investigators to systematically evaluate emotional tone across millions of tweets. Ahmaud Arbery, Breonna Taylor, and George Floyd were killed on Feb 23, 2020, March 13, 2020, and May 25, 2020, respectively.

Nationally, the percentage of tweets referencing African American people that were classified as negative declined from 49% in early November to 34% in early June, a 32% decrease. This decline, however, was short-lived, with negative sentiment rising again in the weeks following George Floyd's murder. In tandem, the study observed a temporary rise in the percentage of tweets referencing Black people that were positive, lasting from the end of May to early June. Similar patterns were observed across the four U.S. regions. For instance, in the South, negative Black sentiment declined from 51% in early November to 36% in early June, and in the Northeast, from 45% to 29% during the same time period.

While quantitative analysis revealed temporary shifts in racial sentiment, qualitative analysis uncovered deeper narratives centered on collective reflection and the desire for lasting social change. From a random sample of 1,500 tweets posted before (November 1, 2019, to February 22, 2020) and after (May 26 to June 30, 2020) the three killings, for a total of 3,000 tweets, several central themes emerged. These included discussions of race and racism conveyed in either positive tones (e.g., affirmations; hope and optimism about racial equality; 14%) or negative tones (e.g., racist labeling; 38%), calls to action addressing systemic racism (e.g., vote; petitions; 18%), and counter-narratives opposing race-related change (e.g., focused on violence of the protests; 6%).

Although posts before and after the killings featured expressions of cultural pride, affirmation, and empowerment, the post-event period reflected heightened hope and optimism toward racial equality. Many social media users described a growing awareness of systemic injustice and engaged in deeper self-reflection around issues of power and privilege. One user wrote, "I am a White disabled woman yet never realized how privileged I've been until the past 3–4 weeks of listening, reading, and learning Black history." Additionally, there were also expressions of hope for the future: "I'm seriously emotional. I'm so grateful for all the protesters all over the world. This is the first time I feel valuable and needed in society. I am not Black. I'm a POC. I finally don't feel alone in this fight. I have an abundance of HOPE we can evolve and heal united." Most notably, after the killings, we observed tweets that were calls to action addressing systemic racism. These tweets included posts calling for action against police brutality, participating in protests, signing petitions, voting, and standing in solidarity with the Black community in their fight for social justice. At the same time, some users posted counter-narratives that focused on protest-related violence, "Black-on-Black" crime, and critiques that issues of race were being exaggerated or politicized.

The integration of quantitative and qualitative methods in this paper illuminated shifts in racial sentiment and discussions related to racism and police brutality in the United States. One year following George Floyd's murder, 30 U.S. states passed laws focused on police reform and oversight. Among these, 16 states implemented restrictions or bans on neck restraints, and 10 introduced new mandates or increased funding for body-worn cameras (Eder et al. 2021). Real-time tracking of public sentiment toward race can help identify key moments when policy agendas are more likely to shift. When such windows of opportunity are leveraged for concrete reforms or programmatic initiatives, the resulting impact may endure even after public attention to issues of racial injustice declines (Figure 6.1).

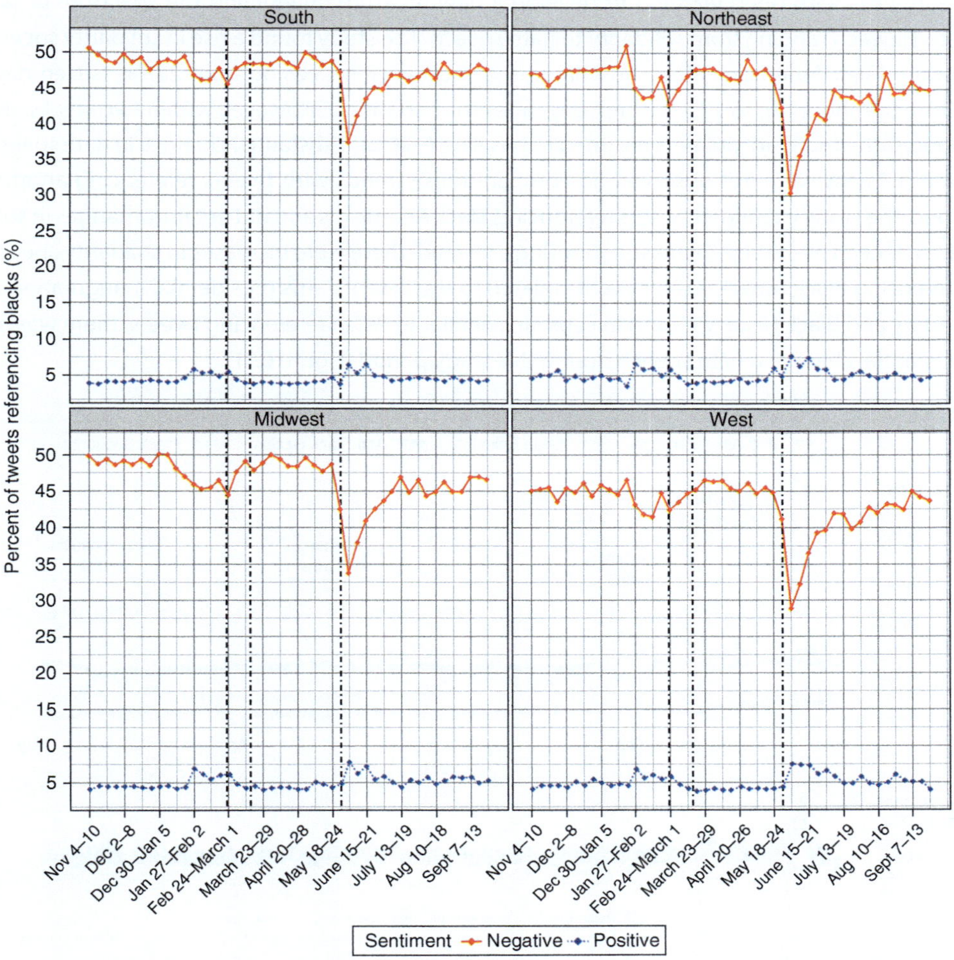

Figure 6.1 Weekly trends in percent of tweets referencing Black people that are negative and positive by U.S. region, November 2019–September 2020. Vertical lines represent the dates of the killings of Ahmaud Arbery (Feb 23), Breonna Taylor (March 13), and George Floyd (May 25).
Source: Nguyen et al. (2021) / National Library of Medicine.

CASE STUDY 3. ATLANTA SPA SHOOTINGS

On March 16, 2021, a White man entered three Atlanta-based massage parlors and killed eight women, six of whom were Asian American. This tragedy sparked widespread public outrage and grief, reigniting discussions about anti-Asian racism and intersectional vulnerability in the United States. Criss et al. (2023) conducted a mixed-methods study to examine themes related to race and racism as well as temporal trends in expressions of hate speech and solidarity before and after the shootings.

A random 1% sample of publicly available tweets from January to April 2021 was collected using the Twitter Streaming API. Tweets were in English, from the United States, and used one or more 518 race-related keywords. According to the keywords used, tweets were classified by racial/ethnic reference, with the study focusing on those referencing Asian or Black Americans. The final dataset included 708,933 tweets.

Quantitatively, the study employed a novel measure integrating faceted item response theory (IRT) with deep learning to develop a new measure quantifying the spectrum of targeted speech ranging from solidarity to hate speech. The study found a rise in solidarity speech toward Asian Americans after the Atlanta spa shootings, increasing from 22.7% (seven days before the shooting) to 27.2% (three days after the shootings). However, within two weeks, the proportion of solidarity tweets returned to baseline (~20%). Substantial changes in hate speech toward Asians were not observed. To compare these trends with tweets referencing another group, the study examined tweets referencing Black Americans and did not find changes in solidarity speech after the Atlanta spa shootings. Instead, there were increases in solidarity speech referencing Black Americans for events related to the Biden/Harris presidential inauguration in January and Black History Month in February. Similar to Asian referencing tweets, there was no substantial change in hate speech during this study period (Figure 6.2).

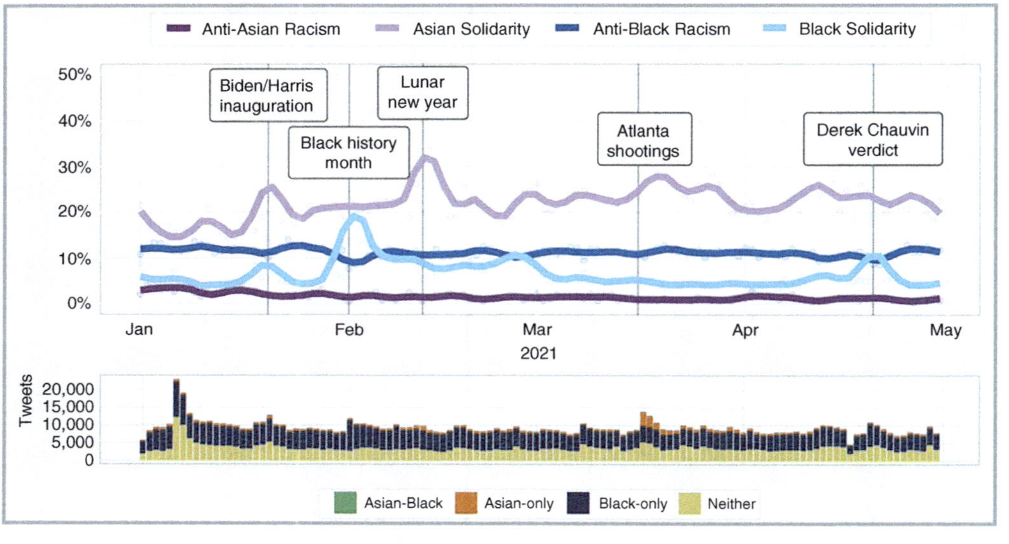

Figure 6.2 Impactful events, estimated rates of racism-related and solidarity messages on Twitter, and tweet volume from January to April 2021, stratified by tweets containing Asian and Black keywords. Asian-Black denotes that tweets include both Asian and Black keywords. Solidarity speech was defined as hate speech scores <−3, and racist speech was defined as hate speech scores >0.5.
Source: Criss et al., 2023 / Frontiers Media SA / CC BY 4.0.

To gain a deeper understanding of online discourse during this period, a qualitative content analysis was conducted on a random sample of 1,000 tweets preceding the shootings (January 1 to March 15, 2021) and 2,000 tweets after the shootings (March 17 to March 28, 2021), for a total of 3,000 tweets. Themes that emerged included expressions of solidarity with the Asian community (4% before the shootings; 17% after); condemnation of the shooting (9% after); discussions of racism (10% before; 18% after); intersectional vulnerabilities related to age, race, and gender (4% before; 6% after); and the relationship between Asian and Black struggles against racism (5% before; 7% after).

Consistent with the quantitative trend of increasing expressions of solidarity as assessed by the machine learning model, the qualitative content analysis revealed a rise in tweets expressing sympathy and support. Some posts suggested ways to support Asians during this time, such as frequenting Asian-owned businesses and providing transportation to friends who felt unsafe using public transportation.

Discussions of racism were present both before and after the shootings, but became more prevalent in the latter period. These included posts calling out Asian-related racism, discussions of historic racism reflected in government policies, and long-standing stereotypes. Relatedly, a subset of posts related to the intersectional racial violence noted the recent attacks on elderly Asians, Asian women, and elderly Asian women. Several posts also expressed the continual denial or downplaying of racism against Asian people.

The content analysis further revealed discussions about the shared and unique struggles of Black and Asian communities in confronting racism. There were discussions related to friction or lack of perceived support between Asian and Black people. This included calls for unity and solidarity between Black and Asian Americans and posts highlighting the role of white supremacy as the root cause of inequities.

These studies provide examples of how quantitative and qualitative methods provide complementary information that enriches our understanding of important race-related events.

Opportunities and Pitfalls

Opportunities

Qualitative, quantitative, and mixed-methods research methodologies present unique and complementary capabilities that can be leveraged to reveal synchronous public health insights.

- **Qualitative Research Strengths**
  Qualitative research provides a comprehensive understanding of individual perspectives, behaviors, and motivations. This approach is particularly valuable for gleaning complex social phenomena and context-driven public health perceptions. Techniques such as

interviews, focus groups, and content analysis enable researchers to analyze emerging public health behaviors without predefined variables. Thus, qualitative research is marked by its context-specific adaptability to analyze human experiences, behaviors, and perspectives.

- **Quantitative Research Strengths**
  Quantitative research facilitates large-scale analytical computations, revealing broad public health trends across diverse populations. Moreover, depending upon the representative nature of the sample, quantitative research may be more generalizable to broader populations.
- **Mixed-Methods Research Strengths**
  While quantitative approaches identify large-scale analytical trends, qualitative research reveals the underlying factors contributing to the broad trends, including specific users' perceptions through thematic analysis. Mixed-methods research capitalizes upon the strengths of both qualitative and quantitative research methodologies to investigate a more holistic understanding of public health trends. Triangulation allows for the independent corroboration of research findings, further enhancing scientific credibility, reproducibility, and integrity.

Collectively, qualitative, quantitative, and mixed-methods research studies offer valuable insights to address public health challenges. As social media data continues to expand in both volume and complexity, it is important for researchers to select the most appropriate methodology, remaining mindful of its inherent strengths and limitations. By doing so, scientists can foster heightened scientific rigor, drive public health advancements, and inform targeted policy interventions.

Pitfalls

Although qualitative and mixed-methods social media research can reveal real-time public health insights, there are notable limitations.

- **Qualitative Research Limitations**
  Due to the lack of predefined variables, qualitative research can be subjective in nature, susceptible to the perspectives of the researchers. Strategies such as double-coding and group consensus can help minimize the potential impact of individual biases on the findings, ensuring that each qualitative code is independently corroborated by distinct researchers. Additionally, social media datasets are dynamic and often noisy, making it challenging due to data oversaturation and the ever-changing nature of social media content.
- **Quantitative Research Limitations**
  Quantitative analyses rely on statistical models to analyze human behavior and interactions, which may neglect the nuanced richness of diverse digital experiences. Furthermore, while social media embodies an untapped source of big data, certain demographic populations may

be underrepresented or overrepresented in digital platforms, which may not correlate with the general population. Researchers must remain vigilant of the data biases and oversimplifications to ensure the generalizability of quantitative research findings.

- **Mixed-Methods Research Limitations**
  Integrating qualitative and quantitative research methods offers unique advantages but has several challenges as well. Primarily, combining qualitative and quantitative data methodologies can be difficult, particularly since each method contains its own unique assumptions, analytical frameworks, and constraints. Given the complexity and size of social media datasets, mixed-methods analyses can be research-intensive. Furthermore, the findings from qualitative and quantitative research methodologies may not always corroborate one another, contributing to conflicting conclusions and interpretations.

Therefore, each research methodology brings its unique strengths and limitations. By being cognizant and adopting complementary approaches, researchers can mitigate the potential risks while upholding scientific integrity to harness social media data's richness and discover cornerstone public health findings.

KEY POINTS AND TAKEAWAYS

- **Differentiate between qualitative and quantitative research methodologies and identify strengths and limitations.**
  Qualitative research is distinguished by its context-driven, interpretative, and adaptive nature, fostering the exploration of emerging public health research trends. While it may reveal in-depth insights to investigate underlying factors that contribute to public health trends, it remains vulnerable to researcher bias, high background noise, and misinterpretation. In contrast, quantitative research is broadly defined by its analytical computations and statistical modeling, decomposing broad public health trends into more scalable and accessible data visualizations. However, quantitative methodologies remain susceptible to sampling bias and potential oversimplification.
- **Explain the complementary integration of mixed-methods research techniques.**
  Mixed-methods research harnesses the complementary strengths of both quantitative and qualitative methodologies to holistically investigate public health research questions. Additionally, triangulation allows for independent research findings to corroborate across studies.
- **Highlight real-world applications of qualitative, quantitative, and mixed-methods research studies.**
  The chapter has enumerated diverse real-world social media research studies, highlighting how mixed-methods methodologies can be used to investigate

themes of hostility, discrimination, resilience, and solidarity among minority demographic groups. This integration enables researchers to both measure broad patterns and capture the human narratives driving them.

Conclusion

This chapter outlined foundational social media methodologies, including qualitative, quantitative, and mixed-methods approaches. While each technique has unique strengths and weaknesses, the fusion of qualitative and quantitative methods allows for a more comprehensive analysis of large-scale digital discussions. Overall, the practical guidance and real-world studies underscore the complementary nature of qualitative and quantitative methods and offer a framework for future social media research. The strategic use of diverse methodologies ensures more robust research findings and invaluable insights into emerging public health concerns and complex social dynamics.

References

Askew, D. A., Foley, W., Kirk, C., & Williamson, D. (2021). "I'm outta here!": a qualitative investigation into why Aboriginal and non-Aboriginal people self-discharge from hospital. *BMC Health Services Research, 21*(1), 907. doi:10.1186/s12913-021-06880-9

Aspers, P., & Corte, U. (2019). What is qualitative in qualitative research. *Qualitative Sociology, 42*, 139–160. doi:10.1007/s11133-019-9413-7

Busetto, L., Wick, W., & Gumbinger, C. (2020). How to use and assess qualitative research methods. *Neurological research and practice, 2*, 14. doi:10.1186/s42466-020-00059-z

Criss, S., Nguyen, T. T., Michaels, E. K., Gee, G. C., Kiang, M. V., Nguyen, Q. C., Norton, S., Titherington, E., Nguyen, L., Yardi, I., Kim, M., Thai, N., Shepherd, A., & Kennedy, C. J. (2023). Solidarity and strife after the Atlanta spa shootings: a mixed methods study characterizing Twitter discussions by qualitative analysis and machine learning. *Frontiers in public health, 11*, 952069. doi:10.3389/fpubh.2023.952069

Eder, S., Keller, M.H., and Migliozzi, B. (2021). As new police reform laws Sweep across the U.S., some ask: are they enough? *The New York Times*. https://www.nytimes.com/2021/04/18/us/police-reform-bills.html (accessed 6 June 2025).

Nguyen, T. T., Criss, S., Michaels, E. K., Cross, R. I., Michaels, J. S., Dwivedi, P., Huang, D., Hsu, E., Mukhija, K., Nguyen, L. H., Yardi, I., Allen, A. M., Nguyen, Q. C., & Gee, G. C. (2021). Progress and push-back: how the killings of Ahmaud Arbery, Breonna Taylor, and George Floyd impacted public discourse on race and racism on Twitter. *SSM Population Health, 15*, 100922. doi:10.1016/j.ssmph.2021.100922. PMID: 34584933; PMCID: PMC8455860

O'Brien, B. C., Harris, I. B., Beckman, T. J., Reed, D. A., & Cook, D. A. (2014). Standards for reporting qualitative research: a synthesis of recommendations. *Academic Medicine, 89*(9), 1245–1251. doi:10.1097/ACM.0000000000000388

Richardson, D. M., & Nuru-Jeter, A. M. (2012). Neighborhood contexts experienced by young Mexican-American women: enhancing our understanding of risk for early childbearing. *Journal of Urban Health: Bulletin of the New York Academy of Medicine, 89*(1), 59–73. doi:10.1007/s11524-011-9627-9

Scharrer, E., & Ramasubramanian, S. (2021). *Quantitative Research Methods in Communication: The Power of Numbers for Social Justice* (1st ed.). Routledge. doi:10.4324/9781003091653

Snelson, C. L. (2016). Qualitative and mixed methods social media research: a review of the literature. *International Journal of Qualitative Methods, 15*(1). (Original Work Published 2016). doi:10.1177/1609406915624574

CHAPTER 7

USING SOCIAL MEDIA TO MEASURE CULTURAL RACISM AND EXAMINE PHYSICAL HEALTH OUTCOMES

Thu T. Nguyen[1], Penchala Sai Priya Mullaputi[1], and Quynh C. Nguyen[2]
[1]Department of Epidemiology and Biostatistics, School of Public Health, University of Maryland, College Park, MD, USA
[2]National Institute of Nursing Research (NINR), National Institutes of Health (NIH), Bethesda, MD, USA

LEARNING OBJECTIVES

1. Define cultural racism
2. Discuss potential ways to use social media to measure cultural racism
3. Examine the relationship between social media-derived measures of cultural racism and other measures of racial bias, racial attitudes, and hate
4. Present applied studies examining social media-derived cultural racism and health

Overview

Social media holds promising potential to meaningfully contribute to the understanding and reduction of health inequities. Research has demonstrated the need to move beyond individual-level determinants to better understand structural and cultural phenomena that impact health outcomes. One important area of research includes the role of bias in creating and perpetuating health inequities. Yet, much of the existing research on discrimination often relies heavily on self-reported incidents, tends to focus on single dimensions of discrimination, and inadequately considers structural and cultural forms of discrimination.

While social media has emerged as both a manifestation and a major purveyor of hatred and stigma toward marginalized identities, it is also an untapped source of support, counter-hate, resilience, and community capital. In this chapter, we provide specific illustrative examples to demonstrate how researchers may capture norms, biases, and beliefs to create area-level measures of cultural racism as well as track its associations with policies, hate crimes, and health inequities.

Cultural Racism

In prior research, we highlighted cultural racism as a critical driver of health inequities (Nguyen et al. 2023). Cultural racism is the infusion of the ideology of racial hierarchy into the values, language, imagery, symbols, and unstated assumptions of the larger society (D. R. Williams et al. 2019) and is expressed through media, stereotyping, and norms within society. Cultural racism also manifests in policies, programs, and institutional practices (Hicken et al. 2021). It forms the context that enables and reinforces other dimensions of racism including individual, internalized, and structural racism (Michaels et al. 2023).

Cultural racism has traditionally been measured through community members' attitudes toward other groups (McConnell and Leibold 2001). However, survey-based approaches can be time-consuming, expensive, and prone to self-report biases. In contrast, social media provides a complementary data source for assessing social and cultural norms, attitudes, and beliefs toward minoritized groups. Unlike structured surveys, social media discussions capture a free-flowing exchange of ideas and information that are not prompted by specific research questions. The relative anonymity of online environments often encourages individuals to express views they might withhold in face-to-face interactions (Suler 2004). In the following sections, we present applied examples that utilize social media to measure cultural racism.

Applied Examples of Using Social Media to Study Cultural Racism

Social media provides an invaluable lens into cultural racism, offering insights into the norms, attitudes, and beliefs that shape societal dynamics. These platforms reveal the clash between societal values and entrenched biases, making cultural racism—from microaggressions to overt hate speech—visible in real time. At the same time, they serve as arenas for advocacy and resistance, reflecting broader societal tensions and helping researchers uncover exclusionary patterns and opportunities for meaningful change.

Several studies have used social media to track real-world consequences of cultural racism. For instance, anti-Black and anti-LGBTQIA+ sentiment on social media has been correlated with a rise in hate crimes, illustrating how online cultural racism can translate into physical violence (Bozhidarova et al. 2023). Wei and colleagues found that spikes in social media-derived negative racial sentiment toward Asians were associated with increases in anti-Asian hate crimes in New York City. Conversely, positive sentiment of tweets referencing Asian Americans was associated with a decrease in anti-Asian hate crimes in the same month (Wei et al. 2024), although this association was not statistically significant after covariate adjustment. Notably, another study from 2015 to 2018 found no significant association, pointing to the complexity of these relationships (Nguyen et al. 2021).

As depicted by digital studies on cultural racism, social media platforms are not neutral spaces. Algorithms that curate content often perpetuate stereotypes, reducing complex identities to simplistic and harmful portrayals. For instance, research into platforms like TikTok has revealed how Latinx identities are compressed into narrow stereotypes (Lutz and Aragon 2024) and how Black creators face systemic biases that suppress their content (G. Williams 2023). Despite these challenges, marginalized groups harness social media as a mechanism of resistance, countering misrepresentation and building communities of solidarity and resilience.

Social media also serves as a space for exposing and documenting the everyday realities of racism. Users share personal stories of microaggressions and subtle acts of discrimination, offering an unfiltered glimpse into lived realities. Research by Gunturi et al. (2024) delves deeper into this phenomenon, analyzing the language used in these posts to uncover how racism operates in digital spaces (Gunturi et al. 2024). The study distinguishes between posts that perpetuate racism and those that recount personal experiences of discrimination. By exploring these patterns, the research provides valuable insights into how racism is expressed and experienced.

One key area of exploration is how social media amplifies social movements and molds public narratives. Hashtags like #BlackLivesMatter and #StopAsianHate have sparked global conversations, fostering a thriving environment for justice, solidarity, and resistance to oppression. By analyzing the themes and sentiments expressed through such hashtags, scholars gain critical insights into the interplay between digital discourse and societal change (Tong et al. 2022). Social media serves as both a reflection and a shaper of cultural norms, enabling researchers to identify and address patterns of cultural racism in digital and real-world contexts.

The following case studies illustrate how social media data can be leveraged to examine cultural racism and its downstream consequences, particularly in relation to hate speech and population health. Together, these examples demonstrate the measurable impact of online racial sentiment on real-world disparities.

CASE STUDY 1. A DECADE OF TWEETS: EXAMINING ONLINE RACE-RELATED DISCUSSIONS

Several social media platforms have been in existence for nearly two decades, with Facebook launching in 2004 and X (formerly known as Twitter) emerging in 2006 (Esteban Ortiz-Ospina 2019). As the number of users has exponentially increased, and platforms have added more functionality for both users and researchers, it is an exciting time to examine long-term temporal trends on social media. Leveraging the Twitter Academic Research application programming interface (API), Nguyen and colleagues collected 55,844,310 publicly available race-related tweets between 2011 and 2021. Over this 10-year period, there was a 16.5% increase in negative sentiment at the national level. Tweets referencing Black and Middle Eastern individuals exhibited the highest proportions of negative sentiment (Nguyen et al. 2024; Figure 7.1).

The figure also highlights fluctuations in racial sentiment that correspond to major national events with variation in salience by racial or ethnic group. For example, during 2018, national conversations erupted around the border wall, and a spike in the proportion of negative tweets referencing Latinx individuals was observed (Figure 7.1). Conversely, during the summer of 2020, there was a decline in negative sentiment toward Black individuals, corresponding to Black Lives Matter protests following the killings of Breonna Taylor, Ahmaud Arbery, and George Floyd.

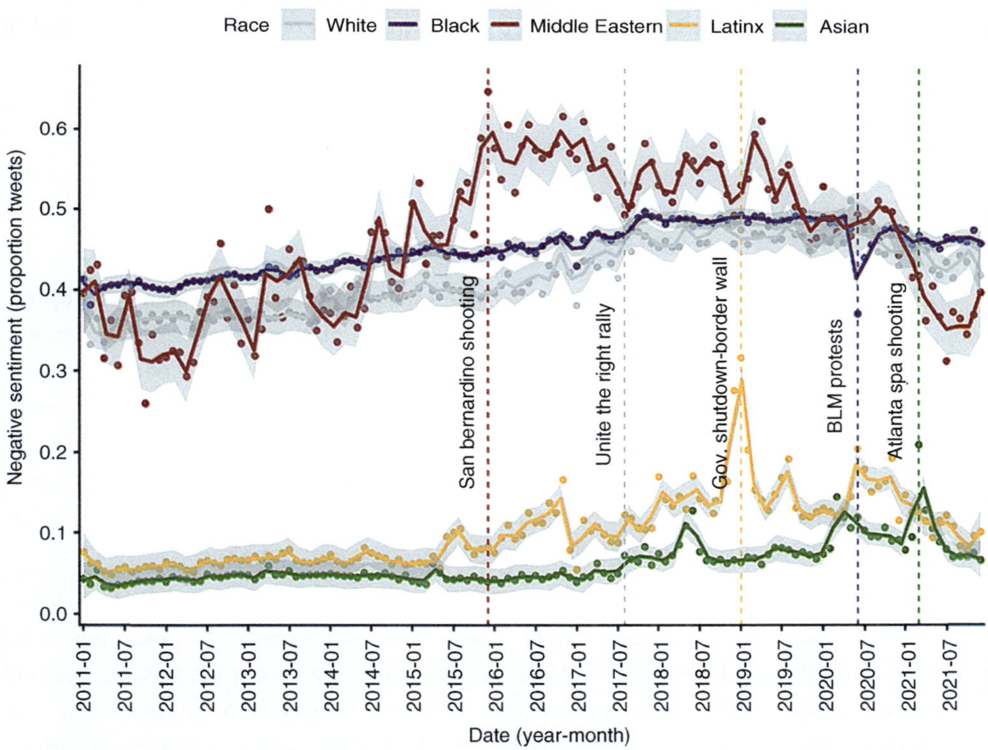

Figure 7.1 Proportion of tweets referencing specific racial and ethnic groups that are negative from 2011 to 2021.
Source: Nguyen et al. (2024) / with permission from Elsevier.

CASE STUDY 2. COMPARISON OF OUR SOCIAL MEDIA-DERIVED MEASURES WITH EXISTING MEASURES OF PREJUDICE, IMPLICIT, AND EXPLICIT RACIAL BIAS

In a related study, Nguyen and colleagues compared social media-derived racial sentiment measures with traditional survey-based and experimental measures of racial bias. These included racial prejudice questions from the General Social Survey (GSS) and implicit and explicit racial bias measures from Project Implicit. The GSS is a nationally representative survey of U.S. noninstitutionalized adults aged 18 and older, conducted biennially since 1972 (NORC 2006). Project Implicit hosts the largest collection of surveys on racial bias, with approximately 26 million tests taken. Participation is voluntary and self-selected. The implicit racial bias test measures automatic, unconscious racial bias, while the explicit racial bias test measures racial attitudes that participants are willing to report; both are publicly available online (Morin 2015).

Nguyen and colleagues found that respondents living in a state with 10% higher negative sentiment in tweets referencing Black people were less likely to endorse that disparities between Black and White Americans in terms of jobs, income, and housing were due to discrimination. Instead, they were more likely to state that such disparities were due to a lack of will. Additionally, these respondents exhibited higher measures of both implicit and explicit racial bias (Nguyen et al. 2021).

CASE STUDY 3. SOCIAL MEDIA AND HATE SPEECH

Mondal and colleagues conducted a large-scale systematic analysis of 512 million Twitter posts and 27.55 million Whisper posts, an anonymous social media platform, to investigate patterns of hate speech (Mondal et al. 2017). Unlike other social media platforms, Whisper allows users to post content without revealing personally identifiable information. Due to this anonymity, users are more likely to engage in online disinhibition, openly sharing details they might not have otherwise shared in alternative settings (Lapidot-Lefler and Barak 2012). Thus, this anonymous social media platform presents a unique environment to investigate online hate speech. Overall, this study characterized online hate speech based on four properties:

1. **Primary Target**: In contrast to other studies that used hate keywords, this study leveraged sentence structure to detect hate speech (Kwok and Wang 2013). Although it did not identify all hate speech beyond the scope of certain sentence structures, this method allowed for the analysis of diverse hate speech targets. Targets were categorized by race, ethnicity, gender, class, sexual orientation, disability, behavior, physical characteristic, and religion.
2. **Anonymity**: A lexicon lookup approach was used to detect whether an X handle contained a personal name or was anonymous. Hate speech related to race or sexual orientation are more likely to be anonymous compared to other categories, such as physical characteristic hate speech.

3. **Geography**: Since the dataset only contained English posts, the three countries with the highest number of posts were analyzed: the United States, Canada, and the United Kingdom. There was a higher prevalence of racist hate speech in U.S. posts (20%) compared to Canada (13%) and the United Kingdom (13%). In addition, sexist hate speech in U.K. posts (14%) was nearly double that in the United States (8%) and Canada (7%).
4. **Context**: In order to investigate the context for each hate speech post, the supporting text surrounding the hate speech expression was examined through a WordTree visualization. Researchers found that the context tended to intensify the hate expression by providing evidence or justification in support of the hate statement.

The researchers proposed a framework for classifying hate speech in social media posts that can be valuable in guiding future work in this area. Their work highlights the importance of further exploration of online hate speech, both to better understand public sentiment and to facilitate the development of strategies to monitor and mitigate hate speech.

In addition to shaping public discourse, online racial sentiment has tangible links to health outcomes. Below, we present case studies that demonstrate how social media-derived measures of cultural racism relate to maternal, cardiovascular, and behavioral health.

CASE STUDY 4. ASSOCIATIONS OF NEGATIVE RACIAL SENTIMENT AND HEALTH OUTCOMES

Birth Outcomes

Using a dataset of 55,844,310 race-related tweets from 2011 to 2021, a study investigated whether area-level racial sentiment was associated with adverse birth outcomes. Maternal stress is a known risk factor for adverse birth outcomes, as it can impact immune function, other physiological systems, and maladaptive coping mechanisms such as smoking and alcohol consumption (Wadhwa et al. 2001; Williams et al. 2019 Alhusen et al. 2016). The researchers hypothesized that areas with greater negative racial sentiment may indicate greater hostility toward racial and ethnic minorities.

The researchers merged sentiment scores derived from Twitter with U.S. natality files over the same period to examine the relationship between state-level sentiment of tweets referencing racial and ethnic minorities and birth outcomes. Findings revealed that mothers residing in states in the top tertile of negative racial sentiment had an 8% higher incidence of low birth weight and a 5% higher incidence of preterm birth compared to mothers living in states in the bottom tertile of negative racial sentiment. This relationship was consistent for the total population as well as racial and ethnic minority mothers, indicating that negative racial sentiment was related to worse birth outcomes for the population as a whole (Nguyen et al. 2023).

Cardiovascular Outcomes

Prior research has also found that individuals living in states with the highest levels of negative sentiment toward racial/ethnic minorities had higher prevalence of coronary heart disease and other cardiovascular disease outcomes. Specifically, negative racial sentiment in tweets referencing racial or ethnic minorities was related to a higher prevalence of hypertension, diabetes, obesity, stroke, and myocardial infarction. Conversely, positive racial sentiment was associated with a reduction in the prevalence of cardiovascular disease (CVD) outcomes (Huang et al. 2020).

Alcohol Use Severity

In a pilot study, Keum and Cano surveyed 322 Black, Latinx, and Asian emerging adults (mean age 23.3) to examine how perceived online racism relates to alcohol use severity. They measured online racism using the Perceived Online Racism Scale, depressive symptoms using the patient health questionnaire-9 (PHQ-9), anxiety symptoms using the generalized anxiety disorder-7 (GAD-7), and coping-related drinking motives, then conducted a multigroup path analysis to test sequential mediation. Across all groups, higher online racism was indirectly linked to greater alcohol use severity through the pathway of increased depressive/anxiety symptoms and stronger coping-related drinking motives. A significant direct effect (not mediated by depressive/anxiety symptoms or coping-related drinking motives) of online racism on alcohol use remained for Latinx and Asian participants, but not for Black participants, highlighting the role of mental health and coping processes in these associations (Keum and Ángel Cano 2023).

Opportunities and Pitfalls

This chapter presented key examples of how cultural racism can be measured using social media data. There remains ample opportunity for continued innovation and methodological development in this area. Many of the existing studies rely primarily on text analysis and often examine one identity in isolation. Future work can develop more sophisticated models to analyze image and video data, which have become integral components of the social media landscape. Furthermore, individuals exist not only within a single identity but also across multiple, simultaneous identities. Delving into the complicated ways bias can show up for intersecting identities by race, gender, sexual orientation, disability, age, and many others is critically needed.

KEY POINTS AND TAKEAWAYS

- **Define cultural racism.**
  Cultural racism is the infusion of racial hierarchy into societal values, language, imagery, and norms, and is systematically perpetuated through media, stereotypes, and institutional practices. Cultural and structural racism are interconnected, mutually reinforcing health inequities.
- **Discuss potential ways to use social media to measure cultural racism.**
  Social media allows for an open exchange of ideas and presents a valuable data source for assessing social and cultural norms, attitudes, and beliefs toward minority groups. In particular, sentiment analysis, hashtag and

keyword tracking, geotemporal mapping, and mixed-methods social media studies allow for the investigation of real-time, collective attitudes across diverse populations.

- **Examine the relationship between social media-derived measures of cultural racism and other measures of racial bias, racial attitudes, and hate.**
  - We found that increasing negative racial sentiment was associated with an array of health outcomes.
  - Hate crimes represent an extreme form of discrimination and are inconsistently associated with negative racial sentiment, which may be a related but distinct concept.
  - Social media data can be integrated with other sources of data to develop a comprehensive understanding of the impact of cultural racism on diverse communities and health disparities.
- **Present applied studies examining social media-derived cultural racism and health.**
  A growing body of studies has highlighted the significant impact of social media-derived cultural racism on the health and well-being of marginalized communities. By collecting social media data over many years, investigators have revealed patterns of racial sentiment across different groups over time. Studies found historic events were particularly salient for specific groups, such as the Black Lives Matter movement for African Americans, the border wall discussions for Latinx Americans, and the COVID-19 pandemic for Asians Americans.

Conclusion

This chapter demonstrates that cultural racism is not only embedded in institutions and everyday interactions, but also deeply woven into the fabric of our digital lives. From the overt hate speech found on anonymous platforms to the ambient racial sentiment captured in millions of tweets, social media offers an unprecedented window into the norms, narratives, and biases that shape public discourse. Yet these patterns are not confined to the screen. We demonstrated how negative racial sentiment online correlates with real-world harms, from spikes in hate crimes to measurable impacts on birth outcomes, cardiovascular health, and substance use. These findings highlight that digital expressions of racism are not abstract; they are embodied, with consequences that ripple across communities and generations.

As social media continues to evolve, so too must our methods for capturing and confronting cultural racism in these spaces. By leveraging digital data responsibly, we can deepen our understanding of the social environments that shape health and, ultimately, advance more equitable futures.

References

Alhusen, J. L., Bower, K. M., Epstein, E., & Sharps, P. (2016). Racial discrimination and adverse birth outcomes: an integrative review. *Journal of Midwifery & Women's Health, 61*(6), 707–720.

Bozhidarova, M., Chang, J., Ale-Rasool, A., et al. (2023). Hate speech and hate crimes: a data-driven study of evolving discourse around marginalized groups, *2023 IEEE International Conference on Big Data (BigData)*, Sorrento, Italy, 2023, pp. 3107–3116, 10.1109/BigData59044.2023.10386312.

Gunturi, U.S., Kumar, A., Ding, X., and Rho, E.H. (2024). Linguistically differentiating acts and recalls of racial microaggressions on social media. In *Proceedings of the ACM on Human-Computer Interaction, 8(CSCW1)*, Association for Computing Machinery (ACM), New York, NY, USA, pp. 1–36.

Hicken, M. T., Miles, L., Haile, S., & Esposito, M. (2021). Linking history to contemporary state-sanctioned slow violence through cultural and structural racism. *The ANNALS of the American Academy of Political and Social Science, 694*(1), 48–58.

Huang, D., Huang, Y., Adams, N., Nguyen, T. T., & Nguyen, Q. C. (2020). Twitter-characterized sentiment towards racial/ethnic minorities and cardiovascular disease (CVD) outcomes. *Journal of Racial and Ethnic Health Disparities, 7*(5), 888–900.

Keum, B. T., & Ángel Cano, M. (2023). Online racism, depressive and anxiety symptoms, coping-related drinking motives, and alcohol use severity among Black, Latina/o/x, and Asian emerging adults. *Addictive Behaviors, 136*, 107468. doi:10.1016/j.addbeh.2022.107468. Epub 2022 Aug 24. PMID: 36087497

Kwok, I., & Wang, Y. (2013). Locate the hate: detecting tweets against blacks, *27*(1), 1621–1622.

Lapidot-Lefler, N., & Barak, A. (2012). Effects of anonymity, invisibility, and lack of eye-contact on toxic online disinhibition. *Computers in Human Behavior, 28*(2), 434–443.

Lutz, N. and Aragon, C. (2024). "We're not all construction workers": algorithmic compression of Latinidad on TikTok. In *Proceedings of the ACM on Human-Computer Interaction, 8(CSCW2)*, Association for Computing Machinery (ACM), New York, NY, USA, pp. 1–31.

McConnell, A. R., & Leibold, J. M. (2001). Relations among the implicit association test, discriminatory behavior, and explicit measures of racial attitudes. *Journal of Experimental Social Psychology, 37*(5), 435–442.

Michaels, E. K., Lam-Hine, T., Nguyen, T. T., Gee, G. C., & Allen, A. M. (2023). The water surrounding the iceberg: cultural racism and health inequities. *Milbank Quarterly, 101*(3), 768–814. doi:10.1111/1468-0009.12662. Epub 2023 Jul 12. PMID: 37435779; PMCID: PMC10509530

Mondal, M., Silva, L.A., and Benevenuto, F. (2017). A measurement study of hate speech in social media, pp. 85–94 (accessed 8 July 2025).

Morin, R. (2015). Exploring racial bias among biracial and single-race adults: The IAT. https://www.zotero.org/google-docs/?6i386p (accessed 8 July 2025).

Nguyen, T. T., Huang, D., Michaels, E. K., Glymour, M. M., Allen, A. M., & Nguyen, Q. C. (2021). Evaluating associations between area-level Twitter-expressed negative racial sentiment, hate crimes, and residents' racial prejudice in the United States. *SSM-Population Health, 13*, 100750.

Nguyen, T. T., Merchant, J. S., Criss, S., Makres, K., Gowda, K. N., Mane, H., Yue, X., Hswen, Y., Glymour, M. M., & Nguyen, Q. C. (2023). Examining twitter-derived negative racial sentiment as indicators of cultural racism: Observational associations with preterm birth and low birth weight among a multiracial sample of mothers, 2011–2021. *Journal of Medical Internet Research, 25*, e44990.

Nguyen, T. T., Merchant, J. S., Yue, X., Mane, H., Wei, H., Huang, D., Gowda, K. N., Makres, K., Najib, C., Nghiem, H. T., Li, D., Drew, L. B., Hswen, Y., Criss, S., Allen, A. M., & Nguyen, Q. C. (2024). A decade of Tweets: visualizing racial sentiments towards minoritized groups in the United States between 2011 and 2021. *Epidemiology, 35*(1), 51–59.

NORC, G. (2006). General social survey. University of Chicago: *NORC*. https://www.zotero.org/google-docs/?6i386p (accessed 8 July 2025).

Ortiz-Ospina, E. (2019). The rise of social media. https://www.usatoday.com/story/tech/2022/07/25/when-was-facebook-created/10040883002/ (accessed 3 August 2025).

Suler, J. (2004). The online disinhibition effect. *Cyberpsychology & Behavior, 7*(3), 321–326.

Tong, X., Li, Y., Li, J., Bei, R., & Zhang, L. (2022). What are people talking about in# BackLivesMatter and# StopAsianHate? Exploring and categorizing Twitter topics emerged in online social movements through the Latent Dirichlet Allocation Model. In *Proceedings of the 2022 AAAI/ACM Conference on AI, Ethics, and Society* (pp. 723–738).

Wadhwa, P. D., Culhane, J. F., Rauh, V., & Barve, S. S. (2001). Stress and preterm birth: Neuroendocrine, immune/inflammatory, and vascular mechanisms. *Maternal and Child Health Journal, 5*, 119–125.

Wei, H., Hswen, Y., Merchant, J. S., Drew, L. B., Nguyen, Q. C., Yue, X., Mane, H., & Nguyen, T. T. (2024). From tweets to streets: observational study on the association between Twitter sentiment and anti-Asian hate crimes in New York City from 2019 to 2022. *Journal of Medical Internet Research, 26*, e53050.

Williams, G. (2023). Black content creators' responses and resistance strategies on TikTok. *arXiv Preprint arXiv:2312.12727*. https://www.zotero.org/google-docs/?ql3XpI (accessed 3 August 2025).

Williams, D. R., Lawrence, J. A., & Davis, B. A. (2019). Racism and health: evidence and needed research. *Annual Review of Public Health, 40*(1), 105–125.

CHAPTER 8

SOCIAL MEDIA, DISABILITY, AND CHRONIC AND RARE ILLNESSES: EXPLORING DIGITAL HEALTH ACROSS DIVERSE POPULATIONS

Katrina Makres[1], Elizabeth Dennard[1], Amrutha S. Alibilli[1], Vidur Jain[1], Alaa Sharaf[1], Quynh C. Nguyen[2], and Thu T. Nguyen[1]
[1]Department of Epidemiology and Biostatistics, School of Public Health, University of Maryland, College Park, MD, USA
[2]National Institute of Nursing Research (NINR), National Institutes of Health (NIH), Bethesda, MD, USA

LEARNING OBJECTIVES

1. Evaluate existing literature on the relationship between social media use and health outcomes among individuals living with chronic conditions, disabilities, and rare illnesses
2. Highlight key strengths and limitations in research on social media use within diverse populations
3. Identify critical data gaps and propose recommendations for future research to advance the field

Overview

The widespread integration of social media into everyday life has shaped how individuals access health information, seek peer support, and construct both personal and collective identities. For individuals living with chronic health conditions and disabilities, these platforms can serve as important tools that bridge gaps in traditional healthcare systems by facilitating peer support, enabling self-management, and fostering participation in online communities that transcend geographic barriers. At the same time, social media presents new risks, including the spread of misinformation, accessibility limitations, and harmful social comparisons that can manifest through negative online experiences. This chapter examines how diverse populations, including individuals with chronic conditions, physical and intellectual disabilities, and rare illnesses, interact with social media platforms in ways that impact their health outcomes. It explores the facilitators who promote meaningful digital participation, the barriers that impede equitable access, and the implications for mental and physical health. Finally, the chapter highlights critical gaps in existing research and outlines directions for future inquiry aimed at building a more inclusive, informed, and supportive digital health environment.

Introduction

While social media has dramatically increased global connectivity, its perceived accessibility benefits are not universal. Populations such as individuals with rare or chronic diseases and individuals with mental or physical disabilities are often overlooked. Despite the growing role of social networking platforms in everyday life, there remains a dearth of literature on their impact on these marginalized populations. This chapter addresses that gap by synthesizing existing knowledge, identifying critical research limitations, and outlining future directions to illuminate this topic.

Populations of Focus: Chronic Illness, Disability, and Rare Illness

Chronic Illness

Chronic diseases are the leading cause of disability and mortality in the United States, accounting for an estimated $4.9 trillion in annual healthcare costs (CDC 2024). Conditions such as cardiovascular disease, cancer, and diabetes mellitus are classified as chronic when they persist for more than one year and significantly hinder long-term health or activities of daily living. Some chronic conditions, including cardiovascular disease and type 2 diabetes, are preventable and manageable through lifestyle modifications such as a balanced, nutritious diet, regular physical activity, and smoking cessation. Research has underscored social media as a valuable resource for health information dissemination, peer support, and self-expression, empowering individuals to manage both disease symptoms and daily life. However, significant challenges persist, including the spread of misinformation, reluctance among patients to discuss social media use with healthcare providers, and variability in the quality of research in this evolving field. There is a need for more rigorous research to fully understand the role of social media in chronic disease surveillance and management. Overall, social media plays a multifaceted role for individuals managing chronic disease; it can positively influence mental health outcomes, foster peer support networks, and provide avenues for shaping digital identities.

Disability

Physical disability (PD) refers to long-term impairments that limit one or more major physical functions, including mobility, coordination, or stamina. Common conditions include spinal cord injuries, muscular dystrophy, multiple sclerosis, cerebral palsy, and amputations resulting from severe injuries. According to the World Health Organization, approximately one in six people worldwide live with a physical or intellectual disability—many of whom face systemic barriers to social connection, healthcare access, and digital participation (WHO 2022). For individuals living with PD, these barriers can profoundly affect both mental health and social inclusion, extending across offline and online contexts. Contributing factors include mobility limitations, public stigma, lack of emotional support, inaccessible platform design, and underrepresentation in both healthcare systems and digital spaces.

Intellectual disability (ID) refers to neurodevelopmental conditions that impair two domains: cognitive functioning (e.g., learning, problem-solving, and judgment) and adaptive functioning, which encompasses conceptual (e.g., language, reading, writing, and memory), social (e.g., empathy and social judgment), and practical skills (e.g., independence, financial management, recreation; APA 2024). Approximately 1–3% of the global population (roughly 200 million people) live with an ID, including 6.5 million individuals in the United States. Causes include genetic syndromes (e.g., Down syndrome, Fragile X syndrome, Prader–Willi syndrome, and Williams syndrome), illness (e.g., meningitis, whooping cough, and measles), or head trauma, brain malformation, maternal disease, birth complications, and environmental exposures (e.g., alcohol, tobacco, radiation, and heavy metals; APA 2024; Cleveland Clinic 2023). Prevalence is notably higher in low-income countries, with estimates of 16.41 cases per 1,000 people (APA 2024; Cleveland Clinic 2023; Special Olympics 2018). Evidence suggests that people with ID are at increased risk of social isolation and often maintain smaller social networks than the general population. Moreover, they are less likely to have access to computers, the internet, and social media platforms (Caton & Chapman 2016). Barriers to internet access may stem from financial, social, and educational inequities, as well as constraints on caregiver expertise, time, and attitudes, as well as individual cognitive, physical, and sensory impairments.

Rare Illness

Globally, millions of individuals live with at least one of over 7,000 classified rare illnesses (Esparcia et al. 2015; Subirats et al. 2018; Bi et al. 2020; Miller et al. 2021). Examples include amyotrophic lateral sclerosis (ALS), a neurodegenerative disorder that has become a global research priority, and sickle cell disease (SCD), a genetic blood disorder considered rare but remains a significant public health concern (Chaudhary & Kumar 2025). For those with rare illnesses, receiving timely diagnoses and adequate healthcare services remains a persistent challenge (Bi et al. 2020; Miller et al. 2021). Social media platforms provide numerous opportunities for connection, peer support, and advocacy, particularly in contexts where patients may be geographically isolated (Yamaguchi & Queralt-Rosinach 2020). Evidence suggests these platforms can mitigate negative mental health outcomes such as anxiety and depression and, in some cases, contribute to improved management of illness-related symptoms such as chronic pain and sensory deficits (Subirats et al. 2018; Bi et al. 2020).

Facilitators of Social Media Engagement

Social and Emotional Support

Social media platforms have become critical spaces of connection for individuals, providing opportunities for friendships, social inclusion, and a sense of belonging (Lui et al. 2021). For people with IDs, several systematic and scoping reviews underscore these benefits. Van Alem et al. (2025) reviewed 21 unique qualitative studies and identified three recurring themes in social media use: establishing new connections, maintaining existing ones, and cultivating belonging. These experiences enhanced user inclusion, autonomy, and empowerment, ultimately supporting mental health and well-being (van Alem et al. 2025). Similarly, Anderson et al. (2023) reported that social media facilitated enjoyment, self-esteem, and the ability for individuals to shape online identities and disclose disability status on their own terms. A review by Glencross et al. (2021) further emphasized that friendship and social connection were the most commonly reported benefits of social media use, accounting for 33% of all identified benefits in their review. Collectively, these findings highlight the role of social media in strengthening social support and emotional resilience among people with ID.

For adolescents with chronic diseases, platforms such as Facebook are often used to find community and connect with peers through private groups (De Nardi et al. 2020). These groups allow individuals to share their unique lived experiences, find solace in shared challenges, and reduce feelings of loneliness and isolation. Importantly, smaller online communities such as forums and chat rooms provide spaces for sensitive conversations that may not occur on mainstream platforms. Stetten et al. (2019) observed that individuals with physical disabilities often engage across multiple platforms, using Facebook for information sharing, forums for emotional expression, and chat rooms for real-time interaction. The anonymity of these platforms enables more open discussion of mental health struggles. Joo et al. (2022) found that participation in peer support programs not only reduced loneliness but also fostered a sense of belonging and family, with peer mentors themselves reporting emotional fulfillment from helping others. Likewise, Kim and Zhu (2020) found that mobile social networking applications (MSNAs) enhanced psychological well-being by enabling meaningful online friendships.

For individuals with rare illnesses, who are often geographically dispersed, social media is particularly vital for reducing isolation and facilitating peer-to-peer support (Schumacher et al. 2014; Yamaguchi & Queralt-Rosinach 2020). Online communities provide opportunities for users to exchange medical information and offer socioemotional support (Coulson et al. 2007; Haller et al. 2018; Gow et al. 2020; Knepper & Arrington 2020). For example, Esparcia et al. (2015) found that community participation helped users feel understood and less isolated in coping with their illness.

Anonymity, meanwhile, encourages judgment-free sharing of sensitive experiences (Coulson et al. 2007; Albright et al. 2016). Some proponents for social media peer support advocate for the involvement of medical professionals in these groups to ensure that peer-exchanged information is accurate and safe (Haller et al. 2018). Online support has also extended to caregivers: Nicholas et al. (2012) reported that online groups for fathers of children with rare diseases helped them cope with the stress of their caretaking responsibilities.

In addition to individuals with rare illnesses, online support groups have demonstrated benefits for other vulnerable populations, including individuals with mental illnesses. Townsend et al. (2012) found that people often sought digital support groups in response to fear of hospitalization, concerns about medication, and financial barriers to care. In contrast to structured medical environments, these groups allow participants to express experiences freely and seek peer support. Lawlor and Kirakowski (2014) further highlighted that users shared personal narratives, treatment concerns, and emotional struggles in ways that promoted empathy and mutual aid. A systematic review of studies on social connectedness interventions for adults with chronic conditions found approximately 56.3% reported positive outcomes, including improved depressive symptoms and better glycemic control (Wright et al. 2023).

Finally, digital health communities represent a broader form of online support, extending beyond peer-to-peer interaction. Such communities often incorporate forums, resource libraries, and networking opportunities for patients, caregivers, and healthcare providers (Eysenbach et al. 2004). These communities may be open-access bulletin boards or closed networks requiring approval for participation (Green et al. 2020). By facilitating inclusive environments where information, empathy, and practical guidance can circulate, both individual well-being and collective resilience can be reinforced.

Digital Identity

In addition to strengthening social support, social media enables individuals to construct and express digital identities. By creating uniquely identifiable profiles and sharing user-generated content, individuals can publicly articulate perspectives and experiences (Lui et al. 2021). For adolescents with chronic diseases, social media offers a means to present themselves as a "normal part of society" while sharing both positive and negative experiences with peers who have similar conditions (De Nardi et al. 2020). This duality of online connection and offline challenges supports identity construction while mitigating the sense of alienation adolescents often experience due to their chronic illness.

For many people with disabilities, digital identity is also shaped through gaming and virtual platforms. Virtual environments such as Second Life,

Gather.town, and ZEPETO allow individuals to customize avatars in ways that either conceal, reveal, or selectively express aspects of disability (Park & Kim 2022). For example, a player with a hearing impairment may design an avatar with a cochlear implant to signal communication needs. While there is no uniform consensus on whether to display or conceal disability online, the vast majority agree that online games and spaces should support diverse representation of the disability spectrum by providing a wide range of customizable features and avatars.

Video-sharing platforms such as TikTok and Bilibili have further expanded opportunities for identity expression among people with physical disabilities (Huang & Wang 2023). Creators have cited many reasons for producing both short- and long-form videos. For some, these platforms provide emotional support and help meet social needs by connecting with others online. Others use video content to raise awareness about disabilities, challenge common stereotypes, or share practical information and experiences. In some cases, content creation also generates income, contributing to financial independence and enhancing self-esteem and self-worth. However, video creation by people with disabilities has risks. Creators have reported exposure to discrimination, harassment, and online violence. Some also describe compulsive video production, which can exacerbate anxiety and interfere with rehabilitation (Huang & Wang 2023). Studies also suggest that emotional support, while present in some online communities, is often less consistently available than informational or instrumental support (Duplaga & Szulc 2019; Lee and Cho 2019; Lal et al. 2022). This gap can leave users feeling unsupported during vulnerable moments of distress.

Inclusion and Empowerment

Social media also fosters inclusion and empowerment, a multidimensional concept encompassing competence, self-determination, and meaningful participation (Bizzotto et al. 2025). Prior research suggests that empowerment from online interactions enables individuals with chronic conditions to engage more actively in clinical consultations and communicate more effectively with healthcare professionals. A systematic review found that approximately 24% of cross-sectional studies reported an association between empowerment gained through peer interactions on social media and increased patient participation in clinical consultations (Kjærulff et al. 2023). Empowerment can also strengthen treatment adherence, improve patient–physician relationships, and enhance advocacy in clinical decision-making (Lui et al. 2021). Importantly, empowerment is not limited to active posting. Lawlor & Kirakowski (2014) found that both active contributors and "lurkers" in online support groups for mental illness reported empowerment benefits. Liu and Wang (2021) examined how online health communities empower individuals with mental illnesses by increasing self-efficacy, encouraging continued use of online resources, and facilitating access to social support. Similar trends are documented in rare disease communities, where empowerment manifests as "better informed, enhanced social well-being, greater confidence in relationship[s] with physicians, greater acceptance of illness, greater [confidence] in treatment, greater optimism and control, [and] improved self-esteem" (Nieroba & Larysz 2020). Digital inclusion further enhances empowerment by decreasing isolation and expanding social capital. Park (2024) demonstrated that smartphone use increased life satisfaction among individuals with physical disabilities, providing access to networks, information, and services that support autonomy. This digital inclusion, along with the ability to independently manage communication, scheduling, and daily tasks, supported a sense of autonomy, an important contributor to psychological well-being.

Research and Education

While the majority of this chapter has focused on patient-driven uses of social media—such as building communities, sharing experiences, and advocating for change, these platforms also hold significant value for researchers. Beyond serving as spaces for peer connection, social media can function as a rich data source and a powerful recruitment tool for public health studies to advance scientific knowledge. Social media analytics can be leveraged as cost-effective complements to traditional public health surveillance methods (Lui et al. 2021). Large-scale data is valuable for identifying populations at risk of various diseases in addition to understanding health practices, dietary habits, and lifestyle behaviors in real time. Applying big data analytics to social media data reveals significant promise for determining chronic disease risk factors, improving diagnostic accuracy, enhancing patient outcomes, guiding treatment plans, and promoting diverse clinical trial recruitment. For instance, a randomized trial recruited cancer survivors and evaluated a Facebook-based physical activity intervention, which led to significant weight loss and increased vigorous exercise (Valle et al. 2013). Similarly, Lawlor and Kirakowski (2014) noted that researchers studying mental health disorders leveraged existing online groups to expedite the recruitment process (Lawlor & Kirakowski 2014).

Clinical research is necessary to advance treatments and cures for illnesses, but it often presents difficulties in achieving results. One of the most difficult aspects of clinical research is reaching the target accruals. Applequist et al. (2020, 2023) reported that 32% of clinical trials closed prematurely due to accrual challenges, often stemming from limited funding or geographically dispersed participants. Social media offers a cost-effective means of disseminating trial information, thereby improving enrollment (Applequist et al. 2020, 2023). While clinical data provide valuable insights into diagnoses, treatments, and measurable health outcomes, social media complements them by capturing patients' quality of life, symptoms, and lived experiences often absent from traditional sources (Miller et al. 2021). For example, Yamaguchi & Queralt-Rosinach (2020) used X (formerly Twitter) to collect patient histories for ALS and multiple sclerosis (MS) directly from users' timelines. By finding posts before and after diagnosis, the study demonstrated that social media could capture patient-centric details, such as symptom progression and daily functioning, which are often missing from clinical records. Such findings highlight how social media can enrich understanding of patient quality of life and complement clinical data. However, when gathering data, it is important to think about social media limitations. This data may lack representation, could contain bias, and findings may not generalize to the wider community at large (Miller et al. 2021). Future public health research can leverage social media data for disease surveillance, management, and health disparities research, emphasizing integrated data collection and analysis in combining both traditional and nontraditional data sources.

Barriers to Supportive and Accessible Online Environments

Misinformation

One of the most significant concerns regarding health information on social media is the rapid dissemination of misinformation. Because anyone can post online, not all content is reliable, raising concerns about credibility and the ability of users to critically evaluate information (Bizzotto et al. 2025). A mixed-methods study integrating a Facebook survey with qualitative interviews explored patients' and physicians' perspectives about the benefits and risks of using social media for disease self-management (Dudina & Judina 2023). Patients described the benefits of peer-to-peer expertise and the exchange of personal disease anecdotes but acknowledged risks such as the spread of unverified information and the potential loss of anonymity. Physicians, in contrast, expressed broad mistrust of social media, citing misinformation and the influence of unqualified "digital experts," whose falsehoods can undermine both patient safety and physicians' professional authority. Furthermore, patients are often reluctant to transparently express which health advice they acquired from social media, so healthcare professionals are largely unaware of patients' vulnerability to misinformation (Kjærulff et al. 2023). To illustrate how misinformation circulates in practice, recent studies have examined the quality of mental health content on newer platforms such as TikTok.

CASE STUDY 1. TIKTOK AND ATTENTION-DEFICIT/HYPERACTIVITY DISORDER: A CROSS-SECTIONAL STUDY OF SOCIAL MEDIA CONTENT QUALITY (YEUNG ET AL. 2022 / NATIONAL LIBRARY OF MEDICINE)

As social media becomes more accessible and used for mental health information, it is critical to evaluate the quality of content, especially on emerging platforms such as TikTok. Yeung et al. (2022) analyzed 100 videos tagged "#adhd" (Attention-Deficit/Hyperactivity Disorder), which had an average of 2.8 million views and 31,175 shares per video. Of these, 89 were created by individuals without healthcare expertise. Using the Patient Education Materials Assessment Tool for Audiovisual Materials (PEMAT-A/V) and the *Journal of the American Medical Association* (JAMA) benchmark criteria, the researchers found that while videos scored high on understandability (PEMAT-A/V score of 94.3%), they scored poorly on actionability (PEMAT-A/V scores of 14.3%) and credibility (average JAMA score of 1.3). Content analysis showed that 52% of the videos were classified as misleading, most often through oversimplification or misclassification of ADHD symptoms. Personal story videos attracted the highest engagement despite their variable accuracy. Overall, this study underscores the risks of widespread misinformation on emerging platforms and highlights the need for improved content moderation and greater involvement of healthcare professionals in digital spaces.

Cyberbullying and Privacy Concerns

People with chronic illnesses who share their experiences online are disproportionately targeted by cyberbullying, including harassment, ridicule of physical symptoms, and public shaming of medical or lifestyle decisions (Alhaboby et al. 2023; Al-Turif & Al-Sanad 2023). Such victimization not only causes emotional distress, but it is also associated with exacerbating depression, anxiety, and stress. These psychological effects can, in turn, worsen physical health, hinder self-management, and reduce quality of life. Privacy concerns add another layer of risk. Given the limited number of individuals with rare diseases and their unique lived experiences, they are at a heightened risk of being identified through social media and online support groups, especially in small, close-knit communities where unique disease characteristics make anonymity harder to maintain, heightening the possibility of digital exploitation (Gow et al. 2020).

Accessibility

Alongside risks of exploitation, accessibility for vulnerable populations remains a pressing concern. A recent evaluation of social media platforms found that for accessibility (e.g., keyboard navigation, image alt text/alt descriptions, video captioning, compatibility), Facebook scored 86%, followed by X at 78%, Instagram at 70%, and Snapchat at 62% (Khasawneh 2024). While adaptive tools—such as screen readers, sip-and-puff devices that translate breathing actions into commands, and voice-command interfaces—have expanded opportunities for online engagement (Lapierre et al. 2024), many platforms still fail to fully accommodate diverse needs. Critical accessibility features, including screen reader compatibility, consistent captioning for videos, and user-friendly layouts (e.g., eye tracking or sip-and-puff controls), are often inconsistent. Interfaces may remain cluttered or unintuitive for users with cognitive impairments, and integration with assistive technologies is rarely seamless. Affordability and digital literacy further limit adoption, particularly in underserved communities (Sweet et al. 2020). The high cost of adaptive tools such as head-tracking mouse pointers exacerbates the financial burden on individuals with disabilities.

Despite these limitations, social media platforms and virtual environments have become essential resources. eHealth enables remote consultations, prescription management, and specialist care without travel. Tele-rehabilitation delivers therapy and adaptive exercises from home, while virtual classrooms open opportunities for learning and community engagement. Together, these tools can reduce physical and logistical barriers, foster self-reliance, and help prevent social exclusion for people with disabilities.

Data Gaps and Future Directions

Despite growing interest in digital inclusion and social media use among individuals with chronic illness, disability, and rare diseases, important data gaps remain across the literature, which limit the implementation of inclusive digital practices. First, much of the evidence on the benefits of social support and digital inclusion is based on cross-sectional reviews. While informative, these studies cannot establish temporal associations between variables (Tough et al. 2017; Kim & Zhu 2020; Park 2024). Second, a critical data gap includes the limited geographic distribution and cultural diversity across existing studies. Evidence on peer support and online communities is promising but highly context-specific, with limited generalizability across cultural, socioeconomic, and geographic settings (Stetten et al. 2019; Joo et al. 2022). Community- and health-based interventions remain concentrated in high-income countries, producing a gap in understanding the needs and solutions for low-resource environments (Martin Ginis et al. 2021; Bhattarai & Smedema 2023; Gréaux et al. 2023).

Third, although adaptive technologies are well-documented, evidence on long-term adoption, affordability, and sustainability remains scarce, especially among marginalized communities (Manzoor & Vimarlund 2018; Lapierre et al. 2024). Research on rare diseases has largely focused on the role of support groups and on how social media can be leveraged for recruitment and patient monitoring during clinical trials. However, less attention has been given to capturing the broader, long-term experiences of these patients, and longitudinal evidence remains limited (Park & Kim 2022; Huang & Wang 2023). Fourth, emerging research on digital identity and creative expression highlights new opportunities but also underscores risks such as discrimination and fragile online support networks. A critical data gap in this field includes the underreporting of study participant disability and illness severity. For example, in a systematic review by van Alem et al. (2025), only 7 out of 21 identified qualitative studies explicitly stated participant disability severity; most focused on mild-to-moderate ID, with only one including individuals with multiple or severe disabilities. This underreporting restricts the generalizability of findings. Finally, research remains imbalanced in focus. Most studies emphasize the risks of social media (e.g., accessibility barriers, cyberbullying, exploitation), while fewer explore its potential benefits, such as social connection, empowerment, and self-esteem. In addition, inconsistent reporting of demographics and outcomes makes it difficult to compare findings across studies. Addressing these data gaps will require more representative sampling strategies that capture the heterogeneity of populations discussed in this chapter, along with the use of diverse study designs that reflect the varied online experiences of those living with chronic illness, disability, and rare illness. Additionally, it is critical to incorporate global perspectives, especially from underrepresented countries, to capture the diversity of digital experiences. A more inclusive evidence base can inform digital policies, accessible platform design, and effective support strategies for individuals with chronic illnesses, disabilities, or rare diseases.

Conclusion

This chapter underscores the dual role of social media: as a facilitator of inclusion and empowerment and as a source of significant challenges for individuals living with chronic illness, disability, and rare diseases. Facilitators such as social and emotional support, digital identity construction, and empowerment opportunities highlight the potential of these platforms to reduce isolation, foster resilience, and enhance participation in both healthcare and broader social life. Social media also provides novel opportunities for research and education, offering insights into lived experiences, supporting clinical recruitment, and advancing more patient-centered approaches. At the same time, barriers such as misinformation, cyberbullying, privacy risks, and accessibility limitations temper these benefits and risk widening existing health disparities. Addressing these issues will require inclusive digital policies, accessible platform design, and stronger collaborations among healthcare professionals, researchers, and technology developers. Ultimately, social media represents a powerful yet unequal tool for shaping health outcomes. Harnessing its potential while mitigating its risks will be essential for fostering equitable, supportive, and health-centered digital environments.

References

Albright, K., Walker, T., Baird, S., Eres, L., Farnsworth, T., Fier, K., Kervitsky, D., Korn, M., Lederer, D. J., McCormick, M., Steiner, J. F., Vierzba, T., Wamboldt, F. S., & Swigris, J. J. (2016). Seeking and sharing: why the pulmonary fibrosis community engages the web 2.0 environment. *BMC Pulmonary Medicine, 16*, 4. doi:10.1186/s12890-016-0167-7

van Alem, J. L. L., Frielink, N., & Embregts, P. J. C. M. (2025). Social internet use by people with intellectual disabilities: a systematic review and thematic synthesis of qualitative studies. *Journal of Intellectual Disability Research: JIDR, 69*(4), 243–264. doi:10.1111/jir.13211

Alhaboby, Z. A., Evans, H., Barnes, J., & Short, E. (2023). The impact of cybervictimization on the self-management of chronic conditions: lived experiences. *Journal of Medical Internet Research, 25*, e40227. doi:10.2196/40227

Al-Turif, G. A. R., & Al-Sanad, H. A. R. (2023). The repercussions of digital bullying on social media users. *Frontiers in Psychology, 14*, 1280757. doi:10.3389/fpsyg.2023.1280757

American Psychiatric Association (2024). What is intellectual disability? https://www.psychiatry.org:443/patients-families/intellectual-disability/what-is-intellectual-disability (accessed 20 August 2025).

Anderson, S., Araten-Bergman, T., & Steel, G. (2023). Adults with intellectual disabilities as users of social media: a scoping review. *British Journal of Learning Disabilities, 51*(4), 544–564. doi:10.1111/bld.12534

Applequist, J., Burroughs, C., Ramirez, A., Merkel, P. A., Rothenberg, M. E., Trapnell, B., Desnick, R. J., Sahin, M., & Krischer, J. P. (2020). A novel approach to conducting clinical trials in the community setting: utilizing patient-driven platforms and social media to drive web-based patient recruitment. *BMC Medical Research Methodology, 20*(1), 58. doi:10.1186/s12874-020-00926-y

Applequist, J., Burroughs, C., Merkel, P. A., Rothenberg, M., Trapnell, B., Desnick, R., Sahin, M., & Krischer, J. (2023). Direct-to-consumer recruitment methods via traditional and social media to aid in research accrual for clinical trials for rare diseases: comparative analysis study. *Journal of Medical Internet Research, 25*(1), e39262. doi:10.2196/39262

Bhattarai, M., & Smedema, S. M. (2023). Improving health of persons with disabilities living in poverty: a scoping review. *Rehabilitation Counselors and Educators Journal, 12*(1). doi:10.52017/001c.37747

Bi, Q., Shen, L., Evans, R., Zhang, Z., Wang, S., Dai, W., & Liu, C. (2020). Determining the topic evolution and sentiment polarity for albinism in a Chinese online health community: machine learning and social network analysis. *JMIR Medical Informatics, 8*(5), e17813. doi:10.2196/17813

Bizzotto, N., de Bruijn, G.-J., & Schulz, P. J. (2025). Clusters of patient empowerment and mental health literacy differentiate professional help-seeking attitudes in online mental health communities users. *Health Expectations: An International Journal of Public Participation in Health Care and Health Policy, 28*(1), e70153. doi:10.1111/hex.70153

Caton, S., & Chapman, M. (2016). The use of social media and people with intellectual disability: a systematic review and thematic analysis. *Journal of Intellectual and Developmental Disability, 41*(2), 125–139. doi:10.3109/13668250.2016.1153052

CDC (2024). About chronic diseases. chronic disease. https://www.cdc.gov/chronic-disease/about/index.html (accessed 20 August 2025).

Chaudhary, A., & Kumar, V. (2025). Rare diseases: a comprehensive literature review and future directions. *Journal of Rare Diseases, 4*(1). doi:10.1007/s44162-025-00099-6

Cleveland Clinic (2023). Intellectual disability: supporting strengths & adapting to challenges. *Cleveland Clinic*. https://my.clevelandclinic.org/health/diseases/25015-intellectual-disability-id (accessed 20 August 2025).

Coulson, N. S., Buchanan, H., & Aubeeluck, A. (2007). Social support in cyberspace: a content analysis of communication within a Huntington's disease online support group. *Patient Education and Counseling, 68*(2), 173–178. doi:10.1016/j.pec.2007.06.002

De Nardi, L. D., Trombetta, A., Ghirardo, S., Genovese, M. R. L., Barbi, E., & Taucar, V. (2020). Adolescents with chronic disease and social media: a cross-sectional study. *Archives of Disease in Childhood, 105*(8), 744–748. doi:10.1136/archdischild-2019-317996

Dudina, V., & Judina, D. (2023). The use of social media in the self-management of chronic diseases: views of patients and doctors. *The European Journal of Public Health, 33*(Suppl 2), ckad160.1133. doi:10.1093/eurpub/ckad160.1133

Duplaga, M., & Szulc, K. (2019). The association of internet use with wellbeing, mental health and health behaviours of persons with disabilities. *International Journal of Environmental Research and Public Health, 16*(18), 3252. doi:10.3390/ijerph16183252

Esparcia, A. C., Villafranca, P. L., & Ballester, C. C. (2015). La comunicación en la red de pacientes con enfermedades raras en España. *Revista Latina de Comunicación Social, 70*, 673–688. doi:10.4185/RLCS-2015-1065

Eysenbach, G., Powell, J., Englesakis, M., Rizo, C., & Stern, A. (2004). Health related virtual communities and electronic support groups: systematic review of the effects of online peer to peer interactions. *BMJ, 328*(7449), 1166. doi:10.1136/bmj.328.7449.1166

Glencross, S., Mason, J., Katsikitis, M., & Greenwood, K. M. (2021). Internet use by people with intellectual disability: exploring digital inequality—a systematic review. *Cyberpsychology, Behavior, and Social Networking, 24*(8), 503–520. doi:10.1089/cyber.2020.0499

Gow, J., Moffatt, C., & Blackport, J. (2020). Participation in patient support forums may put rare disease patient data at risk of re-identification. *Orphanet Journal of Rare Diseases, 15*(1), 226. doi:10.1186/s13023-020-01497-3

Gréaux, M., Moro, M. F., Kamenov, K., Russell, A. M., Barrett, D., & Cieza, A. (2023). Health equity for persons with disabilities: a global scoping review on barriers and interventions in healthcare services. *International Journal for Equity in Health, 22*(1), 236. doi:10.1186/s12939-023-02035-w

Green, B. M., Van Horn, K. T., Gupte, K., Evans, M., Hayes, S., & Bhowmick, A. (2020). Assessment of adaptive engagement and support model for people with chronic health conditions in online health communities: combined content analysis. *Journal of Medical Internet Research, 22*(7), e17338. doi:10.2196/17338

Haller, J., David, M. P., Lee, N. E., Shalin, S. C., & Gardner, J. M. (2018). Impact of pathologist involvement in Sarcoma and rare tumor patient support groups on Facebook: a survey of 542 patients and family members. *Archives of Pathology & Laboratory Medicine, 142*(9), 1113–1119. doi:10.5858/arpa.2017-0408-OA

Huang, S., & Wang, Y. (2023). How people with physical disabilities can obtain social support through online videos: a qualitative study in China. *International Journal of Environmental Research and Public Health, 20*(3), 2423. doi:10.3390/ijerph20032423

Joo, J. H., Bone, L., Forte, J., Kirley, E., Lynch, T., & Aboumatar, H. (2022). The benefits and challenges of established peer support programmes for patients, informal caregivers, and healthcare providers. *Family Practice, 39*(5), 903–912. doi:10.1093/fampra/cmac004

Khasawneh, M. A. S. (2024). Accessibility matters: investigating the usability of social media platforms for individuals with motor disabilities. *Studies in Media and Communication, 12*(2), 1–11. doi:10.11114/smc.v12i2.6615

Kim, H.-C., & Zhu, Z.-Y. (2020). Improving social inclusion for people with physical disabilities: the roles of mobile social networking applications (MSNA) by disability support organizations in China. *International Journal of Environmental Research and Public Health, 17*(7), 2333. doi:10.3390/ijerph17072333

Kjærulff, E. M., Andersen, T. H., Kingod, N., & Nexø, M. A. (2023). When people with chronic conditions turn to peers on social media to obtain and share information: systematic review of the implications for relationships with health care professionals. *Journal of Medical Internet Research, 25*(1), e41156. doi:10.2196/41156

Knepper, K. N. K. and Arrington, M. I. (2020). Social support and coping in an online PHPV forum. | *EBSCOhost.* https://openurl.ebsco.com/contentitem/gcd:146314721?sid=ebsco:plink:crawler&id=ebsco:gcd:146314721 (accessed 5 September 2025).

Lal, S., Tremblay, S., Starcevic, D., Mauger-Lavigne, M., & Anaby, D. (2022). Mental health problems among adolescents and young adults with childhood-onset physical disabilities: a scoping review. *Frontiers in Rehabilitation Sciences, 3*. doi:10.3389/fresc.2022.904586

Lapierre, N., Huet-Fiola, C., Labrie, D., Vincent-Blouin, E., Côté, C., Gagnon, M., Rhéaume, N., Laberge, J., Best, K. L., & Routhier, F. (2024). Digital platforms to facilitate physical activities for people with physical or sensory disabilities: a scoping review. *Disability and Health Journal, 17*(3), 101626. doi:10.1016/j.dhjo.2024.101626

Lawlor, A., & Kirakowski, J. (2014). Online support groups for mental health: a space for challenging self-stigma or a means of social avoidance? *Computers in Human Behavior, 32*, 152–161. doi:10.1016/j.chb.2013.11.015

Lee, H. E., & Cho, J. (2019). Social media use and well-being in people with physical disabilities: influence of SNS and online community uses on social support, depression, and psychological disposition. *Health Communication, 34*(9), 1043–1052. doi:10.1080/10410236.2018.1455138

Liu, J., & Wang, J. (2021). Users' intention to continue using online mental health communities: empowerment theory perspective. *International Journal of Environmental Research and Public Health, 18*(18), 9427. doi:10.3390/ijerph18189427

Lui, C.-W., Wang, Z., Wang, N., Milinovich, G., Ding, H., Mengersen, K., Bambrick, H., & Hu, W. (2021). A call for better understanding of social media in surveillance and management of noncommunicable diseases. *Health Research Policy and Systems, 19*(1), 18. doi:10.1186/s12961-021-00683-4

Manzoor, M., & Vimarlund, V. (2018). Digital technologies for social inclusion of individuals with disabilities. *Health and Technology, 8*(5), 377–390. doi:10.1007/s12553-018-0239-1

Martin Ginis, K. A., van der Ploeg, H. P., Foster, C., Lai, B., McBride, C. B., Ng, K., Pratt, M., Shirazipour, C. H., Smith, B., Vásquez, P. M., & Heath, G. W. (2021). Participation of people living with disabilities in physical activity: a global perspective. *Lancet (London, England), 398*(10298), 443–455. doi:10.1016/S0140-6736(21)01164-8

Miller, E. G., Woodward, A. L., Flinchum, G., Young, J. L., Tabor, H. K., & Halley, M. C. (2021). Opportunities and pitfalls of social media research in rare genetic diseases: a systematic review. *Genetics in Medicine: Official Journal of the American College of Medical Genetics, 23*(12), 2250–2259. doi:10.1038/s41436-021-01273-z

Nicholas, D. B., Chahauver, A., Brownstone, D., Hetherington, R., McNeill, T., & Bouffet, E. (2012). Evaluation of an online peer support network for fathers of a child with a brain tumor. *Social Work in Health Care, 51*(3), 232–245. doi:10.1080/00981389.2011.631696

Nieroba, E., & Larysz, D. (2020). The internet as an additional source of information on rare illness. A Facebook support group for parents of children with craniosynostosis as a case study. *Polish Annals of Medicine, 27*(1), 53–58. doi:10.29089/2019.19.00078

Park, E.-Y. (2024). The relation among smartphone use, social capital, and life satisfaction in individuals with physical disabilities. *Current Psychology, 43*(13), 11538–11545. doi:10.1007/s12144-023-05275-9

Park, J., & Kim, S. (2022). How do people with physical disabilities want to construct virtual identities with avatars? *Frontiers in Psychology, 13*. doi:10.3389/fpsyg.2022.994786

Schumacher, K. R., Stringer, K. A., Donohue, J. E., Yu, S., Shaver, A., Caruthers, R. L., Zikmund-Fisher, B. J., Fifer, C., Goldberg, C., & Russell, M. W. (2014). Social media methods for studying rare diseases. *Pediatrics, 133*(5), e1345–e1353. doi:10.1542/peds.2013-2966

Special Olympics (2018). Intellectual disabilities. *SpecialOlympics.Org*. https://www.specialolympics.org/about/intellectual-disabilities (accessed 1 September 2025).

Stetten, N. E., LeBeau, K., Aguirre, M. A., Vogt, A. B., Quintana, J. R., Jennings, A. R., & Hart, M. (2019). Analyzing the communication interchange of individuals with disabilities utilizing Facebook, discussion forums, and chat rooms: qualitative content analysis of online disabilities support groups. *JMIR Rehabilitation and Assistive Technologies, 6*(2), e12667. doi:10.2196/12667

Subirats, L., Reguera, N., Bañón, A. M., Gómez-Zúñiga, B., Minguillón, J., & Armayones, M. (2018). Mining Facebook data of people with rare diseases: a content-based and temporal analysis. *International Journal of Environmental Research and Public Health, 15*(9), 1877. doi:10.3390/ijerph15091877

Sweet, K. S., LeBlanc, J. K., Stough, L. M., & Sweany, N. W. (2020). Community building and knowledge sharing by individuals with disabilities using social media. *Journal of Computer Assisted Learning, 36*(1), 1–11. doi:10.1111/jcal.12377

Tough, H., Siegrist, J., & Fekete, C. (2017). Social relationships, mental health and wellbeing in physical disability: a systematic review. *BMC Public Health, 17*(1), 414. doi:10.1186/s12889-017-4308-6

Townsend, L., Gearing, R. E., & Polyanskaya, O. (2012). Influence of health beliefs and stigma on choosing internet support groups over formal mental health services. *Psychiatric Services (Washington, DC), 63*(4), 370–376. doi:10.1176/appi.ps.201100196

Valle, C. G., Tate, D. F., Mayer, D. K., Allicock, M., & Cai, J. (2013). A randomized trial of a Facebook-based physical activity intervention for young adult cancer survivors. *Journal of Cancer Survivorship: Research and Practice, 7*(3), 355–368. doi:10.1007/s11764-013-0279-5

WHO (2022). Mental health. *World Health Organization*. https://www.who.int/news-room/fact-sheets/detail/mental-health-strengthening-our-response (accessed 23 September 2025).

Wright, P. J., Raynor, P. A., Bowers, D., Combs, E. M., Corbett, C. F., Hardy, H., & Patel, K. (2023). Leveraging digital technology for social connectedness among adults with chronic conditions: a systematic review. *Digital Health*, *9*, 20552076231204746. doi:10.1177/20552076231204746

Yamaguchi, A., & Queralt-Rosinach, N. (2020). A proof-of-concept study of extracting patient histories for rare/intractable diseases from social media. *Genomics & Informatics*, *18*(2), e17. doi:10.5808/GI.2020.18.2.e17

Yeung, A., Ng, E., & Abi-Jaoude, E. (2022). TikTok and attention-deficit/hyperactivity disorder: a cross-sectional study of social media content quality. *Canadian Journal of Psychiatry. Revue Canadienne De Psychiatrie*, *67*(12), 899–906. doi:10.1177/07067437221082854

CHAPTER 9

SOCIAL MEDIA AND MENTAL HEALTH

Thu T. Nguyen[1], Junaid S. Merchant[1], Katrina Makres[1], Elizabeth Dennard[1], Shaniece Criss[2], and Quynh C. Nguyen[3]

[1]Department of Epidemiology and Biostatistics, School of Public Health, University of Maryland, College Park, MD, USA

[2]Department of Health Sciences, Furman University, Greenville, SC, USA

[3]National Institute of Nursing Research (NINR), National Institutes of Health (NIH), Bethesda, MD, USA

LEARNING OBJECTIVES

1. Evaluate the literature on the relationship between social media and mental health outcomes across diverse populations
2. Highlight key opportunities and pitfalls in studying the intersection of social media use and mental health
3. Identify critical data gaps and propose recommendations to guide future researchers

Overview

Social media platforms play a critical role in shaping mental health outcomes across diverse populations. However, their impact is complex and multifaceted, often varying widely based on age, gender, sexual orientation, and lived experience. This chapter provides a comprehensive overview of the varied research designs employed across existing literature to investigate the mental health impacts of social media on uniquely affected populations, including adolescents, older adults, and members of the LGBTQ+ community. By examining both qualitative and quantitative methodologies, this chapter highlights how researchers have approached groups' with distinct lived experiences. Additionally, this chapter synthesizes current findings, critically evaluates methodological strengths and limitations, and highlights significant data gaps within the field. Overall, this chapter provides practical recommendations and evidence-informed guidance for advancing future research in this evolving field.

Social Media and Youth Mental Health

Cognitive Effects of Social Media Use

Adolescence represents a critical window for cognitive development, marked by dramatic neurobiological, emotional, and behavioral changes. As social media increasingly becomes a central part of young people's daily lives, researchers have investigated how platforms such as Instagram, Snapchat, and TikTok affect adolescent cognition. A growing body of interdisciplinary literature reveals that social media's influence on cognition is nuanced—sometimes minimal, sometimes profound—depending on the individual, intensity of use, and developmental stage. Flannery et al. (2024) conducted a longitudinal neuroimaging study linking adolescent brain function to addiction-like social media use (ASMU). Their findings propose a neurodevelopmental model in which adolescents exhibit heightened sensitivity to social rewards—such as likes, comments, and shares—due to increased activity in brain regions like the medial prefrontal cortex, hippocampus, and posterior cingulate cortex. This neural hypersensitivity to social feedback can lead to craving and loss of control, mimicking addiction mechanisms traditionally associated with substances. This study revealed that adolescents with higher initial neural responses to social incentives were more likely to report ASMU symptoms two years later. A longitudinal decrease in neural responsiveness—indicative of desensitization or "tolerance"—suggests that the brain requires more frequent or intense stimulation over time to achieve the same reward response. This trajectory mirrors the pattern seen in other addictive behaviors and offers insight into how prolonged social media engagement may rewire the adolescent brain's reward circuitry. Notably, the study highlights that depressive symptoms were more likely to appear in girls exhibiting high ASMU, raising important questions about gender-specific vulnerability.

While Flannery et al. (2024) focused on the developmental neuroscience behind social media addiction, Stieger and Wunderl (2022) presented a contrasting picture through a large-scale behavioral study. Analyzing data from over 12,000 adolescents in Austria, they examined whether social media use impacts core cognitive functions—such as intelligence, spatial reasoning, and information processing. Using psychometric testing and random-forest machine learning models, they found that daily active or passive use of social media, even problematic use, had negligible associations with cognitive test performance. Rather, demographic variables like age and gender explained more variance in cognitive outcomes than social media use. The findings indicate that cognitive detriments are not inevitable and that the perceived harms of screen time may be overstated, especially in relation to traditional cognitive domains.

Another critical and less frequently discussed cognitive domain is cognitive social capital, referring to individuals' perceived trust, shared values, and mutual understanding within social networks. Petersen and Johnston (2015) studied how Facebook and Twitter influence this construct among South African university students. Their findings suggest that while social media fosters networked communication and access to diverse viewpoints, it also risks reinforcing echo chambers that limit exposure to differing ideas. For adolescents, whose cognitive development includes the formation of abstract thought and ethical reasoning, overexposure to like-minded content may reduce opportunities for cognitive challenge and diminish critical thinking skills. Additionally, the reward structures of social media prioritize instant popularity over deep engagement, which may further hinder the development of critical thinking skills.

In sum, the cognitive effects of social media on adolescents are multifaceted. Large-scale data (Stieger and Wunderl 2022) suggest a modest impact on traditional cognitive abilities, while neuroimaging research (Flannery et al. 2024) illustrates how social media may influence brain development and symptoms of addiction. Cognitive disruptions related to distraction, multitasking, and sleep loss (Bryant 2018) indicate that even if IQ scores remain unaffected, the quality and depth of thinking and learning may be altered. Finally, changes in social cognition and critical thinking (Petersen and Johnston 2015) underline the importance of media literacy in navigating an increasingly digital world. Social media is neither inherently harmful nor cognitively benign; its impact depends on how it is used, by whom, and at what stage of development.

Youth Behavior, Internet Access, and Mental Health

The ubiquity of social media has sparked considerable debate regarding its impact on adolescent mental health outcomes. Concerns about the rising youth mental health crisis, alongside increased social media use, prompted the Office of the Surgeon General (2023) to issue an advisory on the effects of social media on youth mental health, citing current evidence on the potential harms and benefits for adolescents. This section synthesizes the existing literature on the multifaceted relationship between social media and youth mental health, considering both direct and indirect effects, as well as the complexities of measuring and interpreting these associations. Two major themes have emerged: (1) patterns of social media use, and (2) the nature of content exposure among adolescents. This section also highlights documented mechanisms and recommendations before summarizing existing challenges and opportunities for future research.

Research linking social media and mental health builds on prior studies that examined screen time as a primary exposure of interest among adolescents and young adults. Population-level studies have shown that excessive screen time—commonly defined as more than one hour per day on any screen (e.g., TV, computers, smartphones, etc.)—is associated with lower psychological well-being and increased risk of depression and anxiety, particularly among adolescents compared to younger children (Twenge and Campbell 2018; Oswald et al. 2020; Nagata et al. 2024). However, systematic reviews have yielded mixed findings and identified smaller effect sizes (i.e., weaker relationships) than originally reported in earlier studies (Orben and Przybylski 2019; Ferguson et al. 2022; Nagata et al. 2024).

Notably, some studies have demonstrated positive associations between internet use and well-being, suggesting that different forms of digital media may have varying effects on mental health (Liu et al. 2024; Vuorre and Przybylski 2024). These conflicting findings have motivated more rigorous research to identify specific factors distinguishing social media's impact on mental health from general screen time measures (Orben and Przybylski 2019; Ferguson et al. 2022).

The simultaneous rise of smartphones, internet access, and social media platforms over the past two decades has drastically altered youth behavior and screen time habits. Historically, the dominant form of youth screen-based leisure had been cable television. As recently as 2015, nearly half of U.S. teens reported watching live television daily, while just over a third of teens reported watching online videos daily (Rideout and Robb 2019; Vogels and Gelles-Watnick 2023). By 2019, these patterns shifted with under a quarter of U.S. teens watching live television daily, while 69% were watching online videos on platforms like YouTube (Rideout and Robb 2019). This trend has been attributed to increased smartphone ownership, with current estimates suggesting that over 40% of 8–12-year-olds (i.e., tweens) own smartphones. Although most social media platforms set a minimum user age of 13, engagement among younger users is increasing (Rideout et al. 2022; HHS 2023). Approximately 18% of 8–12-year-olds report using platforms such as Snapchat, Instagram, Facebook, Discord, and Reddit, while 64% report watching online videos daily (American Academy of Pediatrics 2023). Unlike the relatively passive consumption of television, social media is often tailored to one's personal interests and is highly interactive (Anderson and Jiang 2018). Thus, the growing prevalence of PSMU has been attributed to how these platforms are designed to maximize user engagement, which can encourage excessive use, promote behavioral dysregulation, and underlie different mechanisms contributing to negative mental health outcomes (5Rights Foundation 2021).

Benefits of Social Media Use: Social Connection, Peer Acceptance, and Creative Expression

Several studies have challenged the notion of a direct link between social media use and adverse teen mental health outcomes, emphasizing the importance of quality of usage as a key driver of this relationship (Orben and Przybylski 2019; Beyens et al. 2020; Plackett et al. 2023). Some research suggests that the timing and context of social media engagement influence its impact on mental well-being. For example, moderate social media use, ranging from almost daily to several times per day, particularly on weekends, is associated with more positive mental health outcomes compared to both nonuse and near-constant use (Przybylski and Weinstein 2017).

CASE STUDY 1. SOCIAL MEDIA USE AND POSITIVE MENTAL HEALTH

A cross-sectional study by Clayborne et al. (2025) examined the association between social media use and positive mental health indicators among 13,113 adolescents from the 2017–2018 Canadian Health Behavior in School-aged Children study. Participants were categorized as non-active (never or at most weekly), active (almost daily to several times a day), intense (almost all the time), or problematic social media users (assessed using the Social Media Disorder Scale). Positive mental health indicators included self-efficacy, self-confidence, life satisfaction, and psychological well-being. This study found that both intense and problematic social media use (PSMU) were linked to lower levels of positive mental health across all indicators, genders, and grade levels. When compared to active social media use, PSMU was associated with lower levels of all positive mental health indicators. Additionally, intense social media use was associated with lower life satisfaction among young girls, and non-active social media use was associated with lower self-confidence among adolescents in grades 9 and 10. Finally, PSMU was associated with lower odds of high positive mental health across all groups. Notably, non-active use was linked to higher self-confidence and life satisfaction across all grades (Clayborne et al. 2025).

These findings suggest that non-problematic social media use can benefit adolescent mental health, whereas problematic use may negatively impact adolescent self-efficacy, self-confidence, life satisfaction, and psychological well-being. Longitudinal research is necessary to investigate how these observed associations change over time and potentially establish temporality between types of social media use and positive and negative mental health outcomes. Additionally, future researchers could examine the mechanisms linking types of social media use with mental health indicators to better inform prevention strategies aimed at strengthening youth mental health.

Importantly, the purpose of social media use matters. Using social media primarily for peer connection and entertainment (e.g., gaming and videos), rather than passive content consumption or self-presentation, is associated with greater well-being (Naslund et al. 2016; Liu et al. 2024; Vuorre and Przybylski 2024). For instance, a large-scale international multiverse analysis of over two million users across 168 countries (2006–2021) examined associations between internet access and multiple measures of well-being and found significant positive associations with life satisfaction, positive experiences, and social well-being (Vuorre and Przybylski 2024). Due to the large number of predictors, outcomes, and subgroups in this analysis, the authors implemented multiverse analyses to examine variability across findings. The results align with existing surveys demonstrating that teens are more likely to self-report positive experiences with social media compared to those who do not have mobile internet access, including increased social connection, creative expression, and feelings of support and acceptance from peers (Bickham et al. 2022; Vogels and Gelles-Watnick 2023).

Problematic Social Media Use (PSMU)

The displacement hypothesis proposes that increased reliance on digital media for leisure reduces time spent on protective mental health behaviors such as physical activity, adequate sleep, and in-person social interactions

(Wang et al. 2019; Oswald et al. 2020). This hypothesis is supported by evidence showing that increased screen time is associated with reduced "green time"—exposure to, or time spent in nature, which has positive impacts on mental health and well-being (Oswald et al. 2020).

CASE STUDY 2. SOCIAL MEDIA USE AND DEPRESSIVE SYMPTOMS

Some studies show that changes in problematic social media use (PSMU) are related to changes in depressive symptoms (Raudsepp and Kais 2019). A longitudinal study by Raudsepp and Kais explored the relationship between PSMU and depressive symptoms among 397 adolescent girls across three time points (2016–2018). Latent growth models were employed to test whether PSMU changes were associated with depressive symptoms and whether baseline PSMU predicted subsequent changes in these symptoms. Results revealed that higher baseline depressive symptoms predicted a greater increase in PSMU, but initial PSMU did not predict changes in depressive symptoms among study participants (Raudsepp and Kais 2019). This study highlights the importance of baseline mental health characteristics when addressing social media use and calls for more representative studies to better understand these complex interactions.

Experimental and quasi-experimental research also provides insight into potential impacts. A natural experiment examining Facebook's staggered rollout across college campuses showed slight increases post baseline in depression and anxiety rates and lowered academic achievement with the availability of the social media platform (Braghieri et al. 2022). Moreover, a couple of small-scale randomized control trials on limiting social media use in young adults have demonstrated reductions in internalizing symptoms and loneliness and improved subjective well-being, highlighting the promise of interventions targeting excessive social media use (Hunt et al. 2018; Allcott et al. 2020). However, despite the importance of these controlled experiments, other studies have challenged this evidence by asserting that current research is unable to support claims regarding the harmful effects of social media use on adolescent internalizing disorders (Ferguson et al. 2022). For example, a meta-analysis of 46 studies by Ferguson and colleagues found numerous methodological weaknesses, including a lack of an analysis plan, protocol pre-registration, and outcome measure variability across included studies. These weaknesses highlight the need for more rigorous study designs, standardized metrics, and longitudinal approaches to better capture the complex interplay between social media use and adolescent mental health.

Harms of Social Media Use: Cyberbullying, Predation, and Discrimination

Developmental researchers have proposed a biopsychosocial model that centers adolescence as a critical period for socio-emotional development that heightens sensitivity to social environments and increases vulnerability to the potential harms of social media (Blakemore and Mills 2014;

Orben et al. 2024). Building on considerable research that has characterized the rapid changes in cognition, biology, and social behavior that occur during adolescence into young adulthood, this framework suggests that social media uniquely influences developmental processes shaping both healthy and unhealthy psychological trajectories (Orben and Przybylski 2019; Orben et al. 2024). For instance, teenagers are often aware of social comparisons and highly driven by the need to fit in with their peers, so the number of likes and followers they accrue provides a new way of quantifying their perceived popularity (Orben et al. 2024; Jeste et al. 2025). Unlike synchronous, face-to-face interaction, social media's public and asynchronous nature amplifies the perceived reward of online social success (e.g., positive comments on a post, post likes, follower requests, etc.), as well as exacerbates the stress of unfulfilled social needs (e.g., no online engagement to a social media post; Orben et al. 2024). Thus, developmental theories provide an explanatory framework for understanding how psycho-social mechanisms link social media exposures to teen mental health outcomes.

The asynchronous and often anonymous nature of social media enables users to express views and engage in behaviors that they are less likely to enact in-person, especially in forums or comment sections that lack moderation—an effect described as online disinhibition (Suler 2004; Prajith and Bhuyan 2025). As social media becomes integral to adolescent social life, it simultaneously opens new avenues for cyberbullying and other forms of identity-based harassment, exclusion, and rumor-spreading that can reach broad audiences (Suler 2004; HHS 2023). Studies have consistently linked experiences of cyberbullying with increased rates of anxiety, depression, and suicidal ideation among teenagers (Kowalski et al. 2014; Hinduja and Patchin 2019). Furthermore, teens who experience cyberbullying are more likely to suffer from low self-esteem, poor academic performance, delayed social development, and other emotional difficulties (Nixon 2014). This may be exacerbated by the persistent and pervasive nature of online interactions, such that victims often feel that there is no safe space, which further intensifies the negative impact of these interactions.

Social media anonymity can also foster predatory behaviors and contribute to the normalization of antagonistic online cultures. Adolescent girls and transgender youth are disproportionately targeted by malicious actors seeking to harass, financially extort, or sexually exploit them, with nearly 60% of preteen and teenage girls reporting unwanted contact from strangers on Instagram and Snapchat (HHS 2023; Nesi et al. 2023). Furthermore, social media environments have also fostered hostility through echo chambers where misogyny, racism, and other forms of aggression are rewarded with engagement, virality, and affirmation from like-minded communities (Jane 2014; Marwick and Caplan 2018). Prolonged exposure to these spaces can desensitize teens to harmful content, entrench aggression as a cultural norm, and create subcultures, such as the "Manosphere," promoting misogyny (Phillips 2015; Marwick and Caplan 2018).

The harms of social media extend beyond overtly negative content. Teen mental health can also be impacted by seemingly positive influencer culture. As platforms evolved from digital spaces designed for social connection and democratized user-generated content to revenue-generating media-serving platforms, there was a simultaneous rise of influencers—individuals who curate content for vast audiences (Adeane and Stasiak 2024). Recent estimates indicate that 72% of teens follow influencers (Faverio and Anderson 2022). Research suggests that teens are increasingly forming parasocial relationships with influencers, which have been linked to addictive behaviors, negative self-comparisons, diminished self-esteem, and heightened symptoms of anxiety (Adeane and Stasiak 2024; Lynde-Smith 2024). For example, exposure to fitness influencers and images of idealized bodies on social media has been linked to eating disorders and body dissatisfaction even among boys (Griffiths et al. 2018; Rodgers et al. 2020; Suhag and Rauniyar 2023; Alzahuf et al. 2024).

Research suggests distinct mechanisms driving this relationship across diverse populations. For example, Instagram usage is associated with body image issues among teen girls (Kleemans et al. 2018), who, along with LGBTQ+ teens, are more likely to be exposed to hate-based content and experience cyberbullying on social media (Angoff and Barnhart 2021; APA 2023; HHS 2023). On the other hand, social media exposure to racial violence negatively impacts Black teens' mental health (Baskin-Sommers et al. 2021; Marshall et al. 2024). Collectively, these findings underscore that social media's psychological risks are not uniformly distributed but vary according to identity, lived experience, and exposure type.

Social Media and the Older Adult Population

With the advent of social media, older generations are increasingly adopting digital networking platforms. Among American adults aged 65 and older, usage has surged nearly fourfold since 2010, now reaching 45% in this age group, the most accelerated growth across all age demographics (Faverio and Anderson 2022). Social media exerts both beneficial and detrimental effects on older adults' mental health. On one hand, it can foster social connections and mitigate isolation. This social engagement is especially important given that one in three older adults experiences chronic social isolation, a factor linked to adverse health outcomes (Gerlach et al. 2024). Social media can also serve as an accessible source of information, provide cognitive stimulation, and facilitate healthy cognitive aging. On the other hand, exposure to hateful content may augment anxiety and depression. Furthermore, technological difficulties can exacerbate the digital divide and heighten cybersecurity risks.

There are a myriad of literature studies investigating the positive impact of social media use on cognitive aging, social connectedness, and life satisfaction. This trend stands in stark contrast to the dearth of such literature studies exploring the positive effects of social media on adolescent mental health, as enumerated previously in the chapter. This section explores the dual potential of social media as both a positive and negative influence on older adults' cognitive health and well-being. It also outlines future directions to enrich the understanding of the evolving dynamic between social media platforms and older adults' mental health.

Impacts of Aging

Aging is often accompanied by a range of limitations that can significantly affect individuals' social engagement and overall well-being. Physically, mobility limitations increase due to conditions such as arthritis, osteoporosis, and loss of hand-eye coordination (Ferrucci et al. 2014). Retirement often results in the loss of professional and social networks and subsequent feelings of isolation (Haris et al. 2014; Iqbal et al. 2016). Furthermore, financial constraints stemming from reduced income can further impede participation in hobbies, travel, and other enriching activities (Meymo and Nyström 2017). Collectively, these physical, social, and financial limitations can result in a cycle of inactivity and social disengagement that undermines emotional health and increases the risk of depression (Nervik et al. 2011; Iqbal et al. 2016). The cumulative effects also heighten the risk of serious mental health concerns, including suicide and depression (Haris et al. 2014).

Social Media's Beneficial Effects

Social media can counteract cognitive decline, promote health, augment socialization, and prevent premature mortality among older adults (Cornejo et al. 2013; Campos et al. 2016; Ugalde et al. 2023; Li et al. 2025). Cao and colleagues (2022) identified key drivers of sustained social media use among this group: self-protection, social motivation, perceived usefulness, and entertainment. As aging amplifies physical and psychological vulnerabilities, including feelings of isolation, social media platforms offer a vital virtual environment for connection and discourse. These digital platforms help mitigate real-world social limitations by fostering a sense of community through shared content and interactive engagement. Additionally, social media serves as a readily accessible source for information, encompassing health, safety, and essential resources.

Social media offers several unique advantages over comparable technological media. Its content is user-generated and user-specific, presenting older adults with substantial independence and empowerment to navigate platforms freely, acquire accessible knowledge, and even curate digital content. Beyond personalization, social media also serves as a comprehensive public forum, encompassing a myriad of themes from political news to public health information, allowing older adults to remain engaged and informed along with rapid societal advancements.

Social media bolsters older adults' emotional well-being by facilitating connection with friends and family despite geographic distances, time constraints, or mobility limitations (Iqbal et al. 2016; Li et al. 2025). The interactive multimedia, images, videos, audio, comments, status updates, and other features simulate traditional communication methods, while facilitating the sharing of memories and reconnection with acquaintances (Haris et al. 2014; Meymo and Nyström 2017).

In addition to promoting social connectedness, social media is a readily accessible source of health information for older adults (Haris et al. 2014). A cross-sectional survey found that approximately 90% of older users reported using social media to learn and disseminate health information (Tennant et al. 2015). They can join online groups to connect with people with similar health concerns, offering information and support (Iqbal et al. 2016). Additionally, information regarding prognosis, symptoms, and treatments is easily accessible and frequently consulted through social media (Parida et al. 2016). Social media presents older adults with a platform to exchange health experiences, manage diseases, and interact with health professionals for general health information. While secure telemedicine is the preferred approach for one-on-one healthcare appointments, social media platforms provide a space for health organizations and clinics to disseminate preventative health information, disease outbreak updates, and other vital information (Merchant et al. 2021).

Challenges for Older Adults in Using Social Media

Despite the significant increase in older adult social media users, this demographic faces unique barriers that limit widespread adoption and sustained engagement. Limited digital literacy can hinder navigation of online environments, while age-related conditions, such as reduced vision, arthritis pain, and memory decline, may further discourage acquisition of new technological skills. Furthermore, extended screen use may contribute to eye strain, and technological expenses can pose financial barriers (Meymo and Nyström 2017; Ugalde et al. 2023).

Lee et al. (2022) identified four primary barriers to older adults' use of social media:

1. **Intrapersonal:** Self-perceptions regarding the futility of learning how to use novel social media platforms
2. **Functional:** Age-related limitations, such as diminished memory, spatial reasoning, and analytical thinking, which deter learning technical skills
3. **Structural:** Financial barriers, including the cost of devices, software, and internet services, that hinder access to digital platforms
4. **Interpersonal:** A lack of individuals who can provide guidance or teach digital skills, coupled with a limited network of online contacts

Together, these factors collectively underscore the barriers that impede older adults' digital engagement on social media, further exacerbating the digital divide.

Social Media's Detrimental Effects

The widespread popularity of social media has paradoxically transformed the digital landscape for older adults. While these platforms have introduced novel avenues for interpersonal communication and social engagement, the feelings of isolation largely remain due to a lack of humanistic, face-to-face interactions. Pervasive online interactions can augment depression, anxiety, and other significant concerns that take a toll on older adults' cognitive and emotional well-being. Despite the platforms' fundamental purpose of social connection, they contribute to information overload and social comparison that may augment feelings of inadequacy and isolation. Moreover, limited safeguards serve as a fertile environment for digital scams and misinformation propagation, particularly threatening to vulnerable populations. These threats not only risk financial security, but they can also heighten sentiments of fear and stress when engaging with online content. Overall, understanding the holistic impact of social media on older adults' physical, mental, and emotional health is crucial to uphold safety and well-being for aging populations.

The COVID-19 pandemic further illuminated these risks. Quarantine measures and social isolation intensified reliance on digital communication, yet older populations continued to experience profound detachment and emotional distress (Vahia IV et al. 2020; Mather and Scommegna 2023). A particular study during the pandemic investigated the correlation between social media usage type: active (posting, commenting, sharing) versus passive (viewing, liking) and depression across racial groups (Chhatwani et al. 2022). The findings revealed that active social media usage was associated with depression for both African American and Caucasian older adults. In contrast, passive social media use was correlated with depression only among African American older adults and not their Caucasian counterparts. This trend highlights the importance of considering racial disparities when assessing the mental health impact of digital networking platforms for older populations.

Internet Scams

In recent years, cyberattacks targeting personal information, financial credentials, and sensitive account data have surged, disproportionately impacting vulnerable populations, such as older adults (Alwanain 2020; Chen et al. 2025). Notably, the most prevalent targets of digital scams are PayPal, Facebook, Microsoft, Netflix, and WhatsApp (Alwanain 2020). Given Facebook's popularity among older users, it is a frequent conduit for phishing scams directed at this demographic (Alwanain 2020; Narayanan et al. 2021).

Older adults are susceptible to cyber scams due to a myriad of factors, including limited digital literacy and technical skills (Alwanain 2020; Narayanan et al. 2021; Chen et al. 2025). Their propensity to trust online information, coupled with cognitive decline, further inhibits their ability to distinguish between legitimate and fraudulent online information (Narayanan et al. 2021; Chen et al. 2025). Those with limited at-home support or without individuals to teach safe social media navigation skills are particularly at risk (Chen et al. 2025). Further escalating the challenges, older populations often have higher credit limits, and there may be a delay in noticing fraudulent charges (Alwanain 2020).

Digital scams impose a profound financial burden on older Americans. In 2019, the Internet Crime Complaint Center received more than 68 000 complaints from victims aged 60 and older, totaling approximately $835 million in reported losses (Alwanain 2020). This figure reflects only documented cases; many incidents remain unreported due to embarrassment or fear of continued harassment (Alwanain 2020). Each year, millions of older Americans fall victim to financial schemes or fraud, underscoring the urgent need for targeted digital literacy and fraud-prevention initiatives (Narayanan et al. 2021).

Misinformation

Misinformation on social media poses a significant threat to older adults, particularly on politically charged topics and health-related misconceptions such as vaccine hesitancy. A 2017 Twitter study of 4.5 million retweeted stories found that false information was 70% more likely to be shared rapidly compared to accurate information (Vosoughi et al. 2018). Furthermore, during the 2016 U.S. presidential election, Americans aged 65 and older were seven times more likely to share fake news on social media compared to younger users (Guess et al. 2019). Falsehoods often gain traction because they present novel or emotionally provocative narratives, especially on sensitive topics such as terrorism, natural disasters, health crises, and economic instability. A qualitative study exploring older adults' perceptions of misinformation found that despite their general awareness of its existence, their failure to detect specific falsehoods often stimulates polarized emotions of fear and anxiety (Vivion et al. 2024). Although the seniors disliked the information overload present on social media platforms and aspired to corroborate the credibility of the information source, it was difficult and time-consuming to cross-reference every online statement. Therefore, social media has far-reaching implications on not only older adults' susceptibility to misinformation but also their unintentional contribution to the broader propagation of falsehoods. These patterns highlight the need for interventions that strengthen source-evaluation skills and reduce exposure to misleading content.

Social Media and the LGBTQ+ Community

Social media has become a vital tool for members of the lesbian, gay, bisexual, transgender, queer or questioning, and other gender and sexual minority (LGBTQ+) communities. Research indicates that LGBTQ+ youth engage with social media and digital communication platforms more frequently than their heterosexual counterparts, granting these platforms substantial influence over their daily experiences (Fisher et al. 2024). While there is no singular way to use social media or define its impact uniformly, these platforms can exert both negative and positive effects on LGBTQ+ individuals (Fisher et al. 2024). This section explores key patterns and challenges that emerge from social media use within this community.

Online Discrimination

Participation in social media exposes all users to the risk of cyberbullying and online harassment. As noted by Escobar-Viera's research team, social media serves as a space where individuals may encounter "rejection, discrimination, bullying, and other negative experiences" (Escobar-Viera et al. 2022). However, members of the LGBTQ+ community are disproportionately subjected to such encounters due to their gender identity and sexual orientation (Abreu and Kenny 2018; McConnell et al. 2017; Fisher et al. 2024). LGBTQ+ youth, in particular, experience rates of cyberbullying and victimization up to three times higher than those of their non-LGTBQ+ peers (Miller 2017; McConnell et al. 2017; Berger et al. 2022). This elevated vulnerability can lead individuals to conceal their identities online (McConnell et al. 2017). Compounding this issue, many LGBTQ+ youth refrain from reporting cyberbullying incidents, possibly due to limited familial support, fear of being outed, or the perception that harassment cannot be stopped (Abreu and Kenny 2018).

Several platform features contribute to susceptibility to discriminatory behavior. For instance, anonymity can lower users' inhibitions, often resulting in more aggression or harmful posts (McConnell et al. 2017). The persistent nature of online content increases the visibility and impact of discriminatory messages, and cyberbullying can transcend digital boundaries, manifesting offline in schools and other community spaces (Abreu and Kenny 2018).

Discrimination Variance within the LGBTQ+ Community

The LGBTQ+ is an umbrella term that encompasses diverse populations with significant variation in lived experiences. Within this broad community, marginalized ethnic queer people may find themselves further isolated or relegated to the periphery (Das and Farber 2020). The intersectionality of race, gender identity, and sexual orientation frequently influences online treatment. For example, transgender people of color who share personal narratives online often encounter intensified discrimination (Das and Farber 2020). Importantly, LGBTQ+ individuals may face hostility not only from cisgender and heterosexual peers but also from within their own community. Social hierarchies and internal biases are reflected in online platforms, where disparities based on gender identity and sexual orientation persist. Transgender and "other" gender youth are more likely to experience online victimization compared to cisgender peers (McConnell et al. 2017). Among cisgender individuals, females who identify as a sexual minority face more discrimination than their male sexual minority counterparts (McConnell et al. 2018). In addition, bisexual individuals, particularly women, receive hate messages from LGBTQ+ peers (Abreu and Kenny 2018; Escobar-Viera et al. 2022). These circumstances are also consistent outside of the queer community, as bisexual youth have higher rates of discrimination than other sexual minority youth from their heterosexual peers, highlighting the pervasive nature of the issue (Abreu and Kenny 2018).

Counteracting Online Discrimination

In response to pervasive online discrimination, many LGBTQ+ individuals adopt proactive strategies to navigate and curate their digital environments. These strategies include hiding, blocking, or downvoting harmful content to influence algorithms (Escobar-Viera et al. 2022). Individuals often exercise caution by screening potential connections before accepting friend requests, including reviewing profiles for any indicators of intolerance or hostility (Berger et al. 2022). Other protective measures include customizing privacy settings, being selective about shared content, and, in some cases, choosing not to disclose one's gender identity or sexual orientation online (McConnell et al. 2017).

Impacts of Discrimination

The effects of online discrimination extend far beyond the initial exposure to a harmful post and significantly impact offline well-being. For LGBTQ+ youth, cyberbullying can reinforce existing negative thoughts and contribute to declines in mental health (Thilakaraj et al. 2024). Empirical evidence indicates that these individuals are at increased risk for a range of adverse outcomes, including suicidal ideation and attempts, low self-esteem, elevated rates of depression, heightened physical aggression, body-image concerns, increased levels of isolation, and decreased grade point average (Abreu and Kenny 2018). In general, individuals who experience discrimination online are more likely to suffer diminished mental and emotional well-being (McConnell et al. 2017). Given the magnitude of harm associated with online discrimination, there is a critical need for policymakers, educators, and digital platform leaders to implement strategies aimed at mitigating this exposure to LGBTQ+ individuals.

Social Media's Impact on Mental Health

Even outside the realm of social media, LGBTQ+ individuals report disproportionately higher rates of mental health challenges, largely due to their elevated exposure to violence and discrimination (Berger et al. 2022). This disparity is even more pronounced among rural queer youth, who often report higher levels of isolation, depression, and suicidality (Escobar-Viera et al. 2022). As previously discussed, cyberbullying exacerbates these outcomes by increasing risk for depression, suicidality, and substance use (Abreu and Kenny 2018; Pordeus et al. 2022; Thilakaraj et al. 2024).

Negative Impacts on Mental Health

While social media can serve as a source of connection and support, excessive use can lead to detrimental psychological effects. LGBTQ+ individuals who frequently turn to social media for online support or identity exploration may develop social media dependency (Hu 2020). Such dependency has been linked to negative impacts on sleep quality, reduced life satisfaction, increased depression, and lower self-esteem (Twenge and Campbell 2018; Hu 2020; Masoed et al. 2021). Furthermore, individuals who disclose their gender identity or sexual orientation online may experience heightened feelings of loneliness offline (Berger et al. 2022). Although social media is often used to seek emotional support, overreliance on digital support networks has also been associated with reduced quality of life (McConnell et al. 2017). Additionally, certain online environments where heteronormative tendencies are reinforced by categorizing users based on perceived characteristics such as education, race, gender, and sexual orientation (Das and Farber 2020). This exclusionary discourse can further marginalize users who do not conform to standards, reinforcing feelings of alienation. Emphasis on the importance of traditional family structures and assimilation into mainstream society can further marginalize queer individuals, particularly those whose identities do not fit into widely accepted categories (Das and Farber 2020). Notably, bisexual people are often excluded from online discussions, leading to feelings of invisibility within both queer and non-queer spaces (Das and Farber 2020).

Positive Impacts on Mental Health

Despite these potential risks, social media also plays a major role in fostering psychological resilience and community support among LGBTQ+ individuals (Berger et al. 2022; Fisher et al. 2024). For many, especially those in rural or socially conservative areas, digital platforms offer vital means of connection (Escobar-Viera et al. 2022). These individuals often find that digital platforms provide a nonconfrontational and affirming environment where they can more easily access emotional support (Escobar-Viera et al. 2022). Research suggests that engaging with LGBTQ+ support networks online is associated with improved mental health outcomes by reducing isolation and fostering a sense of belonging (McConnell et al. 2017; Berger et al. 2022). Social media also plays a crucial role in addressing discrimination by offering spaces for shared experiences and support (Oz et al. 2023). These platforms help individuals process hate and connect with others who share coping strategies and encouragement, particularly benefiting those newly facing such challenges (Miller 2017; Das and Farber 2020).

Finding Solidarity Online

Social media has significantly enhanced the ability of LGBTQ+ individuals to establish meaningful connections within their community. Many users gravitate toward platforms that offer a degree of anonymity, enabling selective disclosure based on comfort and safety (Miller 2017; McConnell et al. 2017; Berger et al. 2022). These digital environments can function as safe spaces, fostering inclusivity and emotional support for the queer community. Notably, a 2021 study found that 70% of LGBTQ+ youth reported access to safe and affirming online spaces, in contrast to only 50% who identified such environments at school and 34% at home (Fisher et al. 2024).

Establishing an Identity

The process of identity formation can be complex and challenging for many individuals, particularly for those who identify as sexual and/or gender minorities. Social media serves as a vital resource for LGBTQ+ youth, offering tools for self-exploration and identity development in a controlled and autonomous environment (Miller 2017; Berger et al. 2022). Given the fluidity of gender and sexual orientation, access to online information and diverse narratives helps provide both language and context for understanding one's experiences (Das and Farber 2020). This contributes to a stronger sense of belonging and self-recognition. Many LGBTQ+ individuals use social media to "test" coming out, gradually disclosing their identity within a small, trusted online network before sharing more broadly (Hu 2020). A 2020 study reported that one in five queer people initially come out through social media, emphasizing the platform's importance for identity expression and connection (Terribili 2022).

Sharing Experiences

Beyond surface-level interaction, social media offers LGBTQ+ individuals opportunities to form deeper connections by sharing personal experiences and seeking advice from peers. This community-driven engagement is particularly significant during incidents of discrimination or cultural events affecting the LGBTQ+ community. Social media functions as a storytelling platform where users exchange guidance pertaining to life, identity, safety, sex, and sexuality (McConnell et al. 2017; Das and Farber 2020; Berger et al. 2022). The ability to share coming-out stories and gender transitions fosters mutual understanding and validation (Das and Farber 2020). Social media also enables connections between individuals who might not ordinarily cross paths, including those from different geographic or social contexts. Moreover, visibility of celebrities who publicly support the queer community or disclose gender and/or sexual orientation can serve as a powerful resource of empowerment on the individual level (Hu 2020; Oz et al. 2023). These digital interactions frequently translate into real-world involvement, as platforms also serve as hubs for promoting virtual and in-person LGBTQ+ events (Terribili 2022).

Online Activism

Social media serves as a powerful medium for disseminating diverse forms of information, including personal updates, political discourse, news, and event coverage (Taylor et al. 2020). Many individuals leverage these platforms to reach large audiences, express concerns, and organize events aimed at amplifying the voices of those impacted by specific laws or policies (Miller 2017; Hu 2020). Politically informed users can share knowledge to educate others, foster awareness, and empower communities at the grassroots level (Hu 2020). Importantly, social media enables participation in activism for individuals unable to be physically present at demonstrations or events, allowing them to show solidarity and contribute to campaigns virtually (Ofori-Parku and Moscato 2018). While these networks offer effective tools for mobilizing supporters, questions remain about whether genuine, systematic change can be executed primarily through online channels (Hu 2020). External factors, such as governmental counter-movements, can influence the momentum of digital activism. Tactics such as physical violence, harassment, doxxing, arrests, and legal actions are frequently used to intimidate activists, deterring real-life action (Earl et al. 2022). Additionally, inherent features of social media can undermine the sustainability of movements. Online trends shift rapidly, and activism that relies heavily on digital engagement can be perceived as transient or performative (Ofori-Parku and Moscato 2018). This phenomenon has given rise to the term "slacktivism," which refers to minimal or symbolic online engagement that fails to translate into meaningful, real-world impact (Dennis and Finotello 2019).

CASE STUDY 3. OZ ET AL. (2023) / WITH PERMISSION OF SAGE PUBLICATIONS LTD

The decision by Turkey's political leaders to withdraw from the Istanbul Convention, a treaty aimed at preventing gender-based violence, sparked significant backlash, particularly among women and the LGBTQ+ community (Amnesty International 2021). In response, many within the LGBTQ+ mobilized online to resist the decision and its implications. Understanding the impact of this movement requires examining the broader social and political context in Turkey, where conservative ideologies dominate, and LGBTQ+ individuals often face discrimination, violence, and censorship (Acconcia et al. 2022). State-sanctioned homophobia, coupled with frequent inflammatory rhetoric by political figures, emboldens online bullying and attacks. Social media platforms are frequently used to threaten, intimidate, and organize hate against LGBTQ+ individuals. As a result, online harassment has escalated in frequency and severity since the government's withdrawal from the convention. Though it is not just the conservative views that make this a fascinating case study, there is also the factor of state and lateral surveillance—citizens monitoring each other's behavior (Andrejevic 2004; Caliskan 2021). These dynamics create an atmosphere of fear and caution, making digital spaces hard to navigate for the LGBTQ+ community.

Despite these risks, activists have continued to engage in online resistance, utilizing hashtag campaigns and other digital tools to coordinate protests, disseminate information, and cultivate solidarity (Goswami 2018; Murthy 2018; Chon and Park 2020). However, such visibility has also made activists targets of government retaliation, including threats of physical violence, political persecution, and punitive actions against family members. LGBTQ+ individuals in Turkey experience social isolation from family and friends. While the movement has garnered scholarly attention, it also illustrates the limitations and dangers of digital resistance under authoritarian regimes.

CASE STUDY 4. DAS AND FARBER (2020) / JOHN WILEY & SONS; IT GETS BETTER (2017)

The *It Gets Better Project,* launched in September 2010, was developed in response to higher suicide rates among lesbian, gay, bisexual, and transgender youth. This initiative invites individuals to upload their personal stories and messages of support to a centralized YouTube channel, offering a powerful medium through which users can connect, find comfort, and share coping strategies related to identity-based discrimination. However, critics have noted that the project perpetuates class-, race-, sex-, and gender-based biases seen throughout society as the project's representatives showcase these "ideals." Many who share their stories or represent the project are cis, White, highly educated, upper-class, and gay, which does not fully represent the LGBTQ+ community.

Nonetheless, the initiative has had a significant impact, as over 70,000 individuals have shared their uplifting stories to support, comfort, and empower LGBTQ+ youth. The program aims to reach LGBTQ+ youth before they reach a point of crisis through fostering community, resilience, and hope. Since its inception, the project has expanded through *It Gets Better EDU*, which includes educational resources, youth ambassadors, and specific yearly programming for students. The organization has also developed a global community to help reach LGBTQ+ youth beyond the United States. This case exemplifies how social media-based activism can extend beyond the digital sphere to produce tangible improvements in mental health, academic engagement, and overall well-being for LGBTQ+ youth.

Conclusion

The relationship between social media use and mental health is highly complex, varying across distinct populations and shaped by individual and group-level factors. While social media offers opportunities for peer support, creative expression, cognitive stimulation, and education, it also presents serious harms, including PSMU, identity-based discrimination, and exposure to misinformation. Numerous studies indicate that the impact of social media on mental health depends on users' identity-based characteristics and engagement activities. For youth, especially racial and gender minority teens, social media serves as an essential space for peer connection, creative expression, and identity affirmation, while also exposing them to identity-based discrimination, social comparison, and PSMU. Comparably, older adults benefit from online social support, peer engagement, and cognitive stimulation but also face age-based harms, including digital scams and misinformation, which can worsen symptoms of depression and anxiety. Additionally, members of the LGBTQ+ community, especially teens and young adults with intersecting identities, experience digital spaces as both sites of empowerment and risk, gaining peer support while also encountering cyberbullying and identity-based discrimination.

The effects of social media use on mental health are moderated by identity-based characteristics and engagement patterns across adolescents, older adults, and members of the LGBTQ+ community. While using social media to connect with peers, foster resilience, and express creativity is often associated with positive mental health outcomes, PSMU, social comparison, and exposure to discriminatory content are often associated with negative mental health outcomes. This evolving context across diverse populations underscores the need for a more comprehensive public health response to enhance platform transparency, foster digital literacy, and create safer online environments (Naslund et al. 2020). Future research must be more representative and interdisciplinary, enabling a deeper understanding of the long-term mental health impacts of social media use across diverse populations. Ultimately, collaborative efforts among stakeholders will enable the identification of protective factors and inform evidence-based interventions that empower users to engage with digital technologies in healthy and supportive ways.

References

5Rights Foundation (2021). Pathways: how digital design puts children at risk. https://5rightsfoundation.com/wp-content/uploads/2021/09/Pathways-how-digital-design-puts-children-at-risk.pdf (accessed 1 September 2025).

Abreu, R. L., & Kenny, M. C. (2018). Cyberbullying and LGBTQ youth: a systematic literature review and recommendations for prevention and intervention. *Journal of Child & Adolescent Trauma, 11*(1), 81–97. doi:10.1007/s40653-017-0175-7

Acconcia, G., Perego, A., & Perini, L. (2022). LGBTQ activism in repressive contexts: the struggle for (in)visibility in Egypt, Tunisia and Turkey. *Social Movement Studies*, 1–19. doi:10.1080/14742837.2022.2070739

Adeane, E., & Stasiak, K. (2024). "It's really hard to strike a balance": the role of digital influencers in shaping youth mental health. *Digital Health, 10*, 20552076241288059. doi:10.1177/20552076241288059

Allcott, H., Braghieri, L., Eichmeyer, S., & Gentzkow, M. (2020). The welfare effects of social media. *American Economic Review, 110*(3), 629–676. doi:10.1257/aer.20190658

Alwanain, M. I. (2020). Phishing awareness and elderly users in social media. *International Journal of Computer Science and Network Security, 20*(9), 114–119.

Alzahuf, S., Ahmed, E., Al-Badwyi, J. A., Alkhalifa, M. A., Albinessa, M. A., Bashandi, A. A., Alanazi, D. M., Alawad, F. H., & Alhodibi, M. (2024). Influence of social media on body image and eating disorder prevalence in adolescents: a cross-sectional Saudi study. *Journal of Advanced Trends in Medical Research, 1*(2), 593. doi:10.4103/ATMR.ATMR_104_24

American Academy of Pediatrics (2023). Age to introduce social media. *American Academy of Pediatrics.* https://www.aap.org/en/patient-care/media-and-children/center-of-excellence-on-social-media-and-youth-mental-health/qa-portal/qa-portal-library/qa-portal-library-questions/age-to-introduce-social-media/ (accessed 3 June 2025).

Amnesty International (2021). Here's why the Istanbul convention saves lives. *Amnesty International.* https://www.amnesty.org/en/latest/news/2021/05/heres-why-the-istanbul-convention-saves-lives/ (accessed 10 March 2026).

Anderson, M. and Jiang, J. (2018). Teens, social media and technology 2018. *Pew Research Center.* https://www.pewresearch.org/internet/2018/05/31/teens-social-media-technology-2018/ (accessed 1 September 2025).

Andrejevic, M. (2004). The work of watching one another: lateral surveillance, risk, and governance. *Surveillance & Society, 2*(4), 3359. doi:10.24908/ss.v2i4.3359

Angoff, H. D., & Barnhart, W. R. (2021). Bullying and cyberbullying among LGBQ and heterosexual youth from an intersectional perspective: findings from the 2017 national youth risk behavior survey. *Journal of School Violence, 20*(3), 274–286. doi:10.1080/15388220.2021.1879099

APA. (2023). *Health Advisory on Social Media Use in Adolescence.* American Psychological Association. https://www.apa.org/topics/social-media-internet/health-advisory-adolescent-social-media-use.pdf

Baskin-Sommers, A., Simmons, C., Conley, M., Chang, S.-A., Estrada, S., Collins, M., Pelham, W., Beckford, E., Mitchell-Adams, H., Berrian, N., Tapert, S. F., Gee, D. G., & Casey, B. J. (2021). Adolescent civic engagement: lessons from Black lives matter. *Proceedings of the National Academy of Sciences, 118*(41), e2109860118. doi:10.1073/pnas.2109860118

Berger, M. N., Taba, M., Marino, J. L., Lim, M. S., & Skinner, S. R. (2022). Social media use and health and well-being of lesbian, gay, bisexual, transgender, and queer youth: systematic review. *Journal of medical Internet research, 24*(9), e38449.

Beyens, I., Pouwels, J. L., van Driel, I. I., Keijsers, L., & Valkenburg, P. M. (2020). The effect of social media on well-being differs from adolescent to adolescent. *Scientific Reports, 10*(1), 10763. doi:10.1038/s41598-020-67727-7

Bickham, D., Hunt, E., Bediou, B., and Rich, M. (2022). Adolescent media use: attitudes, effects, and online experiences. *Boston Children's Hospital Digital Wellness Lab.* https://digitalwellnesslab.org/team/michael-rich/ (accessed 1 September 2025).

Blakemore, S. J., & Mills, K. L. (2014). Is adolescence a sensitive period for sociocultural processing? *Annual Review of Psychology, 65*(1), 187–207. doi:10.1146/annurev-psych-010213-115202

Braghieri, L., Levy, R., & Makarin, A. (2022). Social media and mental health. *American Economic Review, 112*(11), 3660–3693. doi:10.1257/aer.20211218

Bryant, A. (2018). The effect of social media on the physical, social emotional, and cognitive development of adolescents. *Merrimack ScholarWorks.* https://scholarworks.merrimack.edu/honors_capstones/37/ (accessed 1 September 2025).

Caliskan, O. (2021). Digital pride on the streets of the internet: Facebook and Twitter practices of the LGBTI movement in Turkey. *Sexuality & Culture, 25*(4), 1447–1468. doi:10.1007/s12119-021-09818-9

Campos, W., Martinez, A., Sanchez, W., Estrada, H., Castro-Sánchez, N. A., & Mujica, D. (2016). A systematic review of proposals for the social integration of elderly people using ambient intelligence and social networking sites. *Cognitive Computation, 8,* 529–542.

Cao, C., Li, D., Xu, Q., & Shao, X. (2022). Motivational influences affecting middle-aged and elderly users' participation intention in health-related social media. *International Journal of Environmental Research and Public Health, 19.* doi:10.3390/ijerph191811240

Chen, H., He, M., Xu, X., & Atkin, D. (2025). Examining older adults' vulnerability to online health scams: insights from routine activity theory. *Frontiers in Public Health, 13,* 1585851.

Chhatwani, M., Mishra, S. K., & Rai, H. (2022). Active and passive social media usage and depression among the elderly during COVID-19: does race matter? *Behaviour & Information Technology, 42*(2), 215–226. doi:10.1080/0144929X.2022.2045359

Chon, M. G., & Park, H. (2020). Social media activism in the digital age: testing an integrative model of activism on contentious issues. *Journalism & Mass Communication Quarterly, 97,* 72–97.

Clayborne, Z. M., Wong, S. L., Roberts, K. C., Prince, S. A., Gariépy, G., Goldfield, G. S., Janssen, I., & Lang, J. J. (2025). Associations between social media use and positive mental health among adolescents: findings from the Canadian Health Behaviour in School-aged Children Study. *Journal of Psychiatric Research, 181,* 333–339. doi:10.1016/j.jpsychires.2024.11.071

Cornejo, R., Tentori, M., & Favela, J. (2013). Enriching in-person encounters through social media: a study on family connectedness for the elderly. *International Journal of Human-Computer Studies., 71*(9), 889–899. doi:10.1016/j.ijhcs.2013.04.001

Das, S., & Farber, R. (2020). User-generated online queer media and the politics of queer visibility. *Sociology Compass, 14*(9), e12824.

Dennis, J., & Finotello. (2019). *Beyond Slacktivism.* Springer International Publishing.

Earl, J., Maher, T. V., & Pan, J. (2022). The digital repression of social movements, protest, and activism: a synthetic review. *Science Advances, 8*(10), eabl8198.

Escobar-Viera, C. G., Choukas-Bradley, S., Sidani, J., Maheux, A. J., Roberts, S. R., & Rollman, B. L. (2022). Examining social media experiences and attitudes toward technology-based interventions for reducing social isolation among LGBTQ youth living in rural United States: an online qualitative study. *Frontiers in Digital Health, 4,* 900695.

Faverio, M. and Anderson, M. (2022). For shopping, phones are common and influencers have become a factor – especially for young adults. https://policycommons.net/artifacts/3176984/for-shopping-phones-are-common-and-influencers-have-become-a-factor/3975479/ (accessed 1 September 2025).

Ferguson, C. J., Kaye, L. K., Branley-Bell, D., Markey, P., Ivory, J. D., Klisanin, D., Elson, M., Smyth, M., Hogg, J. L., McDonnell, D., Nichols, D., Siddiqui, S., Gregerson, M., & Wilson, J. (2022). Like this meta-analysis: screen media and mental health. *Professional Psychology: Research and Practice, 53*(2), 205–214. doi:10.1037/pro0000426

Ferrucci, L., Baroni, M., Ranchelli, A., Lauretani, F., Maggio, M., Mecocci, P., & Ruggiero, C. (2014). Interaction between bone and muscle in older persons with mobility limitations. *Current Pharmaceutical Design, 20*(19), 3178–3197. doi:10.2174/13816128113196660690

Fisher, C. B., Tao, X., & Ford, M. (2024). Social media: a double-edged sword for LGBTQ+ youth. *Computers in Human Behavior, 156*, 108194.

Flannery, J. S., Burnell, K., Kwon, S.-J., Jorgensen, N. A., Prinstein, M. J., Lindquist, K. A., & Telzer, E. H. (2024). Developmental changes in brain function linked with addiction-like social media use two years later. *Social Cognitive and Affective Neuroscience, 19*(1). doi:10.1093/scan/nsae008

Gerlach, L. B., Solway, E. S., & Malani, P. N. (2024). Social isolation and loneliness in older adults. *JAMA, 331*(23), 2058. doi:10.1001/jama.2024.3456

Goswami M.P. (2018). Social media and hashtag activism. *Liberty Dignity and ChangeinJournalism.*https://www.researchgate.net/profile/Manash-Goswami-2/publication/326655352_Social_Media_and_Hashtag_Activism/links/5c9dc10a6fdcc494fdf72b8/Social-Media-and-Hashtag-Activism.pdf (accessed 1 September 2025).

Griffiths, S., Murray, S. B., Krug, I., & McLean, S. A. (2018). The contribution of social media to body dissatisfaction, eating disorder symptoms, and anabolic steroid use among sexual minority men. *Cyberpsychology, Behavior, and Social Networking, 21*(3), 149–156. doi:10.1089/cyber.2017.0375

Guess, A., Nagler, J., & Tucker, J. (2019). Less than you think: prevalence and predictors of fake news dissemination on Facebook. *Sci. Adv., 5*, eaau4586. doi:10.1126/sciadv.aau4586

Haris, N., Majid, R.A., Abdullah, N., and Osman, R. (2014). The role of social media in supporting elderly quality daily life. In *2014 3rd international conference on User science and engineering (i-USEr)* (pp. 253–257). IEEE.

HHS. (2023). *Social Media and Youth Mental Health [The U.S. Surgeon General's Advisory]*. U.S. Department of Health and Human Services: Office of the Surgeon General.

Hinduja, S., & Patchin, J. W. (2019). Connecting adolescent suicide to the severity of bullying and cyberbullying. *Journal of School Violence, 18*(3), 333–346. doi:10.1080/15388220.2018.1492417

Hu, L. (2020). Analysis of LGBTQ groups and movements based on social media. In *2020 3rd International Conference on Humanities Education and Social Sciences (ICHESS 2020)* (pp. 21–25). Atlantis Press.

Hunt, M. G., Marx, R., Lipson, C., & Young, J. (2018). No more FOMO: limiting social media decreases loneliness and depression. *Journal of Social and Clinical Psychology, 37*(10), 751–768. doi:10.1521/jscp.2018.37.10.751

Iqbal, S., Ahsan, K., Hussain, M. A., & Nadeem, A. (2016). Social media as assistive technology for elderly. *Journal of Basic & Applied Sciences, 12*, 211–222.

It Gets Better Project (2017). About. It gets better; it gets better. https://itgetsbetter.org/about/ (accessed 5 October 2025).

Jane, E. A. (2014). 'Back to the kitchen, cunt': speaking the unspeakable about online misogyny. *Continuum, 28*(4), 558–570. doi:10.1080/10304312.2014.924479

Jeste, D. V., Smith, J., Lewis-Fernández, R., Saks, E. R., Na, P. J., Pietrzak, R. H., Quinn, M., & Kessler, R. C. (2025). Addressing social determinants of health in individuals with mental disorders in clinical practice: review and recommendations. *Translational Psychiatry, 15*(1), 1–10. doi:10.1038/s41398-025-03332-4

Kleemans, M., Daalmans, S., Carbaat, I., & Anschütz, D. (2018). Picture perfect: the direct effect of manipulated Instagram photos on body image in adolescent girls. *Media Psychology, 21*(1), 93–110. doi:10.1080/15213269.2016.1257392

Kowalski, R. M., Giumetti, G. W., Schroeder, A. N., & Lattanner, M. R. (2014). Bullying in the digital age: a critical review and meta-analysis of cyberbullying research among youth. *Psychological Bulletin, 140*(4), 1073–1137. doi:10.1037/a0035618

Lee, S., Lohrmann, D. K., Luo, J., & Chow, A. (2022). Frequent social media use and its prospective association with mental health problems in a representative panel sample of US adolescents. *Journal of Adolescent Health, 70*(5), 796–803. doi:10.1016/j.jadohealth.2021.11.029

Li, S., Yin, Y., & Yunus, M. M. (2025). Elderly people in the digital cultural environment: social media use, environmental stress, and intergenerational interaction. *Environment-Behaviour Proceedings Journal, 10*(31), 433–439.

Liu, D., Baumeister, R. F., & Yang, C.-C. (2024). A meta-analysis on the relationship between the use of electronic media and psychological well-being. *Emerging Trends in Drugs, Addictions, and Health, 4,* 100162. doi:10.1016/j.etdah.2024.100162

Lynde-Smith, J. (2024). How social media influencers affect mental health. *Challenge What's Possible.* https://challenge.carleton.ca/social-media-influencers-affect-mental-health/ (accessed 5 October 2025).

Marshall, I. C., Hammer, L. A., Springfield, C. R., & Bonfils, K. A. (2024). Activism in the digital age: the link between social media engagement with Black lives matter-relevant content and mental health. *Psychological Reports, 127*(5), 2220–2244. doi:10.1177/00332941221146706

Marwick, A. E., & Caplan, R. (2018). Drinking male tears: language, the manosphere, and networked harassment. *Feminist Media Studies, 18*(4), 543–559. doi:10.1080/14680777.2018.1450568

Masoed, E. S., Omar, R. A. E. A. T., Magd, A. N. A. E., & Elashry, R. (2021). Social media addiction among adolescents: its relationship to sleep quality and life satisfaction. *International Journal of Research in Paediatric Nursing, 3*(1), 69–78.

Mather, M. and Scommegna, P.2023). Today's research on aging: how COVID-19 protections affected older adults' mental health. *PRB.* https://www.prb.org/resources/todays-research-on-aging-how-covid-19-protections-affected-older-adults-mental-health/ (accessed 5 October 2025).

McConnell, E. A., Clifford, A., Korpak, A. K., Phillips, G., 2nd, & Birkett, M. (2017). Identity, victimization, and support: Facebook experiences and mental health among LGBTQ youth. *Computers in Human Behavior, 76,* 237–244. doi:10.1016/j.chb.2017.07.026

Merchant, R. M., South, E. C., & Lurie, N. (2021). Public health messaging in an era of social media. *JAMA, 325*(3), 223–224. doi:10.1001/jama.2020.24514

Meymo, S., & Nyström, K. (2017). Why do elderly not use social media? An investigation of the elderly's attitudes to HCI. https://doi.org/10.13140/RG.2.2.11842.48323

Miller, R. A. (2017). "My voice is definitely strongest in online communities": students using social media for queer and disability identity-making. *Journal of College Student Development, 58*(4), 509–525.

Murthy, D. (2018). Introduction to social media, activism, and organizations. *Social Media+ Society, 4*(1), 2056305117750716. doi:10.1177/2056305117750716

Nagata, J. M., Al-Shoaibi, A. A. A., Leong, A. W., Zamora, G., Testa, A., Ganson, K. T., & Baker, F. C. (2024). Screen time and mental health: a prospective analysis of the Adolescent Brain Cognitive Development (ABCD) Study. *BMC Public Health, 24,* 2686. doi:10.1186/s12889-024-20102-x

Narayanan, V., Robertson, B.W., Hickerson, A., et al. (2021). Securing social media for seniors from information attacks: modeling, detecting, intervening, and communicating risks. In *2021 Third IEEE International Conference on Trust, Privacy and Security in Intelligent Systems and Applications (TPS-ISA)* (pp. 297–302). IEEE.

Naslund, J. A., Aschbrenner, K. A., Marsch, L. A., & Bartels, S. J. (2016). The future of mental health care: peer-to-peer support and social media. *Epidemiology and Psychiatric Sciences, 25*(2), 113–122. doi:10.1017/S2045796015001067

Naslund, J. A., Bondre, A., Torous, J., & Aschbrenner, K. A. (2020). Social media and mental health: benefits, risks, and opportunities for research and practice. *Journal of Technology in Behavioral Science, 5*(3), 245–257. doi:10.1007/s41347-020-00134-x

Nervik, T., Dahl, Y., and Kofod-Petersen, A. (2011). The value of role models in design of social media for elderly. In *23rd International Conference of the European Federation for Medical Informatics,* Oslo, Norway.

Nesi, J., Mann, S., & Robb, M. B. (2023). *Teens and Mental Health: How Girls Really Feel About Social Media.* Common Sense Media.

Nixon, C. L. (2014). Current perspectives: the impact of cyberbullying on adolescent health. *Adolescent Health, Medicine and Therapeutics, 5,* 143–158. doi:10.2147/AHMT.S36456

Office of the Surgeon General. (2023). Social media and youth mental health: The U.S. Surgeon General's advisory. U.S. Department of Health and Human Services. https://www.hhs.gov/surgeongeneral/priorities/youth-mental-health/social-media/index.html

Ofori-Parku, S. S., & Moscato, D. (2018). Hashtag activism as a form of political action: a qualitative analysis of the #BringBackOurGirls campaign in Nigerian, UK, and US press. *International Journal of Communication, 12,* 23.

Orben, A., & Przybylski, A. K. (2019). The association between adolescent well-being and digital technology use. *Nature Human Behaviour, 3*(2), 173–182. doi:10.1038/s41562-018-0506-1

Orben, A., Meier, A., Dalgleish, T., & Blakemore, S.-J. (2024). Mechanisms linking social media use to adolescent mental health vulnerability. *Nature Reviews Psychology,* 1–17. doi:10.1038/s44159-024-00307-y

Oswald, T. K., Rumbold, A. R., Kedzior, S. G. E., & Moore, V. M. (2020). Psychological impacts of "screen time" and "green time" for children and adolescents: a systematic scoping review. *PLOS ONE, 15*(9), e0237725. doi:10.1371/journal.pone.0237725

Oz, M., Yanik, A., & Batu, M. (2023). Under the shadow of culture and politics: understanding LGBTQ social media activists' perceptions, concerns, and strategies. *Social Media + Society, 9*(3), 20563051231196554.

Parida, V., Mostaghel, R., & Oghazi, P. (2016). Factors for elderly use of social media for health-related activities. *Psychology & Marketing, 33*(12), 1134–1141.

Petersen, C., & Johnston, K. (2015). The impact of social media usage on the cognitive social capital of University Students. *International Journal of an Emerging*

Transdiscipline, 18. https://inform.nu/Articles/Vol18/ISJv18p001-030Petersen1522.pdf

Phillips, W. (2015). *This Is Why We Can't Have Nice Things: Mapping the Relationship Between Online Trolling and Mainstream Culture*. The MIT Press.

Plackett, R., Sheringham, J., & Dykxhoorn, J. (2023). The longitudinal impact of social media use on UK adolescents' mental health: longitudinal observational study. *Journal of Medical Internet Research, 25*(1), e43213. doi:10.2196/43213

Pordeus, M. P., Mesquita, S. M. S., & Pordeus, C. L. V. (2022). Virtual bullying: psycho-emotional causes and consequences in adolescent's victims of cyberbullying. *Research, Society and Development, 11*(5), e55011528686.

Prajith, N., & Bhuyan, B. (2025). The role of online anonymity in fostering self-expression: an analysis of individual and contextual dynamics. *International Journal of Indian Psychology, 13*(1). doi:10.25215/1301.014

Przybylski, A. K., & Weinstein, N. (2017). A large-scale test of the Goldilocks hypothesis: quantifying the relations between digital-screen use and the mental well-being of adolescents. *Psychological Science, 28*(2), 204–215. doi:10.1177/0956797616678438

Raudsepp, L., & Kais, K. (2019). Longitudinal associations between problematic social media use and depressive symptoms in adolescent girls. *Preventive Medicine Reports, 15*, 100925. doi:10.1016/j.pmedr.2019.100925

Rideout, V. and Robb, M. B. (2019). The common sense census: media use by Tweens and Teens, 2019 | Common Sense Media. *Common Sense Media*. https://www.commonsensemedia.org/research/the-common-sense-census-media-use-by-tweens-and-teens-2019 (accessed 9 October 2025).

Rideout, V., Peebles, A., Mann, S., and Robb, M. B. (2022). The common sense census: media use by Tweens and Teens, 2021. *Common Sense Media*. https://www.commonsensemedia.org/research/the-common-sense-census-media-use-by-tweens-and-teens-2021 (accessed 9 October 2025).

Rodgers, R. F., Slater, A., Gordon, C. S., McLean, S. A., Jarman, H. K., & Paxton, S. J. (2020). A biopsychosocial model of social media use and body image concerns, disordered eating, and muscle-building behaviors among adolescent girls and boys. *Journal of Youth and Adolescence, 49*(2), 399–409. doi:10.1007/s10964-019-01190-0

Stieger, S., & Wunderl, S. (2022). Associations between social media use and cognitive abilities: results from a large-scale study of adolescents. *Computers in Human Behavior, 135*, 107358. doi:10.1016/j.chb.2022.107358

Suhag, K., & Rauniyar, S. (2023). Social media effects regarding eating disorders and body image in young adolescents. *Cureus, 16*(4), e58674. doi:10.7759/cureus.58674

Suler, J. (2004). The online disinhibition effect. *CyberPsychology & Behavior, 7*(3), 321–326. doi:10.1089/1094931041291295

Taylor, J. K., Lewis, D. C., & Haider-Markel, D. P. (2020). LGBTQ policy and fragmented federalism in the US. *State and Local Government Review, 52*(4), 255–265.

Tennant, B., Stellefson, M., Dodd, V., Chaney, B., Chaney, D., Paige, S., & Alber, J. (2015). Ehealth literacy and web 2.0 health information seeking behaviors among baby boomers and older adults. *Journal of Medical Internet Research, 17*(3), e70. https://www.jmir.org/2015/3/e70. doi:10.2196/jmir.3992

Terribili, M. D. (2022). Surveying the LGBTQ population(s) through social media, *11*(21), 456–457. doi:10.15167/2279-5057/AG2022.11.21.1361

Thilakaraj, D., Ajay, G.S., and Namboothiri, L. V. (2024). Detecting E-bullying in social media platform with stacked BiLSTM approach. In *2024 Third International Conference on Smart Technologies and Systems for Next Generation Computing (ICSTSN)* (pp. 1–6). IEEE.

Twenge, J. M., & Campbell, W. K. (2018). Associations between screen time and lower psychological well-being among children and adolescents: evidence from a population-based study. *Preventive Medicine Reports, 12,* 271–283. doi:10.1016/j.pmedr.2018.10.003

Ugalde, C., Acosta, M. I., & Carvallo, J. P. (2023). Social media usage by elderly: application of technology acceptance model. *Brazilian Journal of Development, 9*(1), 5902–5918.

Vahia, IV, Jeste, D. V., & Reynolds, C. F. (2020). Older adults and the mental health effects of COVID-19. *JAMA, 324*(22), 2253–2254. doi:10.1001/jama.2020.21753

Vivion, M., Reid, V., Dubé, E., Coutant, A., Benoit, A., & Tourigny, A. (2024). How older adults manage misinformation and information overload – a qualitative study. *BMC Public Health, 24,* 871. doi:10.1186/s12889-024-18335-x

Vogels, E.A. and Gelles-Watnick, R. (2023). Teens and social media: key findings from Pew Research Center surveys. *Pew Research Center.* https://www.pewresearch.org/short-reads/2023/04/24/teens-and-social-media-key-findings-from-pew-research-center-surveys/ (accessed 9 October 2025).

Vosoughi, S., Roy, D., & Aral, S. (2018). The spread of true and false news online. *Science, 359*(6380), 1146–1151. doi:10.1126/science.aap9559

Vuorre, M., & Przybylski, A. K. (2024). A multiverse analysis of the associations between internet use and well-being. *Technology, Mind, and Behavior, 5*(2: Summer 2024), 65–75. doi:10.1037/tmb0000127

Wang, C., Li, K., Kim, M., Lee, S., & Seo, D.-C. (2019). Association between psychological distress and elevated use of electronic devices among U.S. adolescents: results from the youth risk behavior surveillance 2009-2017. *Addictive Behaviors, 90,* 112–118. doi:10.1016/j.addbeh.2018.10.037

CHAPTER 10

SOCIAL MEDIA AS SENTINEL INFORMATION TO DETECT EMERGING NOVEL ILLICIT DRUG TRENDS

Yulin Hswen[1] and Thu T. Nguyen[2]

[1]The Artificial Intelligence Interdisciplinary Institute at Maryland (AIM), College of Computer, Mathematical, and Natural Sciences (CMNS), Department of Epidemiology and Biostatistics, School of Public Health, University of Maryland, College Park, MD, USA

[2]Department of Epidemiology and Biostatistics, School of Public Health, University of Maryland, College Park, MD, USA

LEARNING OBJECTIVES

1. Understand how to utilize crowd-sourced data to analyze drug dynamics
2. Analyze the role of socioeconomic, demographic, and geographic data in identifying disparities in access to addiction
3. Develop policy recommendations based on quantitative analysis of real-time and population-level data to address systemic barriers to drug treatment access

Overview

Social media platforms have become important tools in the surveillance of illicit substance use, offering real-time insights into emerging drug trends such as xylazine (Spadaro et al. 2023; Heidari et al. 2025), nicotine pouches (e.g., Zyn; Shao et al. 2022), vaping (Hswen and Brownstein 2019; Hswen et al. 2021), as well as resurging substances like cocaine (Hswen et al. 2021; Castillo-Toledo et al. 2024). Unlike traditional epidemiological approaches that rely on retrospective surveys, emergency department data, or law enforcement methods such as undercover drug purchases, social media offers a dynamic "social sentinel" system (Nsoesie et al. 2016). These systems enable rapid, geographically specific monitoring of conversations, behaviors, and patterns related to substance use by leveraging features such as geotagging and spatial metadata. While traditional surveys may be susceptible to social desirability bias, social media often captures more authentic expressions of behavior due to its perceived anonymity (Fisher 1993; Haimson et al. 2021). This anonymity allows users to share their beliefs, actions, and experiences, including among underrepresented demographic groups such as younger individuals or those engaged in illicit activities.

Platforms such as Instagram, Reddit, TikTok, and X (formerly known as Twitter) serve as early indicators of evolving drug trends, shedding light on novel methods of use, slang terminology, and regional patterns of dissemination (Deluca et al. 2012; Kazemi et al. 2017; Hswen et al. 2020). Through techniques such as keyword tracking, hashtag analysis, and crawling algorithms, researchers can identify substances gaining traction before they escalate into public health crises (Hswen et al. 2020). This innovative approach complements traditional data sources by offering timely, authentic, and scalable insights that can inform public health interventions and harm reduction strategies.

Concepts

Social media platforms serve as transformative tools for real-time monitoring of illicit substance use, offering several advantages over traditional surveillance methods. Timeliness is a key advantage, as social media enables the near-instantaneous detection of emerging drug trends (Li et al. 2022). For instance, platforms like Reddit and online forums are able to uncover discussions of novel uses or mixtures of vaping products, sudden spikes in mentions of recurring substances (e.g., ketamine), or the emergence of new slang for cocaine that may serve as early indicators of potential public health threats (Wu et al. 2022; McGregor et al. 2024). The granularity of social media data further enhances its utility. User-generated content includes information about drug preparation methods, dosages, and combinations—insights that are invaluable for refining clinical guidelines and developing targeted harm reduction strategies (Balsamo et al. 2021).

Moreover, social media platforms enable geographically specific insights through geospatial metadata, ranging from precise coordinates (e.g., latitude and longitude) to broader location indicators such as city and state tags (Wei et al. 2024). For example, integrating location data from Twitter posts with demographic information from Census datasets can reveal nuanced trends, such as distinguishing patterns of drug use between urban and rural areas or identifying demographic groups at elevated risk (Hswen et al. 2020). This capability allows for geographically tailored interventions that are more effective in addressing localized substance use issues (Hswen et al. 2020).

In addition, artificial intelligence (AI)-driven analytics applied to social media data provide powerful predictive capabilities. Crawling algorithms can track hashtag trends, sentiment, and user interactions on platforms such as Instagram to forecast the spread of emerging substances. For example, these tools can help identify and predict the rise of new substances or dangerous combinations, such as fentanyl mixed with xylazine (tranq), before they become widespread, enabling proactive public health measures (Dunn et al. 2025). Together, the rapid detection, detailed insights, and predictive analytics afforded by social media make it a critical component of modern substance use surveillance and intervention.

Generative AI—particularly large language models (LLMs) based on transformer architectures—offers significant potential to enhance this monitoring (Vaswani et al. 2023; Kotkondawar et al. 2024). These models excel at detecting complex linguistic patterns, including slang, euphemisms, and novel terminology that frequently emerge in discussions of illicit or newly synthesized substances (Al-Ghannam et al. 2024). These strengths enable researchers to identify and characterize evolving drug use patterns and dangerous combinations more rapidly and accurately than traditional keyword- or rule-based surveillance methods.

Another important application of generative AI lies in the creation of synthetic data. When used responsibly, synthetic datasets can preserve user privacy in research on sensitive topics such as illicit drug use (Giuffrè and Shung 2023). These datasets can supplement existing data by addressing missingness, augmenting rare events, and providing test cases for model validation, thereby enhancing the robustness and generalizability of predictive models (Abay et al. 2019). However, these methods must be employed cautiously. Synthetic data should not aim to replicate or replace authentic individual voices but rather serve as a privacy-preserving tool, particularly important when working with marginalized or criminalized populations.

Case Studies: Crowdsourcing Online Black Market Pricing to Understand Supply and Demand of Drug Diversion

CASE STUDY 1. USING CROWDSOURCED DATA TO UNDERSTAND DRUG DIVERSION (LEGAL TO ILLEGAL USE OF PRESCRIPTION DRUGS)

The opioid epidemic remains a pressing public health crisis in the United States. In 2022, there were 81,806 opioid-involved overdose deaths, marking the highest number recorded to date. As of 2021, approximately 2.5 million adults aged 18 or older were living with opioid use disorder (Dowell 2024). These figures underscore the ongoing severity of the opioid crisis nationwide. Among the pharmacological treatments for opioid dependency, buprenorphine has emerged as a highly effective option, offering lower abuse potential and a safer profile compared to other opioids (Shulman et al. 2019). However, access to buprenorphine is often hindered by systemic barriers such as insufficient insurance coverage, limited provider availability, and geographic disparities (Lagisetty et al. 2019).

As a result, individuals seeking buprenorphine for opioid addiction treatment may resort to the illicit market, obtaining the medication outside of regulated channels (Yokell et al. 2011). This phenomenon, known as drug diversion, refers to the transfer of legally prescribed substances from their intended recipient to another individual for unauthorized use. Although illegal, diversion reflects unmet treatment needs and mirrors broader economic patterns (Inciardi et al. 2007). Consistent with formal markets, black market exchanges operate on the principles of supply and demand (Smith 1937; Frank et al. 2021).

This case study examines the use of crowdsourced data from black market drug pricing websites to analyze buprenorphine pricing and gain insights into drug diversion (Hswen et al. 2020). It also demonstrates how to integrate population-level data from sources such as the U.S. Census to analyze temporal, socio-spatial, and seasonal factors that influence these dynamics. This approach provides a perspective on how to use crowdsourced black market pricing data to understand the dynamics of the supply–demand equilibrium within the context of buprenorphine diversion.

Exploring Social Determinants of Illicit Buprenorphine Supply and Demand

Objective: To develop a comprehensive framework for using crowdsourced platforms to analyze trends in the illicit drug market. This case study places an emphasis on buprenorphine, addressing complex ethical considerations, leveraging statistical techniques to validate data, and exploring the impact of information on public health policy strategies.

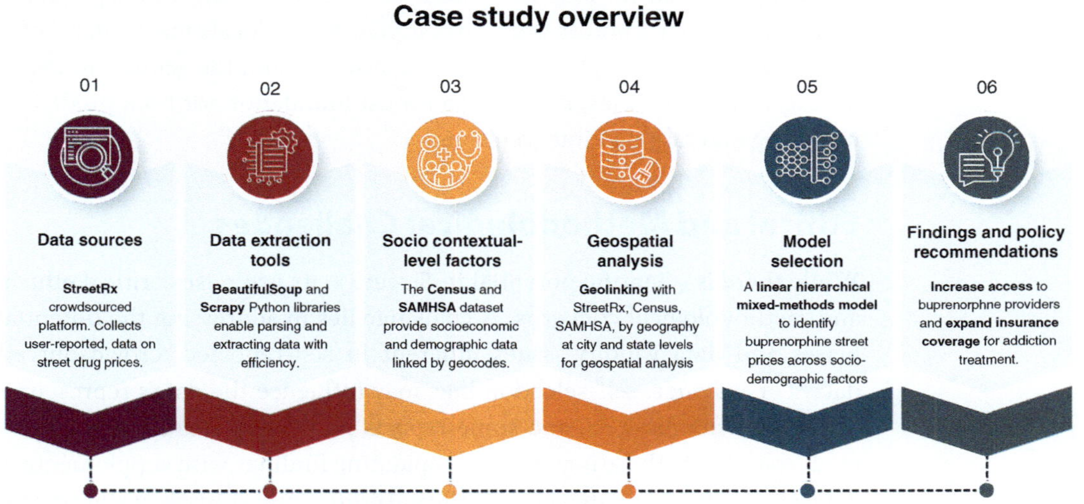

Step 1: Selection of Data Sources

StreetRx is a unique, crowdsourced platform that collects anonymized, user-reported information on prices paid for illicit drugs (Dasgupta et al. 2013). The platform captures essential details such as price per dosage or unit, geographic location of black-market transactions, and temporal trends through time-stamped submissions. By offering granular, real-world insights into the dynamics of drug markets, StreetRx facilitates an in-depth analysis of supply, demand, and accessibility. Unlike traditional surveillance methods that rely on institutional data or retrospective studies, StreetRx offers real-time, user-driven data that addresses critical gaps in understanding the complexities of illicit drug markets. This platform is particularly valuable for examining substances such as buprenorphine, where market behaviors directly impact public health strategies and policy development.

Scientific Advantages of Crowdsourced Platforms

Crowdsourced platforms such as StreetRx offer several notable advantages for the scientific analysis of drug market trends. The granularity of the data is a significant benefit as it provides detailed information about individual transactions that reveal subtle variations in market behavior. For example, it can highlight region-specific differences in buprenorphine pricing, allowing researchers to identify areas where access to legal medication-assisted treatment is inadequate. Another major advantage is the platform's real-time reporting, which enables continuous monitoring of rapid market shifts. This feature is critical for understanding how external factors, such as policy changes or supply chain disruptions, influence drug availability and pricing. Furthermore, crowdsourced data collection is cost-effective, reducing the need for resource-intensive fieldwork while still capturing a broad range of data points from diverse geographic locations. By democratizing data collection, platforms like StreetRx expand the scope and depth of research possibilities, providing a robust foundation for both predictive modeling and targeted interventions.

Ethical and Methodological Challenges

While there is scientific potential in StreetRx, its use raises critical ethical and methodological concerns. A challenge lies in addressing the potential biases and data validity issues inherent in self-reported, crowdsourced data. For instance, self-selection bias may influence the data's representativeness of submissions, and some reports may be inaccurate or exaggerated. To mitigate these issues, cross-validating findings with supplementary datasets can further enhance reliability. Additionally, the risk of stigmatization must be carefully considered. Public dissemination of findings should emphasize structural factors, such as systemic healthcare inequalities, rather than attributing behaviors to individuals. This approach ensures that research outcomes are framed in a way that promotes understanding and health for all rather than reinforcing stereotypes.

Applications of Real-Time Data in Public Health Research

The real-time data provided by StreetRx enhances public health research and intervention strategies. First, the ability to detect shifts in market dynamics promptly allows public health agencies to take preemptive actions. For instance, aspike in buprenorphine prices might indicate restricted access through legal channels, prompting efforts to improve the availability of medication-assisted treatment in affected regions. Second, fine-grained geospatial analysis enabled by the platform's geographic data provides insights into localized patterns of black-market street activity. Advanced spatial models can help identify high-risk regions that require targeted policy interventions or resource allocation.

Real-time data also supports the integration of predictive analytics into public health strategies. For example, geospatial modeling of buprenorphine pricing data can uncover regional disparities that inform targeted interventions. Integrating such analyses within a broader socio-economic and policy framework ensures that research findings are both actionable and equitable. This comprehensive approach not only enhances the practical relevance of the research but also contributes to the development of more effective and inclusive public health strategies. By modeling StreetRx data, researchers can forecast emerging trends, such as the introduction of new substances or shifts in user preferences. These predictive capabilities allow policymakers to anticipate challenges and respond proactively. Furthermore, real-time data enables researchers to evaluate the impact of regulatory changes on the illicit drug market. For example, expanding access to medication-assisted treatment may reduce reliance on black-market sources, and the effects of such policies can be monitored and assessed over time using StreetRx data.

Step 2: Data Extraction Tools

Data extraction is a critical component of online data analysis, particularly for platforms containing dynamic information such as StreetRx. For this purpose, Python offers a robust ecosystem of libraries tailored to different scales and complexities of data extraction tasks. The BeautifulSoup library is effective for parsing and extracting data from HTML and XML documents, making it suitable for static web pages (Richardson 2007). By leveraging the hierarchical structure of web documents, BeautifulSoup enables researchers to identify, extract, and organize specific data points. For example, it can be employed to retrieve pricing information or text elements from basic online tables and lists.

For heavily structured websites, Scrapy serves as a robust framework. This open-source Python library is particularly adept at handling automated crawling tasks. Scrapy enables users to traverse multiple web pages, extracting complex datasets such as time-stamped entries and geographical coordinates with high efficiency (Mitchell 2018). Scrapy's design also supports integration with pipelines for data storage and preprocessing, streamlining workflows from data acquisition to analysis. Together, these tools enable researchers to programmatically extract structured data directly from online platforms, ensuring scalability and reproducibility.

Example Code:
To illustrate the application of these tools, the following Python scripts demonstrate how BeautifulSoup and Scrapy can be used for data extraction.

Example: Using BeautifulSoup for Static Web Pages

```
from bs4 import BeautifulSoup
import requests

# URL of the webpage to scrape
url = 'https://example.com/drug-prices'

# Send an HTTP request to the URL
response = requests.get(url)

# Parse the HTML content of the page
soup = BeautifulSoup(response.text, 'html.parser')

# Extract specific data points (e.g., prices and locations
prices = soup.find_all('span', class_='price')
locations = soup.find_all ('span', class_='location')

# Display extracted data
for price, location in zip(prices, locations):
    print(f'Price: {price.text}, Location: {location.text}
```

Example: Using Scrapy for Dynamic Websites

```
import scrapy

class DrugPriceSpider(scrapy.Spider):
    name = 'drug_price_spider'
    start_urls = ['https://example.com/drug-data']

  def parse(self, response):
        # Extract data fields from the page
        for entry in response.xpath('//div[@class="drug-en
            yield {
                'price': entry.xpath('.//span[@class="pric
                'location': entry.xpath('.//span[@class="l
                'date': entry.xpath('.//span[@class="date"
            }

# To run the spider: execute the command 'scrapy crawl dru
```

These code examples illustrate the implementation of Python libraries to extract structured data from static and dynamic web sources. By applying these techniques, researchers can provide a foundation for further analysis, such as examining drug pricing trends.

Step 3: Identifying Social Population Level Factors

Analysis to understand how social determinants affect access to opioid treatment begins with identifying and understanding the data sources that provide insights into illicit drug markets and broader population characteristics. Platforms such as StreetRx offer user-submitted information on variables such as price, quantity, drug formulation, dosage, and location (city and state). These data points enable researchers to examine regional pricing patterns, including variations between brand-name and generic formulations. However, StreetRx data represents only one dimension of the broader context. Integrating population-level datasets, such as the U.S. Census data, provides critical socio-economic, geographic, and demographic context to interpret trends observed in illicit market data.

The Census Dataset

Census data, accessible through the U.S. Census API, offers county-level socioeconomic and demographic insights that complement the crowd-sourced information (Walker 2023). Key elements include

- **Median Income:** This variable provides information on economic disparities that influence individuals' ability to afford prescription medications like buprenorphine (Krieger et al. 2003). Analyzing income data alongside drug pricing trends can highlight areas where financial barriers exacerbate dependence on the black market.
- **Percent Covered by Health Insurance:** Health insurance coverage is a critical determinant of healthcare access (Marmot 2013). This variable allows researchers to explore the relationship between insurance rates and the affordability of prescription drugs, providing insights into systemic gaps in healthcare access.
- **Percent Rurality:** Geographic disparities are often pronounced in rural areas, which typically face shortages of healthcare providers, including buprenorphine prescribers (Cyr et al. 2019). This metric enables the identification of underserved regions where targeted interventions may be required.
- **Percent Racial Composition:** This demographic variable is essential for exploring racial health disparities issues, particularly in relation to racial disparities in opioid treatment access (Goedel et al. 2020).

The Substance Abuse and Mental Health Services Administration (SAMHSA) Dataset

The Substance Abuse and Mental Health Services Administration (SAMHSA) dataset provides a catalog of licensed buprenorphine prescribers. This dataset is instrumental in

Measuring Provider Density: Defined as the number of prescribers relative to the population size within a specific area (Wang et al. 2024). This metric allows researchers to identify regions where the supply of buprenorphine prescribers is insufficient to meet demand. By analyzing provider density in conjunction with buprenorphine black market street pricing, researchers can pinpoint underserved areas and highlight gaps in treatment access.

Evaluating Healthcare Infrastructure: The SAMHSA dataset supports an evaluation of whether existing healthcare infrastructure aligns with population needs (Mark 2023). By integrating this dataset with socioeconomic and demographic variables, it allows researchers to generate evidence-based policy recommendations aimed at addressing systemic disparities. This evaluation includes assessing the geographic distribution of prescribers and determining how effectively they serve communities with high levels of unmet need.

Step 4: Cleaning and Preparing the Data

Data Cleaning

Preparing StreetRx data for analysis begins with identifying and removing incomplete entries. Submissions with missing or incomplete geographic information, such as coordinates or city/state details, are excluded. Given that StreetRx is a crowdsourced platform relying on user-submitted data, variables such as price and quantity are voluntarily reported, which may limit external validity due to the anonymous nature of the entries (DEA 2022a). Nonetheless, the Drug Enforcement Administration (DEA 2025) has documented the utility of social media and online forums for monitoring drug sales and trends in the illicit drug market, lending credibility to these data sources (Dasgupta et al. 2013; DEA 2022b). Submissions with outlier prices far beyond the typical range should be flagged for review or removed to ensure that data reflects actual market conditions and can be confidently used for research purposes.

Geolinking with Census Data

The next step involves geocoding each StreetRx submission to its corresponding U.S. county using tools such as the Census geocode Python library. This process enables integration with Census data, providing a foundation for socioeconomic and demographic analysis. For example, geographic alignment allows for the analysis of income disparities, health insurance coverage, and rurality in relation to drug pricing trends, creating a framework for understanding systemic disparities in treatment access.

Integration of Data Sources

The integration of these datasets creates a multi-level analytical framework. For example, merging StreetRx pricing data with census-derived income levels allows for the identification of economically vulnerable regions where black-market dependence is likely to be higher. Similarly, cross-referencing rurality metrics with provider density from the SAMHSA dataset provides a clearer picture of provider inequities, enabling researchers to pinpoint areas most in need of intervention. This combined approach supports the construction of a comprehensive model that accounts for socioeconomic, demographic, and geographic factors. This approach not only identifies disparities but also informs targeted strategies to improve access to treatment. For instance, understanding the correlation between low insurance coverage and high drug prices can guide efforts to expand insurance programs or subsidize medication costs in high-need areas.

Step 5: Model Selection

Selecting an Appropriate Model

Given the hierarchical structure of the dataset, where individual StreetRx submissions are nested within counties, a linear hierarchical mixed-effects model was selected to analyze the natural logarithm of buprenorphine street prices (Sullivan et al. 1999). This modeling approach was chosen for its capacity to account for both fixed and random effects.

Flexibility in Handling Nested Data: The model accommodates the nested relationships, allowing for recognition that individual submissions are influenced by the broader contextual forces at the county level.

Addressing Variation: The model incorporates both fixed effects, which capture systematic differences across counties, and random effects, which account for unobserved heterogeneity at the county level. This dual approach ensures that the analysis accurately reflects both observed and latent factors influencing drug prices.

Model Specifications

The dependent variable is the natural logarithm of buprenorphine street prices, modeled as a function of socioeconomic, demographic, temporal, health insurance coverage, and drug property variables.

Model Equation

$$\log(\text{price}) \sim \text{time} + \text{race} + \text{drug properties} + \text{socioeconomic factors} \\ + \text{health insurance coverage} + \text{healthcare access}$$

Fixed Effects

- **Socioeconomic Factors:** County-level median income, county percent racial demographics, and county percent with health insurance are included to assess the influence of economic and demographic variables.
- **Temporal Factors:** Year and season of purchase are incorporated to capture temporal variations in pricing (Palamar et al. 2020).
- **Drug Properties:** Variables such as bulk purchasing, combination drugs, brand names, and drug formulations are included to understand their impact on street prices (Caulkins and Reuter 2006).
- **Healthcare Access:** County buprenorphine practitioner density is included as a measure of treatment availability.

Random Effects

To address unobserved county-specific variations, the model includes a random intercept for each county. This random intercept accounts for heterogeneity across counties that is not explained by the fixed effects.

Step 6: Key Findings

The analysis revealed several key insights into the factors influencing street-level buprenorphine prices.

Insurance Coverage: Increasing health insurance coverage was associated with reduced buprenorphine black-market prices. Specifically, for each 1% increase in the insured population, street buprenorphine prices decreased by 0.02%. This finding underscores the role of expanded health insurance in reducing demand for illicit sources of medication.

Temporal Trends: Between 2010 and 2018, street buprenorphine prices declined by an average of 3.05% per year. This downward trend reflected a shifting dynamic in illicit demand, likely influenced by broader changes in healthcare access and opioid treatment policies over time.

Seasonal Patterns: Seasonal variations were observed with prices peaking in the summer. During this period, buprenorphine sold for 22.26% more than in the fall, while spring prices averaged 17.12% higher than fall prices. These findings suggest that seasonal factors, such as demand fluctuations or distribution challenges, significantly impact pricing dynamics.

Demographic Insights: In counties with a higher percentage of White residents, buprenorphine street prices increased by 0.64% for each additional percentage point in the White population. This trend highlights demographic influences on pricing and suggests a potential increase in overdose and demand for opioid treatments such as buprenorphine based on racial demographics.

Step 7: Policy Recommendations

Based on these findings, the following policy recommendations are proposed to mitigate reliance on illicit buprenorphine markets and improve public health outcomes.

Expand Access to Buprenorphine Providers: Increasing the number of healthcare providers authorized to prescribe buprenorphine is crucial, particularly in underserved areas (Haffajee et al. 2018). Initiatives such as increasing funding for medical education and training programs, reducing regulatory barriers to prescribing, and offering incentives for providers to practice in high-need areas can significantly enhance access.

Broaden Insurance Coverage for Addiction Treatment: Expanding insurance policies to cover comprehensive addiction treatment services, including buprenorphine prescriptions, can lower out-of-pocket costs and make legal alternatives accessible and affordable. Advocacy should focus on expanding addiction treatment coverage through state Medicaid programs and employer-sponsored insurance plans (Maclean and Saloner 2019).

Target Resources for Seasonal and Vulnerable Populations

Allocating additional resources during peak demand periods, such as spring and summer, can help address seasonal fluctuations in buprenorphine pricing. Furthermore, resources directed toward vulnerable communities, particularly those with low insurance coverage or socioeconomic disadvantage (Najavits and Hien 2013) and tailored interventions, including mobile clinics and targeted financial assistance, can help address these disparities effectively (Gibson et al. 2014).

Identifying and utilizing diverse data sources is a cornerstone of rigorous public health research. Crowdsourced data, census, and the SAMHSA prescriber dataset collectively provide a nuanced understanding of the illicit drug market and its associated disparities. Applying this structured approach, researchers can generate actionable findings that address systemic barriers to treatment, ultimately contributing to more equitable healthcare outcomes.

DISCUSSION QUESTIONS

Insurance Coverage: *Why does increased health insurance coverage correlate with a reduction in buprenorphine street prices?*
Increased health insurance coverage expands access to legally prescribed buprenorphine, reducing reliance on illicit markets. As more individuals obtain the medication through legitimate channels, black-market demand declines, resulting in lower prices. Additionally, expanded coverage may improve affordability for vulnerable populations, further diminishing the need for street-purchased alternatives.

Temporal Trends: *Which factors might explain the consistent annual decline of 3.05% in street buprenorphine prices from 2010 to 2018?*
The annual decline in street buprenorphine prices can be attributed to several factors, including improved access to opioid treatment programs, policy changes that expanded the availability of buprenorphine, and increasing public awareness about opioid addiction treatment. Additionally, advancements in the healthcare infrastructure and the proliferation of legal prescribers during this period likely contributed to reduced dependence on illicit sources.

Seasonal Patterns: *Why do buprenorphine street prices peak during the summer, with significant decreases over the spring and fall?*
Seasonal price peaks in the summer may be driven by increased demand due to social factors, such as heightened recreational drug use during warmer months or disruptions in legitimate supply chains. Seasonal employment patterns and income variability may also influence purchasing power. Conversely, reduced demand during the fall and spring may reflect shifts in routine healthcare access or reduced mobility.

Demographic Insights: *Why are street buprenorphine prices 0.64% higher in areas with higher density of certain population groups?*
Higher street buprenorphine prices in areas with a higher percentage of White residents may reflect localized demand dynamics, driven by a greater prevalence of opioid use disorders within these populations. These communities also experience higher opioid-related mortality rates compared to other groups, which may increase demand for treatment options such as buprenorphine, thereby influencing street-level pricing.

Opportunities and Pitfalls

Opportunities

- **Behavioral Analysis Through Machine Learning Models**
  Social media data can be leveraged to identify behavioral patterns associated with substance use by training machine learning models on text, images, and video content. For instance, image-recognition algorithms applied to Instagram posts could detect drug paraphernalia or substance use scenes, providing visual evidence of emerging trends.

- **Temporal Dynamics of Drug Slang Evolution**
Social media offers a valuable platform for studying how drug-related slang evolves over time and its role in spreading drug use information. Studies can track the origin and propagation of specific slang terms on platforms. This data could inform public health messaging, enabling outreach campaigns that "decode" slang for broader audiences, including parents, educators, and healthcare professionals.
- **Network Analysis of Influencer Impact on Drug Trends**
Social media influencers can play a critical role in the normalizing or promoting drug use. Researchers can use social network analysis to map influencer networks and their role in spreading drug-related content. For example, analyzing follower networks on X or Instagram could reveal clusters of individuals exposed to drug-related messages, enabling targeted interventions aimed at reducing harmful influence.
- **Exploring Socioeconomic Correlations in Drug Use Trends**
Integrating social media data with socioeconomic datasets enables the exploration of how structural determinants, such as healthcare access or the availability of treatment resources, influence drug trends. For example, analyzing X geotags alongside Census Bureau data and provider availability maps can reveal correlations between reduced access to buprenorphine-prescribing providers and increased mentions of diverted opioids or synthetic alternatives like fentanyl. Similarly, economic downturns or unemployment spikes in specific regions can be linked to increases in discussions about substances such as methamphetamine or counterfeit benzodiazepines, offering targeted opportunities for intervention.
- **Identifying Patterns of Polysubstance Use and Associated Risks**
Social media platforms provide valuable insights into the complex behaviors associated with polysubstance use, where individuals mix multiple drugs for enhanced effects or self-medication. By leveraging tools such as hashtag tracking, user-comment analysis, and sentiment classification, researchers can identify emerging drug combinations and assess their prevalence. For instance, analyzing Reddit discussions or black market forums for terms like "tranq dope" (a combination of fentanyl and xylazine) reveals not only the popularity of these substances but also the context of their use, such as self-reported motivations and risks. These insights can guide harm reduction initiatives, including the development of tailored educational campaigns or resource allocation for high-risk populations.
- **Analyzing Environmental and Contextual Triggers of Substance Use**
Social media data can uncover environmental and situational factors that contribute to substance use. Geotagged content from platforms such as Instagram, X, and TikTok can pinpoint events or locations

associated with increased drug-related activity, such as music festivals, nightlife venues, or public gatherings. Analyzing this data in conjunction with temporal patterns can help identify "hot spots" for drug use and inform preemptive harm reduction strategies, such as deploying overdose prevention teams, providing drug-checking services, or distributing naloxone in these settings. These insights can also inform urban planning and public health policies aimed at mitigating environmental risks.

- **Impact of Policy Changes on Substance Use Trends**
  Social media can be a valuable tool to monitor the impact of policy changes, such as changes in drug classification, which can shift diverging techniques or prescribing limits (Powell et al. 2016; Richard et al. 2016). Researchers can track shifts in purchasing behaviors on black market pricing and assess how policies are inadvertently driving users to different alternatives.

Pitfalls

While social media platforms offer transformative capabilities for real-time monitoring of illicit substance use, several limitations and challenges undermine their reliability and accuracy as surveillance tools:

- **Demographic and Geographic Bias**
  Social media users are not representative of the general population, leading to sampling bias. Younger and urban populations are overrepresented on some social media platforms, while older adults, rural populations, and lower-income groups with limited internet access (digital divide) may have limited engagement. As a result, trends among underrepresented demographics may be missed, skew data, and undermine the generalizability of insights.
- **Patterns in Missing Social Media Data**
  Missing social media data is often not missing at random. Subpopulations with lower digital literacy, limited internet access, or older age demographics may contribute less content, leading to their underrepresentation. In the context of illicit drug use, privacy concerns and stigmatization may discourage certain groups from participating in data collection efforts or may lead them to withhold key information. This can result in the underrepresentation of individuals who are less willing to disclose their involvement in illegal activities, while simultaneously overrepresenting those who are more comfortable sharing such information. This creates a systematic pattern of missingness that can introduce bias and limit the generalizability of findings in public health research.

  However, platforms like StreetRx offer increased anonymity, encouraging disclosure of sensitive information compared to traditional government or public health surveys. By supplementing crowdsourced data with traditional methods of data collection, researchers can address these biases, fill gaps, and ensure that their findings more accurately represent the target population. This combined approach strengthens the validity and generalizability of research outcomes, offering a more comprehensive understanding of behaviors and trends within hard-to-reach populations.

- **Lack of Individual-Level and Causal Data**
  Social media primarily provides observational data that are aggregated to examine overall trends, making it difficult to identify individual-level behaviors or establish causal relationships between trends and substance use outcomes. For example, a spike in mentions of a drug may not correlate directly with increased usage but rather with heightened awareness, media coverage, or misinformation. This lack of causality limits the ability to draw definitive public health conclusions.
- **Ambiguity in Substance Identification**
  Social media discussions often use slang, euphemisms, or vague references, making it challenging to identify specific substances or their chemical compositions. For example, terms like "tranq" or "blue pills" may refer to different substances depending on the context, complicating efforts to track actual drug use patterns.
- **Ethical and Privacy Concerns**
  Using internet and social media data to gain authentic insights into illicit drug use offers valuable opportunities to better understand trends and behaviors. However, this approach raises significant ethical challenges, particularly concerning privacy, consent, and the potential for stigmatizing or punitive consequences. The sensitive nature of the subject, which often involves illegal behaviors, amplifies these concerns, especially for groups that may already experience heightened scrutiny or discrimination.

  To address these issues, it is essential to anonymize and aggregate data to prevent identification or misuse. Ethical frameworks should prioritize safeguarding individuals from harm, ensuring that the analysis focuses on population-level analyses rather than individual analyses. By adopting privacy-first methodologies, researchers can mitigate risks of surveillance and stigmatization while maintaining the integrity of the insights gained from these rich data sources.
- **Geospatial Data Limitations**
  While geotagged social media posts provide valuable geographic insights, such data is sparse and often limited to users who opt into location sharing. This constraint can lead to incomplete or biased spatial analyses, particularly in rural or underserved areas where geotagged content is minimal or absent.

- **Inability to Verify Chemical Composition of Drugs**
  Social media platforms can reveal trends in drug mentions and usage patterns, but cannot provide definitive information about the chemical composition of substances being discussed. This limitation requires complementary data sources, such as chemical lab testing or emergency department toxicology reports, to validate findings.
- **Dynamic and Evolving Nature of Social Media**
  The rapidly changing nature of social media trends, algorithms, and user behaviors complicates long-term surveillance. For instance, platforms may introduce new privacy policies or content moderation practices that restrict access to data, or users may migrate to platforms such as WhatsApp or Discord that enable strict privacy settings that make it challenging to integrate these data into surveillance efforts
- **Signal-to-Noise Ratio**
  Social media contains vast amounts of irrelevant or misleading information, making it challenging to distinguish meaningful signals from background noise. False positives, such as coordinated misinformation campaigns, can distort findings and lead to inaccurate conclusions.

KEY POINTS AND TAKEAWAYS

- **Real-Time Detection Trends**: Social media provides near-instantaneous insights into emerging drug trends, offering early warnings for substances such as xylazine and fentanyl. Furthermore, crowdsourced data provides valuable insights into dynamic trends in drug supply and demand, enabling timely responses.
- **Granular Information**: User-generated content reveals nuanced details about drug preparation, dosages, and combinations, aiding clinical and harm reduction strategies.
- **Geographic Specificity**: Geotagged data on platforms can be used to identify regional trends and at-risk demographics for targeted interventions.
- **Predictive Analytics**: AI tools analyze hashtags and sentiment to forecast the dissemination of novel drugs and combinations, enabling proactive responses.
- **Complementary Insights**: Social media data enhances traditional methods by providing scalable, authentic, and timely surveillance capabilities.
- **Addressing Social Determinants**: Social platform analytics highlight population-based factors, including insurance coverage and provider access. When combined with socioeconomic datasets, social media data informs effective interventions to address community disparities.
- **Adapting Public Health Interventions**: Analyses underscore seasonal, temporal, and geographic variations that are imperative to adapt public health interventions to meet dynamic community needs.

Conclusion

Social media platforms provide a unique lens to analyze trends in drug use, paraphernalia, and dissemination. The digital ecosystem not only provides real-time geospatial insights into illicit purchasing patterns and methods of consumption but also serves as a critical early warning system for emerging drug patterns. Integrating diverse data sources, ranging from crowdsourced data to the SAMHSA prescriber dataset, provides a holistic understanding of the illicit drug market and its associated disparities. Despite their potential, social media and crowdsourced data are not without limitations. With the continued expansion of the digital landscape, it is imperative to implement ethical safeguards to uphold individual users' privacy and confidentiality, especially when handling sensitive personal data. In addition, the dynamic nature of social media data makes it particularly vulnerable to demographic bias, ambiguity, and high background noise. Researchers should be mindful of these limitations when developing conclusions based on social media data trends. Overall, social media's timely, scalable insights can be harnessed to implement targeted public health interventions to mitigate illicit drug use and promote health and well-being. Integrating complementary social media data presents a useful approach for advancing public health research and practice.

References

Abay, N. C., Zhou, Y., Kantarcioglu, M., Thuraisingham, B., & Sweeney, L. (2019). Privacy preserving synthetic data release using deep learning. In M. Berlingerio, F. Bonchi, T. Gärtner, N. Hurley, & G. Ifrim (Eds.), *Machine Learning and Knowledge Discovery in Databases* (pp. 510–526). Springer International Publishing. doi:10.1007/978-3-030-10925-7_31

Al-Ghannam, R., Ykhlef, M., & Al-Dossari, H. (2024). Robust drug use detection on X: ensemble method with a transformer approach. *Arabian Journal for Science and Engineering, 49*(9), 12867–12885. doi:10.1007/s13369-024-08845-6

Balsamo, D., Bajardi, P., Salomone, A., & Schifanella, R. (2021). Patterns of routes of administration and drug tampering for nonmedical opioid consumption: data mining and content analysis of Reddit discussions. *Journal of Medical Internet Research, 23*(1), e21212. doi:10.2196/21212

Castillo-Toledo, C., Fraile-Martínez, O., Donat-Vargas, C., Lara-Abelenda, F. J., Ortega, M. A., Garcia-Montero, C., Mora, F., Alvarez-Mon, M., Quintero, J., & Alvarez-Mon, M. A. (2024). Insights from the twittersphere: a cross-sectional study of public perceptions, usage patterns, and geographical differences of tweets discussing cocaine. *Frontiers in Psychiatry, 15*. doi:10.3389/fpsyt.2024.1282026

Caulkins, J. P., & Reuter, P. (2006). Illicit drug markets and economic irregularities. *Socio-Economic Planning Sciences, 40*(1), 1–14. doi:10.1016/j.seps.2004.08.002

Cyr, M. E., Etchin, A. G., Guthrie, B. J., & Benneyan, J. C. (2019). Access to specialty healthcare in urban versus rural US populations: a systematic literature review. *BMC Health Services Research, 19*(1), 974. doi:10.1186/s12913-019-4815-5

Dasgupta, N., Freifeld, C., Brownstein, J. S., Menone, C. M., Surratt, H. L., Poppish, L., Green, J. L., Lavonas, E. J., & Dart, R. C. (2013). Crowdsourcing black market prices for prescription opioids. *Journal of Medical Internet Research, 15*(8), e2810. doi:10.2196/jmir.2810

Deluca, P., Davey, Z., Corazza, O., Di Furia, L., Farre, M., Flesland, L. H., Mannonen, M., Majava, A., Peltoniemi, T., Pasinetti, M., Pezzolesi, C., Scherbaum, N., Siemann, H., Skutle, A., Torrens, M., van der Kreeft, P., Iversen, E., & Schifano, F. (2012). Identifying emerging trends in recreational drug use; outcomes from the psychonaut web mapping project. *Progress in Neuro-Psychopharmacology & Biological Psychiatry, 39*(2), 221–226. doi:10.1016/j.pnpbp.2012.07.011

Dowell, D. (2024). Treatment for opioid use disorder: population estimates — United States, 2024. MMWR. *Morbidity and Mortality Weekly Report,* 73, 567–574, 10.15585/mmwr.mm7325a1.

Drug Enforcement Administration (DEA), Department of Justice. (2022b). Schedules of controlled substances: rescheduling of buprenorphine from schedule V to schedule III. Final rule. *Federal Register, 67*(194), 62354–62370.

Drug Enforcement Administration (DEA), Department of Justice (2022a). One pill can kill. Social media drug trafficking threat, https://www.dea.gov/onepill (accessed 5 October 2025).

Drug Enforcement Administration (DEA), Department of Justice (2025). Social media directory. https://www.dea.gov/contact-us/social-media-directory (accessed July 20 2025).

Dunn, J., Schifano, F., Dudley, E., Arillotta, D., & Guirguis, A. (2025). From veterinary medicine to illicit drug supply: utilising social media to explore the rising emergence of veterinary medicines in human health. *Brain Sciences, 15*(2), 172. doi:10.3390/brainsci15020172

Fisher, R. J. (1993). Social desirability bias and the validity of indirect questioning. *Journal of Consumer Research, 20*(2), 303. doi:10.1086/209351

Frank, R. G., McGuire, T. G., & Nason, I. (2021). The evolution of supply and demand in markets for generic drugs. *The Milbank Quarterly, 99*(3), 828–852. doi:10.1111/1468-0009.12517

Gibson, B. A., Ghosh, D., Morano, J. P., & Altice, F. L. (2014). Accessibility and utilization patterns of a mobile medical clinic among vulnerable populations. *Health & Place, 28,* 153–166. doi:10.1016/j.healthplace.2014.04.008

Giuffrè, M., & Shung, D. L. (2023). Harnessing the power of synthetic data in healthcare: innovation, application, and privacy. *NPJ Digital Medicine, 6*(1), 186. doi:10.1038/s41746-023-00927-3

Goedel, W. C., Shapiro, A., Cerdá, M., Tsai, J. W., Hadland, S. E., & Marshall, B. D. L. (2020). Association of racial/ethnic segregation with treatment capacity for opioid use disorder in counties in the United States. *JAMA Network Open, 3*(4), e203711. doi:10.1001/jamanetworkopen.2020.3711

Haffajee, R. L., Bohnert, A. S. B., & Lagisetty, P. A. (2018). Policy pathways to address provider workforce barriers to Buprenorphine treatment. *American Journal of Preventive Medicine, 54*(6 Suppl 3), S230–S242. doi:10.1016/j.amepre.2017.12.022

Haimson, O.L., Liu, T., Zhang, B.Z., and Corvite, S. (2021). The online authenticity paradox: what being "Authentic" on social media means, and barriers to achieving it. 10.7302/2631.

Heidari, O., Sugarman, O. K., Winiker, A. K., Gattine, S., Flanagan, V., Razaghi, R., & Saloner, B. K. (2025). Personal experiences with Xylazine and behavior change: a qualitative content analysis of reddit posts. *Journal of Addiction Medicine, 19*(2), 135–142. doi:10.1097/ADM.0000000000001383

Hswen, Y., & Brownstein, J. S. (2019). Real-time digital surveillance of vaping-induced pulmonary disease. *New England Journal of Medicine, 381*(18), 1778–1780. doi:10.1056/NEJMc1912818

Hswen, Y., Zhang, A., & Brownstein, J. S. (2020). Leveraging black-market street buprenorphine pricing to increase capacity to treat opioid addiction, 2010–2018. *Preventive Medicine, 137*, 106105. doi:10.1016/j.ypmed.2020.106105

Hswen, Y., Zhang, A., & Brownstein, J. S. (2021). Estimating the incidence of cocaine use and mortality with music lyrics about cocaine. *NPJ Digital Medicine, 4*(1), 1–6. doi:10.1038/s41746-021-00448-x

Inciardi, J. A., Surratt, H. L., Kurtz, S. P., & Cicero, T. J. (2007). Mechanisms of prescription drug diversion among drug-involved club- and street-based populations. *Pain Medicine (Malden, Mass.), 8*(2), 171–183. doi:10.1111/j.1526-4637.2006.00255.x

Kazemi, D. M., Borsari, B., Levine, M. J., & Dooley, B. (2017). Systematic review of surveillance by social media platforms for illicit drug use. *Journal of Public Health (Oxford, England), 39*(4), 763–776. doi:10.1093/pubmed/fdx020

Kotkondawar, R.R., Sutar, S.R., Kiwelekar, A.W., and Kadam, V.J. (2024). Integrating Transformer-based Language Model for Drug Discovery. In *2024 11th International Conference on Computing for Sustainable Global Development (INDIACom)*, pp. 1096–1101. 10.23919/INDIACom61295.2024.10498263.

Krieger, N., Chen, J. T., Waterman, P. D., Rehkopf, D. H., & Subramanian, S. V. (2003). Race/ethnicity, gender, and monitoring socioeconomic gradients in health: a comparison of area-based socioeconomic measures--the public health disparities geocoding project. *American Journal of Public Health, 93*(10), 1655–1671. doi:10.2105/ajph.93.10.1655

Lagisetty, P. A., Ross, R., Bohnert, A., Clay, M., & Maust, D. T. (2019). Buprenorphine treatment divide by race/ethnicity and payment. *JAMA Psychiatry, 76*(9), 979–981. doi:10.1001/jamapsychiatry.2019.0876

Li, K., Zhou, C., Luo, X., Luo, X. (R.), Benitez, J., & Liao, Q. (2022). Impact of information timeliness and richness on public engagement on social media during COVID-19 pandemic: an empirical investigation based on NLP and machine learning. *Decision Support Systems, 162*, 113752. doi:10.1016/j.dss.2022.113752

Maclean, J. C., & Saloner, B. (2019). The effect of public insurance expansions on substance use disorder treatment: evidence from the Affordable Care Act. *Journal of Policy Analysis and Management: [The Journal of the Association for Public Policy Analysis and Management], 38*(2), 366–393. https://www.ncbi.nlm.nih.gov/pmc/articles/PMC7071834/

Mark, T. L. (2023). The United States must improve its data infrastructure to ensure high-quality mental health care. *Frontiers in Health Services, 3*, 1059049. doi:10.3389/frhs.2023.1059049

Marmot, M. (2013). Universal health coverage and social determinants of health. *The Lancet, 382*(9900), 1227–1228. doi:10.1016/S0140-6736(13)61791-2

McGregor, E., Roper, P., Mueller, T., & Weir, N. (2024). Societal attitudes towards ketamine: a Twitter analysis comparing weekday and weekend content. *Research in Social and Administrative Pharmacy, 20*(2), 224. doi:10.1016/j.sapharm.2023.09.042

Mitchell, R. (2018). Web scraping with Python: collecting more data from the modern web. *O'Reilly Online Learning*. https://www.oreilly.com/library/view/web-scraping-with/9781491985564/ (accessed 1 October 2025).

Najavits, L. M., & Hien, D. (2013). Helping vulnerable populations: a comprehensive review of the treatment outcome literature on substance use disorder and PTSD. *Journal of Clinical Psychology, 69*(5), 433–479. doi:10.1002/jclp.21980

Nsoesie, E. O., Flor, L., Hawkins, J., Maharana, A., Skotnes, T., Marinho, F., & Brownstein, J. S. (2016). Social media as a sentinel for disease surveillance: what does sociodemographic status have to do with it? *PLoS Currents, 8*. doi:10.1371/currents.outbreaks.cc09a42586e16dc7dd62813b7ee5d6b6

Palamar, J. J., Rutherford, C., & Keyes, K. M. (2020). Summer as a risk factor for drug initiation. *Journal of General Internal Medicine, 35*(3), 947–949. doi:10.1007/s11606-019-05176-3

Powell, G. E., Seifert, H. A., Reblin, T., Burstein, P. J., Blowers, J., Menius, J. A., Painter, J. L., Thomas, M., Pierce, C. E., Rodriguez, H. W., Brownstein, J. S., Freifeld, C. C., Bell, H. G., & Dasgupta, N. (2016). Social media listening for routine post-marketing safety surveillance. *Drug Safety, 39*(5), 443–454. doi:10.1007/s40264-015-0385-6

Richard, A. M., Judson, R. S., Houck, K. A., Grulke, C. M., Volarath, P., Inthirany Thillainadarajah, Yang, C., Rathman, J. F., Martin, M. J., Wambaugh, J. F., Knudsen, T. B., Jayaram Kancherla, Mansouri, K., Patlewicz, G., Williams, A. J., Little, S. H., Crofton, K. M., & Thomas, R. S. (2016). Toxcast chemical landscape: paving the road to 21st century toxicology. *Chemical Research in Toxicology, 29*(8), 1225–1251. doi:10.1021/acs.chemrestox.6b00135

Richardson, L. (2007). Beautiful soup documentation. https://sethc23.github.io/wiki/Python/Beautiful_Soup_Documentation.pdf (accessed 1 October 2025).

Shao, Y., Zou, J., Xie, Z., Mayne, R. G., Ossip, D. J., Rahman, I., McIntosh, S., & Li, D. (2022). Perceptions of oral nicotine pouches on reddit: observational study. *Journal of Medical Internet Research, 24*(7), e37071.

Shulman, M., Wai, J. M., & Nunes, E. V. (2019). Buprenorphine treatment for opioid use disorder: an overview. *CNS Drugs, 33*(6), 567–580. doi:10.1007/s40263-019-00637-z

Smith, A. (1937). *The Wealth of Nations (1776) (Vol. 11937). – References – Scientific Research Publishing*. Scientific Research. https://www.scirp.org/reference/referencespapers?referenceid=3687989

Spadaro, A., O'Connor, K., Lakamana, S., Sarker, A., Wightman, R., Love, J. S., & Perrone, J. (2023). Self-reported Xylazine experiences: a mixed-methods study of reddit subscribers. *Journal of Addiction Medicine, 17*(6), 691–694. doi:10.1097/ADM.0000000000001216

Sullivan, L. M., Dukes, K. A., & Losina, E. (1999). An introduction to hierarchical linear modelling. *Statistics in Medicine, 18*(7), 855–888. doi:10.1002/(SICI)1097-0258(19990415)18:7<855::AID-SIM117>3.0.CO;2-7

Vaswani, A., Shazeer, N., Parmar, N., Uszkoreit, J., Jones, L., Gomez, A. N., Kaiser, L., & Polosukhin, I. (2023). Attention is all you need. (No. arXiv:1706.03762). *arXiv*. doi:10.48550/arXiv.1706.03762

Walker, K. (2023). *Analyzing US Census Data: Methods, Maps, and Models in R*. Routledge & CRC Press. https://www.routledge.com/Analyzing-US-Census-Data-Methods-Maps-and-Models-in-R/Walker/p/book/9781032366449

Wang, Y., Hu, T., Roosan, M., et al. (2024). Assessing buprenorphine treatment utilization and SAMHSA data waiver provider distribution in 2021: a real-world analysis in California. 10.21203/rs.3.rs-4676680/v1.

Wei, H., Hswen, Y., Merchant, J. S., Drew, L. B., Nguyen, Q. C., Yue, X., Mane, H., & Nguyen, T. T. (2024). From tweets to streets: observational study on the association between Twitter sentiment and anti-Asian hate crimes in New York City from 2019 to 2022. *Journal of Medical Internet Research*, *26*(1), e53050. doi:10.2196/53050

Wu, D., Kasson, E., Singh, A. K., Ren, Y., Kaiser, N., Huang, M., & Cavazos-Rehg, P. A. (2022). Topics and sentiment surrounding vaping on Twitter and Reddit during the 2019 e-cigarette and vaping use-associated lung injury outbreak: comparative study. *Journal of Medical Internet Research*, *24*(12), e39460. doi:10.2196/39460

Yokell, M. A., Zaller, N. D., Green, T. C., & Rich, J. D. (2011). Buprenorphine and Buprenorphine/Naloxone diversion, misuse, and illicit use: an international review. *Current Drug Abuse Reviews*, *4*(1), 28–41. doi:10.2174/1874473711104010028

CHAPTER 11

SOCIAL MEDIA AND GLOBAL HEALTH

Katrina Makres[1], Yajie Xiong[2], Elizabeth Dennard[1], Penchala Sai Priya Mullaputi[1], and Thu T. Nguyen[1]
[1]Department of Epidemiology and Biostatistics, School of Public Health, University of Maryland, College Park, MD, USA
[2]Department of Sociology, University of Maryland, College Park, MD, USA

LEARNING OBJECTIVES

1. Discuss the different uses of social media for public health worldwide.
2. Discuss how social media research is performed in high-income and low- and middle-income countries.
3. Explore the role of advertisements on social media and their impact on public health.

Overview

Global health research has consistently demonstrated that public health challenges transcend national borders, requiring coordinated international efforts. While global health research has been historically dominated by institutions in high-income countries, there has been a notable shift to address disparities in resource-limited settings (Beaglehole and Bonita 2010). Research institutions specializing in public health are increasingly flourishing in low- and middle-income countries (LMICs), offering invaluable perspectives and contextually relevant solutions to local health priorities.

One expanding frontier in global health is the study of social media's evolving role in public health information dissemination, access, and interpretation. With nearly half of the global population using social media, these platforms' influence extends far beyond personal interactions, shaping public health communication, targeted interventions, and crisis responses (World Population Review 2025). However, this influence is not uniformly distributed across regions due to disparities in technological access, regulatory policies, and cultural contexts. This chapter examines the broad impact of social media on public health with a particular emphasis on key regional differences and their implications for promoting health for all worldwide.

Regional and national factors, such as economic conditions, governmental policies, and cultural preferences, significantly shape social media usage. Although Facebook remains the most prevalent global platform, distinct regional differences are evident (Vincos Blog 2023). Notably, a substantial proportion of global social media users reside in LMICs (Islam et al. 2019), with Asia accounting for the largest share of users (16.98%), followed by Africa (13.92%; World Population Review 2025). In Africa, Facebook continues to be a cornerstone of digital communication and information dissemination (Vincos Blog 2023). Furthermore, in both Latin America and Africa, WhatsApp has emerged as a dominant platform, often serving as the primary means of communication due to its accessible and inexpensive messaging features (Vincos Blog 2023). In contrast, China presents a unique digital ecosystem, where platforms such as WeChat have developed into comprehensive "super apps" that integrate communication, payments, and public service functionalities (Talin 2024). These regional differences impact the distribution and reception of health messages, potentially affecting the efficacy of public health interventions.

While social media facilitates rapid information exchange, it also accelerates the spread of misinformation, posing significant challenges to public health efforts. False health claims, anti-vaccine campaigns, and the promotion of unverified or understudied interventions can rapidly proliferate and undermine public trust in medical authorities. In response, governments are increasingly regulating social media to combat misinformation, as exemplified by Brazil's 2024 temporary ban on X (formerly Twitter) to curtail public health-related misinformation (ET Online 2024). Meanwhile, countries such as China and Iran enforce stringent social media censorship to exert government control over digital public health discourse (ET Online 2024). These divergent regulatory approaches raise critical ethical and practical considerations regarding the delicate balance between safeguarding individual freedom of expression and public health protection.

A foundational question remains: How are these platforms being utilized, and what are their consequential impacts on global public health?

As digital technologies continue to advance, the role of social media in public health is expanding. Researchers are increasingly harnessing social media data to monitor pandemics, analyze public sentiment on health issues, and develop targeted interventions. This chapter will further explore these dynamic interactions and provide a comparative analysis of social media's impact on public health across both high-income and low- and middle-income countries. Furthermore, it will examine the influential role of social media advertising in shaping health behaviors and perceptions, providing a comprehensive perspective on the opportunities and challenges of social media research in global public health research and practice.

Key Concepts/Terms

Low- and middle-income Countries (LMICs): Countries classified by the World Bank as having Gross National Income (GNI) per capita of less than $14,005 USD for the fiscal year 2025

(Metreau et al. 2024). Approximately 60% of the countries in the world are categorized as LMICs (Metreau et al. 2024; Lencucha and Neupane 2022). As of 2023, the majority of Africa (East, Central, West, and Southern) has the largest concentration of LMICs, encompassing 47 countries classified under this group (Metreau et al. 2024).

High-income Countries: Nations with a GNI per capita exceeding 14,006 USD for the fiscal year 2025, as classified by the World Bank (Metreau et al. 2024). These countries represent approximately 40% of the world's nations (Metreau et al. 2024). As of 2023, Europe and Central Asia account for the largest number of high-income countries, totaling 40 nations (Metreau et al. 2024).

Low- and Middle-Income Countries

Global health reflects the complex interplay between a country's wealth, health challenges, and access to technology, all of which shape distinct public health landscapes. In many LMICs, rising burdens of noncommunicable diseases along with persistent communicable threats demand innovative solutions. Social media has emerged as a powerful tool for health communication and education, offering opportunities to bridge information gaps and promote behavior change, despite the persistence of challenges such as digital literacy and unequal access. This section explores how digital platforms are leveraged in low- and middle-income countries to improve public health outcomes, evaluate interventions, and shape policies.

Understanding the Health Landscape in LMICs

In discussions of global economic and health disparities, countries are often categorized as LMICs or high-income nations. While these classifications are primarily based on a country's gross national income, economic status is not the sole differentiating factor. The health of countries varies considerably, and it is essential to consider each nation's health landscape before delving deeper into social media public health research.

By 2030, noncommunicable diseases (NCDs), such as cancer and cardiovascular disease, are projected to become the leading causes of death in LMICs, signaling a significant epidemiological transition (Alwan and Maclean 2009). These conditions not only have high prevalence rates but also often manifest earlier in life, leading to prolonged periods of disability and long-term health impacts (Alwan and Maclean 2009). Individuals from lower socioeconomic classes and other disadvantaged populations are disproportionately impacted, exacerbating health gaps (Alwan and Maclean 2009). Despite the growing prevalence of NCDs, communicable diseases remain a significant concern in LMICs. Diseases such as human immunodeficiency virus (HIV) and tuberculosis are becoming more prevalent in a myriad of countries, underscoring the persistent challenges in infectious disease control (Kaluvu et al. 2022). Despite these challenges, preventative measures can help mitigate the risk of both communicable and noncommunicable diseases. Public health strategies such as awareness campaigns, early testing, and behavioral modifications play a crucial role in disease prevention–all of which can be impacted through social media.

The Role of Social Media in Public Health

A common misconception is that LMICs lack sufficient technological infrastructure to support and implement digital public health interventions. Although LMICs may have limited access to technology in comparison to high-income countries, there have been significant improvements in digital connectivity. This trend can help elucidate the corresponding increase in social media use in LMICs (Hagg et al. 2018). Notably, many regions have experienced "leapfrogging" in technology, adopting newer, cost-effective solutions without following traditional developmental stages (Hagg et al. 2018). While this leapfrogging has contributed to a rapid increase in social media usage, it has also presented significant challenges. Many individuals in LMICs have not historically integrated digital technologies into daily life, and as a result, media literacy remains limited. (Polanco-Levicán and Salvo-Garrido 2022). This critical gap can leave social media users vulnerable to the negative effects of unregulated digital spaces, including the proliferation of misinformation. The widespread dissemination of false or misleading health content represents one key threat to public health.

Despite the growing integration of social media into public health practice, limited evidence exists on how low- and middle-income countries utilize these platforms for public health research and intervention implementation. Documented studies across LMICs have focused on educational programs and initiatives to mitigate negative health outcomes. These initiatives often focus on public health awareness and the spread of misinformation. Ultimately, these programs must be tailored to their intended audience to promote public health knowledge and reach populations in a timely manner (Islam et al. 2019).

Given the rising burden of noncommunicable diseases and associated mortality among young adults in LMICs, it is critical to explore how social media platforms can be leveraged to reach younger populations (Islam et al. 2019). Since younger individuals are more likely to utilize social media platforms, public health advocates and organizations have an opportunity to engage this demographic in real time. Additionally, noncommunicable diseases can be mitigated through the implementation of educational programs and interventions across diverse communities and geographic regions to encourage sustainable behavior change.

Social media campaigns, such as education programs, also allow for the evaluation of public health programs. There are six performance metrics that indicate program efficacy (CDC 2024):

1. **Program Reach:** how many users have been exposed to a given campaign.
2. **Impressions:** how many times a specific post has been viewed.
3. **Engagement Frequency:** how many times users have interacted with a social media post.
4. **Engagement Rate:** proportion of users exposed to a post who interact with the post
5. **URL Clicks:** number of times a social media user clicks on a link.
6. **Followers:** how many users have subscribed to a campaign's main social media account.

These key performance indicators allow researchers to evaluate how many users are viewing public health resources and track key data points across diverse populations and time points.

CASE STUDY 1. STROKE AWARENESS IN NEPAL (TUNKL ET AL., 2023 / NATIONAL LIBRARY OF MEDICINE / CC BY 4.0)

Tunkl's team evaluated the efficacy of a social media education program focused on stroke awareness across multiple social media platforms over six months in Nepal. Stroke awareness was selected as the outcome of interest due to its high mortality rate and the critical importance of timely treatment (Feigin et al. 2021; Emberson et al. 2014). Additionally, Nepali high-school students and individuals living in rural regions are often unable to identify common symptoms of a stroke or the correct treatment response (Pontes-Neto et al. 2008; Thapa et al. 2016; Silwal et al. 2019). The study assessed four core metrics: reach, impressions, engagement, and URL clicks. Study aims centered on feasibility, effectiveness, and identifying best practices. To maximize accessibility, study content was made available in both English and Nepali and incorporated both organic (unpaid promotions) and paid advertisements to compare efficacy. Importantly, researchers ensured that all social media content (text, photos, and videos) was reviewed by medical professionals before dissemination. Results indicated that paid advertisements resulted in 45 times more user impressions than organic social media posts. Additionally, over 250,000 URL clicks were recorded across study time points, indicating high engagement. Ultimately, social media posts were deemed a cost-efficient strategy for promoting stroke awareness among study participants, with a cost per click of 0.01 EUR. Notably, the study did not observe a decrease in engagement over time, indicating a potential for reaching future Nepali social media users. Overall, this case study highlights the viability of using social media as a low-cost, high-impact strategy for promoting stroke awareness in low- and middle-income settings, particularly when content is medically vetted and supported by strategic advertisement.

Expanding the Scope of Social Media Research

Social media serves as an excellent source for bidirectional health communication (Pimmer and Tulenko 2016). Additionally, it allows for building career-based connections and peer support across healthcare organizations (Islam et al. 2019). With an anticipated shortage of roughly 10 million healthcare workers by 2030, social media can play a critical role in narrowing this gap in LMICs by enhancing communication among healthcare professionals and accelerating the delivery of healthcare services (World Health Organization 2025). In 2018, Hagg et al. performed a scoping review to capture LMIC internet use in the context of public health. Topics included global emergency response, disease surveillance, and the facilitation of health-based communication via social media platforms (Hagg et al. 2018).

While researchers in low- and middle-income countries have investigated the efficacy of various social media educational campaigns, additional resources are required to expand the scope of research using social media data. Significant barriers include limited access to raw social media datasets, inadequate funding, and constrained technological infrastructure. Therefore, it is imperative to bridge existing knowledge gaps by broadening the scope of social media research studies, thereby enabling policymakers and public health professionals to make informed, community-oriented decisions and strategically allocate resources.

High-Income Countries

High-income countries exhibit complex public health profiles that offer valuable opportunities for investigation through social media research. In contrast to LMICs, these nations experience a greater incidence of noncommunicable diseases (e.g., cardiovascular disease, cancer, and diabetes) than communicable diseases (Roser et al. 2021). Despite differences in prevalence estimates, both communicable and noncommunicable diseases have been increasing over the last three decades (Roser et al. 2021). Importantly, healthcare disparities persist even within high-resource settings, with low-income populations experiencing a disproportionate share of adverse health outcomes (Roser et al. 2021). While some similarities in disease profiles exist between LMICs and high-income countries, the public health strategies employed in social media research differ significantly.

Research Focus: The Negative Impact of Social Media

In high-income countries, research has largely emphasized social media's deleterious effects on physical and mental health outcomes. In contrast, its utility is viewed as a valuable public health tool in LIMCs. Numerous studies have underscored the influence of social media on suicide rates and body image, often using social media data to analyze the relationship between national characteristics and user health outcomes. For example, Padmanathan et al. (2020) examined the relationship between social media use, economic factors, and youth suicide rates in the following high-income countries: Australia, the United Kingdom, Spain, Poland, Japan, and the Republic of Korea. Their findings indicate that social media interactions, when combined with economic stressors and income inequality, can exacerbate existing mental health challenges among young adults (Padmanathan et al. 2020).

National and Comparative Studies: Understanding Cultural Variations

While country-level studies in high-income countries remain limited, there have been notable efforts to examine the role of social media in public health. Several studies have focused on global challenges, while others have examined country-specific cultural contexts. For example, Liu et al. (2022) conducted a study in Panama City that highlighted the utility of social media for analyzing traffic incidents. The researchers developed a machine learning model to gather and code traffic accident-related posts from Twitter. The model achieved a remarkable precision rate of 92% and an incident classification rate of 97%, with the model's classification capabilities encompassing accidents, obstacles, and general hazards. Although this research was tailored to Panama City's infrastructural needs, this machine learning model holds promise for traffic incident prediction and infrastructural road assessments. Additionally, this methodology has the potential to meet the informational needs of other nations, since traffic accident prevalence estimates continue to rise globally.

An emerging body of literature also seeks to analyze social media usage patterns across diverse populations, with a focus on public health implications. Song et al. (2016) analyzed trust in online health content across the United States, Hong Kong, and Korea. Researchers collected information on how social media users gather health information on these platforms. Their study found that Americans more frequently used expertise-based sites for information, while individuals living in Korea and Hong Kong referenced blogs and more experience-based sites. In addition, cultural norms influenced information-seeking behavior, with Hongkongers and Koreans more likely to research health topics on behalf of relatives compared to Americans. Ultimately, these findings underscore the importance of cultural context in designing digital health behaviors and the need for tailored public health strategies that resonate with target populations.

Shifting Research Priorities: Social Media as a Public Health Tool

Despite advancements in public health tools, research in high-income countries has been relatively slow to explore the constructive role of social media. While the literature often highlights the dangers of misinformation, fewer studies have examined how digital spaces can be leveraged for health promotion, education, and intervention implementation. However, recent shifts in research priorities suggest a growing interest in using social media for public health monitoring. Sentiment analysis, for instance, has emerged as a valuable technique for tracking public opinion on health-related issues. For example, Nguyen et al. (2020) studied how sentiment toward the Asian community in the United States shifted during the COVID-19 pandemic. Their findings demonstrate that social media can serve as a tool for real-time public health monitoring, helping researchers and policymakers better understand and address emerging social issues. While the majority of social media research in high-income countries tends to follow broader analytical approaches, there are examples where studies mirror campaign-based strategies commonly employed in low- and middle-income countries. These efforts often focus on specific diseases and aim to promote behavioral change. Similar to LMICs, findings from high-income countries can inform policymakers by shaping public health strategies, guiding resource allocation, and influencing future research priorities.

Social Media Advertising Laws

Marketing plays a pivotal role in shaping public health by influencing consumer behavior and decision-making. Social media platforms have become central avenues for advertising, largely due to their revenue models, which rely on advertisement placements. These platforms have also transformed the way companies interact with the public, enabling direct interaction and access to large audiences. In contrast to traditional print and visual media, which are subject to strict content regulations, social media advertising operates within a less regulated space (Balkin 2021). In response, regulatory bodies around the world have introduced country-specific legislation to regulate digital advertising.

In the United States, for example, the Federal Trade Commission (FTC) is responsible for creating and evaluating laws concerning advertisements (BENlabs, 2024; Table 11.1). Regulatory bodies consider various factors in advertising practices, including advertisement types, target audience, marketing strategies, and other factors involved in ad production. These factors are essential for establishing clear guidelines that help ensure corporate accountability and protect consumer welfare. Although the FTC's jurisdiction is limited to the United States, its regulatory influence is notable due to the global reach of American companies and the widespread use of U.S.-based social media platforms. Table 11.1 presents examples of regulatory bodies in several countries.

There are notable similarities in social media advertising regulations across different countries. Most regulations emphasize the need for advertisement transparency, requiring that promotional content be clearly disclosed, truthful, and not misleading. Additionally, age-appropriate advertising is a priority, particularly for products with legal

Table 11.1 Advertisement Regulation Agencies

Country	Federal Agency
Australia	Australian Competition and Consumer Commission
Canada	Canadian Code of Advertising Standards
Europe	European Commission
India	Advertising Standards Council of India
United Kingdom	United Kingdom's Advertising Standards Authority

Source: Adapted from BENlabs, 2024.

age restrictions, such as alcohol, tobacco, and vaping. Among these, vaping has become a growing area of concern, as its popularity has surged in recent years, especially among younger individuals. Given that social media is widely used by this demographic, advertisements for vaping products can easily reach and influence a vulnerable audience. Regulations set by federal agencies play a crucial role in mitigating public health risks associated with these products. These regulations vary by country, with some instituting complete bans, while others maintain partial restrictions or lack specific regulations altogether. Table 11.2 provides an overview of social media advertising laws across select countries for alcohol, tobacco, and vaping.

Regulation of Social Media Advertisements and Data Privacy

The regulation of social media advertisements varies globally, with various countries enforcing stringent laws while others maintain minimal or no regulations. Ascertaining specific social media advertisement regulations presents significant challenges due to limited public access to legal information. The lack of legal transparency further complicates efforts to comprehensively assess existing regulatory frameworks.

However, there are some clear patterns regarding how countries regulate social media platforms for age-restricted products. If a particular product is deemed to be illegal within a nation, its advertisements are also subject to a complete ban across all social media platforms. When examining tobacco and vaping regulations specifically, two distinct patterns emerge:

1. Various countries apply identical regulations to vaping as they do to traditional tobacco products.
2. Due to the recent emergence of vaping, other countries have yet to establish specific laws governing its advertisement.

Regardless of the types of regulatory frameworks in place, enforcement on social media platforms poses unique challenges. Digital platforms transcend national borders, making it difficult to completely restrict content.

Table 11.2 Social Media Advertisement Regulations for Alcohol, Tobacco, and Vaping

Country	Alcohol	Tobacco	Vaping
Afghanistan	Complete Ban	Complete Ban	Complete Ban
Australia	X	Complete Ban	Complete Ban
Cambodia	X	Complete Ban	Complete Ban
China	X	X	X
Haiti	—		
Romania		X	X
Russia	Complete Ban	—	—
South Africa	X	Complete Ban	
Sri Lanka	Complete Ban	Complete Ban	
United States of America	X	X	X

Legend and Explanation

- X: Some laws regulate advertisements for this product on social media.
- Complete Ban: Advertising this product is entirely illegal on social media.
- —: No available data on regulations for this product in the country.
- Blank: No specific laws exist regulating how this product is advertised on social media.

Citations from Left to Right, Top to Bottom: (Federal Trade Commission 2014; Adapted from Alcohol Focus Scotland 2017; Lichtenberg 2017; World Health Organization 2019, 2021; Cancer Council Victoria 2019; EUCAM 2022; Morapi and Altini 2022; Campaign for Tobacco-Free Kids 2024; FDA 2024; Liao and Li 2023; Egbe 2023; Hirimuthigodage and Disanayake 2023; Australian Government Department… 2024; Barker et al. 2024; Chandraratne et al. 2024; Popescu et al. 2024; Shao and Luo 2024; Sinorn 2024; Sophorn 2024; Southeast Asia Tobacco…, 2024; Sprint Law 2025)

While regulatory bodies and social media platforms may implement content moderation policies, viral posts and alternative sharing methods can allow prohibited advertisements to reach unintended audiences. Given that vaping poses significant health risks, particularly to younger audiences, it is crucial to implement stricter advertising regulations on social media platforms. Research indicates that exposure to pro-tobacco content on social media influences young individuals by shaping their perceptions that smoking is socially acceptable and desirable (Cancer Council Victoria 2019). These findings underscore the pressing need for regulatory measures that limit youth exposure to harmful advertising and counteract pro-tobacco messaging.

The Impact of Vaping Advertisements on Public Health

In many countries where alcohol, tobacco, and vaping advertisements are regulated but not banned, age-based restrictions define the intended audience. These regulations align with national laws specifying the legal age for drinking, smoking, or purchasing vaping products. Social media platforms are required to comply with these regulations by tracking users' ages and targeting advertisements accordingly (Federal Trade

Commission 2014). However, several challenges undermine the effectiveness of these restrictions:

- **Age Falsification:** Users can falsify their age during account creation, allowing underage individuals to view adult advertisements.
- **Content Bypassing:** Content may bypass platform regulations when users screenshot or screen record an ad and repost it, making it accessible to a broader audience outside its intended age group.
- **Influencer Marketing Challenges:** Influencer marketing presents enforcement difficulties, as promotional content created by influencers is less regulated than official brand advertisements, making it harder for platforms to restrict exposure to underage users.

In some cases, companies circumvent advertising laws by designing rogue advertisements that bypass social media platforms' approval systems. These advertisements are often accessible only for a short period before being flagged and removed (O'Sullivan-Gavin and Amazeen 2016). In a few instances, these advertisements may not explicitly violate national laws but instead contravene platform policies. Each social media platform enforces its own set of advertising rules, making it crucial for companies to understand both national regulations and corresponding platform policies (Cancer Council Victoria 2019). As digital markets and emergent products like vaping evolve rapidly, social media platforms must continuously update their policies to protect users from misleading and harmful advertisements.

The Intersection of Data Privacy and Public Health

Another key factor influencing advertisements on social media is data privacy. Data privacy plays a significant role in shaping user exposure to digital advertisements. For example, when social media platforms sell user data to advertisers, individuals become more susceptible to targeted advertisements for harmful or age-restricted products and are at a higher risk of encountering scams and fraudulent schemes, which can negatively impact financial health.

The European Union's Approach to Data Privacy and Advertisement Regulation

The European Union (EU) has implemented some of the strictest data privacy laws in the world (Nielsen 2024). These regulations are designed to protect users by restricting how companies collect and utilize personal data. Consequently, businesses cannot purchase social media users' data for targeted advertising, making ads less intrusive and less influential on the public. Additionally, the EU's Digital Services Act

(DSA) strengthens user protections by requiring social media platforms to (Larrison 2025):

- Limit the spread of misinformation and hate speech.
- Ban targeted advertisements.
- Undergo annual audits to ensure compliance with regulations.

The EU enforces severe penalties on companies that fail to comply with these laws. For example, Meta was fined $1.3 billion for violating EU data privacy regulations (Larrison 2025). These harsh financial penalties serve as a deterrent, ensuring that major technology corporations adhere to legal standards and prioritize user privacy and protection. While other countries have introduced similar regulations, none are as comprehensive or rigorously enforced as the EU's framework. Moving forward, policymakers must strike a balance between protecting consumers and allowing social media businesses to operate and grow through advertising-based revenue models.

Opportunities and Pitfalls

Despite growing interest, significant gaps remain in this field due to the lack of global social media research. There is a critical need for more research that examines social media trends across diverse populations and countries. Another gap includes the lack of separation between low- and middle-income countries, as they are often coupled into this broad category (Lencucha and Neupane 2022). Low-income countries and middle-income countries differ substantially in terms of resource allocation, economic structure, public health awareness, and cultural factors that influence social media usage. Recent frameworks have proposed more granular income-based classifications, distinguishing between low-income, lower-middle-income, upper-middle-income, and high-income countries (Roser et al. 2021). Social media research aligned with these distinctions would allow for more nuanced analysis and meaningful comparisons. There are numerous opportunities to expand research using social media to investigate current events, temporal trends, and user behavior. Ultimately, further research in this area could better inform regulatory bodies, programs, and interventions.

KEY POINTS AND TAKEAWAYS

- Low- and middle-income countries focus on educational campaigns through social media to positively influence public health.
- High-income countries focus on how social media impacts individual health outcomes.
- Social media advertising influences exposure to harmful advertisements, which vary significantly by country.

Conclusion

Social media is a valuable tool for the scientific community, offering insights that can enhance global understanding of public health. Researchers can leverage social media platforms to analyze diverse populations and gain better insights into the daily lives of individuals, as user-generated content often reflects personal behaviors, attitudes, and health-related concerns. Examining social media trends across distinct geographic regions allows researchers to identify societal patterns in different contexts. While foundational knowledge has been established, significant opportunities remain for advancing research in this area. Such studies have the potential to inform resource allocation strategies and guide the development of effective programs and policies. As social media continues to evolve, so does its potential to shape public health policy, enhance communication strategies, and support equitable global health outcomes.

References

Admin, B.E.N. (2024). The FTC and beyond: Ad disclosure rules around the world. *BENlabs*. https://www.benlabs.com/resources/ad-disclosure-rules-global/ (accessed 9 August 2025).

Alcohol Focus Scotland (2017). Promoting good health from childhood. Reducing the impact of alcohol marketing on children in Scotland. [Report]. *Alcohol Focus Scotland*. https://www.drugsandalcohol.ie/26921/ (accessed 9 August 2025).

Alwan, A., & Maclean, D. R. (2009). A review of non-communicable disease in low- and middle-income countries. *International Health*, *1*(1), 3–9. doi:10.1016/j.inhe.2009.02.003

Australian Government Department of Health, Disability and Ageing (2024). Advertising and sponsorship bans. https://www.health.gov.au/topics/smoking-vaping-and-tobacco/tobacco-control/advertising-bans (accessed 9 August 2025).

Balkin, J.M. (2021). How to regulate (and not regulate) social media. https://www.journaloffreespeechlaw.org/balkin.pd (accessed 21 August 2025).

Barker, H. E., Czaplicki, L., Cui, Y., Shen, R., Nian, Q., Xie, M., & Cohen, J. E. (2024). Exposure to and appeal of tobacco ads and displays in China: a qualitative exploration of Chinese youth perceptions. *Nicotine & Tobacco Research: Official Journal of the Society for Research on Nicotine and Tobacco*, *26*(4), 427–434. doi:10.1093/ntr/ntad192

Beaglehole, R., & Bonita, R. (2010). What is global health? *Global Health Action*, *3*. doi:10.3402/gha.v3i0.5142

Campaign for Tobacco-Free Kids (2024). Sri Lanka legal summary. *Tobacco Control Laws*. https://www.tobaccocontrollaws.org/legislation/sri-lanka (accessed 21 August 2025).

Cancer Council Victoria (2019). Tobacco in Australia: facts & issues: 11.11 internet promotion. https://www.tobaccoinaustralia.org.au/chapter-11-advertising/11-11-internet-promotion (accessed 21 August 2025).

CDC (2024). Job aid: social media campaign evaluation. *Overdose Resource Exchange (ORE)*. https://www.cdc.gov/overdose-resources/php/files/social-media-campaign-evaluation-job-aid.html (accessed 21 August 2025).

Chandraratne, N. K., Negi, N. S., Siyambalapitiya, H., De Seram, S., Selladurai, N., Pieris, K., Rothenstein-Henry, R., & Murukutla, N. (2024). Public opinion on alcohol policies in Sri Lanka. *Frontiers in Public Health, 12.* doi:10.3389/fpubh.2024.1409012

Egbe, C.O. (2023). Social media marketing of electronic cigarettes to youth. https://catherineegbe.com/2023/06/14/social-media-marketing-of-electronic-cigarettes-to-youth/ (accessed 21 August 2025).

Emberson, J., Lees, K. R., Lyden, P., Blackwell, L., Albers, G., Bluhmki, E., Brott, T., Cohen, G., Davis, S., Donnan, G., Grotta, J., Howard, G., Kaste, M., Koga, M., von Kummer, R., Lansberg, M., Lindley, R. I., Murray, G., Olivot, J. M., … Stroke Thrombolysis Trialists' Collaborative Group. (2014). Effect of treatment delay, age, and stroke severity on the effects of intravenous thrombolysis with alteplase for acute ischaemic stroke: a meta-analysis of individual patient data from randomised trials. *Lancet (London, England), 384*(9958), 1929–1935. doi:10.1016/S0140-6736(14)60584-5

ET Online (2024). 10 countries where social media faces the most restrictions – Logging off. *The Economic Times.* https://economictimes.indiatimes.com/nri/latest-updates/10-countries-where-social-media-faces-the-most-restrictions/logging-off/slideshow/113125384.cms (accessed 3 September 2025).

EUCAM (2022). Romania. *European Centre for Monitoring Alcohol Marketing.* https://eucam.info/regulations-on-alcohol-marketing/romania/ (accessed 3 September 2025).

FDA (2024). Advertising and promotion. *U.S. Food and Drug Administration.* https://www.fda.gov/tobacco-products/products-guidance-regulations/advertising-and-promotion (accessed 3 September 2025).

Federal Trade Commission (2014). Self-regulation in the alcohol industry: report of the federal trade commission. https://www.ftc.gov/system/files/documents/reports/self-regulation-alcohol-industry-report-federal-trade-commission/140320alcoholreport.pdf (accessed 3 September 2025).

Feigin, V. L., Stark, B. A., & Johnson, C. O. (2021). Global, regional, and national burden of stroke and its risk factors, 1990–2019: a systematic analysis for the Global Burden of Disease Study 2019. *The Lancet. Neurology, 20*(10), 795–820. doi:10.1016/S1474-4422(21)00252-0

Hagg, E., Dahinten, V. S., & Currie, L. M. (2018). The emerging use of social media for health-related purposes in low and middle-income countries: a scoping review. *International Journal of Medical Informatics, 115,* 92–105. doi:10.1016/j.ijmedinf.2018.04.010

Hirimuthigodage, D. and Disanayake, N. (2023). Indirect promotion of tobacco throughsocialmedia.https://www.ips.lk/wp-content/uploads/2023/06/Indirect-promotion-of-tobacco-through-social-media_ips.pdf]. Institute of Policy Studies of Sri Lanka (accessed 3 September 2025).

Islam, S., Tabassum, R., Liu, Y., et al. (2019). The role of social media in preventing and managing non-communicable diseases in low-and-middle income countries: hope or hype? https://dro.deakin.edu.au/articles/journal_contribution/The_role_of_social_media_in_preventing_and_managing_non-communicable_diseases_in_low-and-middle_income_countries_hope_or_hype_/20774212/2 (accessed 19 September 2025).

Kaluvu, L., Asogwa, O. A., Marzà-Florensa, A., Kyobutungi, C., Levitt, N. S., Boateng, D., & Klipstein-Grobusch, K. (2022). Multimorbidity of communicable and non-communicable diseases in low- and middle-income countries: a systematic review. *Journal of Multimorbidity and Comorbidity, 12*, 26335565221112590. doi:10.1177/26335565221112593

Larrison, B. (2025). Digital advertising regulation in 2025: what marketers need to know. *Basis Technologies*. https://basis.com/blog/digital-advertising-regulation-what-marketers-need-to-know (accessed 19 September 2025).

Lencucha, R., & Neupane, S. (2022). The use, misuse and overuse of the 'low-income and middle-income countries' category. *BMJ Journals*. https://gh.bmj.com/content/7/6/e009067 (accessed 19 September 2025)

Liao, T. and Li, B. (2023). New measures for online advertising in China: what you need to know. https://www.morganlewis.com/pubs/2023/04/new-measures-for-online-advertising-in-china-what-you-need-to-know (accessed 19 September 2025).

Lichtenberg, K. (2017). E-cigarettes: current evidence and policy. *Missouri Medicine, 114*(5), 335–338. https://www.ncbi.nlm.nih.gov/pmc/articles/PMC6140188/

Liu, L., Guevara, A., & Sanchez-Galan, J. E. (2022). Identification and classification of road traffic incidents in Panama City through the analysis of a social media stream and machine learning. *Intelligent Systems with Applications, 16*, 200158. doi:10.1016/j.iswa.2022.200158

Metreau, E., Young, K. E., & Eapen, S. G. (2024). World Bank country classifications by income level for 2024–2025. *World Bank Blogs*. https://blogs.worldbank.org/en/opendata/world-bank-country-classifications-by-income-level-for-2024-2025

Morapi, L. and Altini, N. (2022). In brief: prohibited and controlled advertising in South Africa. *Lexology*. https://www.lexology.com/library/detail.aspx?g=a7b56f50-f5ee-4723-9287-fd4b9c3da8e8 (accessed 19 September 2025).

Nguyen, T. T., Criss, S., Dwivedi, P., Huang, D., Keralis, J., Hsu, E., Phan, L., Nguyen, L. H., Yardi, I., Glymour, M. M., Allen, A. M., Chae, D. H., Gee, G. C., & Nguyen, Q. C. (2020). Exploring U.S. shifts in anti-Asian sentiment with the emergence of COVID-19. *International Journal of Environmental Research and Public Health, 17*(19), 7032. doi:10.3390/ijerph17197032

Nielsen, A. (2024). Social media marketing regulations: what your business can't do. https://joybyte.com/blog/social-media-marketing-regulations (accessed 19 September 2025).

O'Sullivan-Gavin, S. and Amazeen, M.A. (2016). The advertising industry in the social media age: the ethical and legal implications of unsanctioned rogue or "Scam" ads. https://www.academia.edu/25247792/The_Advertising_Industry_in_the_Social_Media_Age_The_Ethical_and_Legal_Implications_of_Unsanctioned_Rogue_or_Scam_Ads (accessed 1 October 2025).

Padmanathan, P., Bould, H., Winstone, L., Moran, P., & Gunnell, D. (2020). Social media use, economic recession and income inequality in relation to trends in youth suicide in high-income countries: a time trends analysis. *Journal of Affective Disorders, 275*, 58–65. doi:10.1016/j.jad.2020.05.057

Pimmer, C., & Tulenko, K. (2016). The convergence of mobile and social media: affordances and constraints of mobile networked communication for health workers in low- and middle-income countries. *Mobile Media & Communication, 4*(2), 252–269. doi:10.1177/2050157915622657

Polanco-Levicán, K., & Salvo-Garrido, S. (2022). Understanding social media literacy: a systematic review of the concept and its competences. *International Journal of Environmental Research and Public Health, 19*(14), 8807. doi:10.3390/ijerph19148807

Pontes-Neto, O. M., Silva, G. S., Feitosa, M. R., de Figueiredo, N. L., Fiorot, J. A., Rocha, T. N., Massaro, A. R., & Leite, J. P. (2008). Stroke awareness in Brazil: alarming results in a community-based study. *Stroke, 39*(2), 292–296. doi:10.1161/STROKEAHA.107.493908

Popescu, C., Turcu, C., and Crețu, R. (2024). Romania enacts law restricting ads for electronic cigarettes and heated tobacco products. *CMS Law-Now.* https://cms-lawnow.com/en/ealerts/2024/07/romania-enacts-law-restricting-ads-for-electronic-cigarettes-and-heated-tobacco-products (accessed 1 October 2025).

Roser, M., Ritchie, H., and Spooner, F. (2021). Burden of disease. *Our World in Data.* https://ourworldindata.org/burden-of-disease (accessed 1 October 2025).

Shao, D. and Luo, Q. (2024). Country comparative guides | China: advertising & marketing. *Country Comparative Guides | the Legal 500.* https://www.legal500.com/guides/chapter/china-advertising-marketing/?export-pdf (accessed 1 October 2025).

Silwal, S., Khadka, S., & Sah, B. K. (2019). Knowledge on stroke among middle aged adult in a community at Ratuwamai, Morang. *Tribhuvan University Journal, 33*(1), 31–42. doi:10.3126/tuj.v33i1.28680

Sinorn, T. (2024). Ministry intensifies e-cigarette ban with new guidelines. *Kiripost.* https://kiripost.com/stories/ministry-intensifies-e-cigarette-ban-with-new-guidelines

Song, H., Omori, K., Kim, J., Tenzek, K. E., Morey Hawkins, J., Lin, W.-Y., Kim, Y.-C., & Jung, J.-Y. (2016). Trusting social media as a source of health information: online surveys comparing the United States, Korea, and Hong Kong. *Journal of Medical Internet Research, 18*(3), e25. doi:10.2196/jmir.4193

Sophorn, P. (2024). Advertisement of alcohol products: determination of procedures, rules, and formalities (Prakas No. 084). *HBS LAW.* https://hbslaw.asia/updates/advertisement-of-alcohol-products-determination-of-procedures-rules-and-formalities-prakas-no-084/ (accessed 1 October 2025).

Southeast Asia Tobacco Control Alliance (2024). Viniton guilty of violating law banning tobacco advertising, says Cambodian court – SEATCA. https://seatca.org/viniton-guilty-of-violating-law-banning-tobacco-advertising-says-cambodian-court/ (accessed 1 October 2025).

Sprint Law (2025). Guide to Australian alcohol advertising laws: 2025th edition. *Sprint Law.* https://sprintlaw.com.au/articles/australian-alcohol-advertising-laws/ (accessed 1 October 2025).

Talin, B. (2024). WeChat explained – understanding the Chinese super app. *MoreThanDigital.* https://morethandigital.info/en/wechat-explained-understanding-the-chinese-super-app/ (accessed 1 October 2025).

Thapa, L., Sharma, N., Poudel, R. S., Bhandari, T. R., Bhagat, R., Shrestha, A., Shrestha, S., Khatiwada, D., & Caplan, L. R. (2016). Knowledge, attitude, and practice of stroke among high school students in Nepal. *Journal of Neurosciences in Rural Practice, 7*(4), 504–509. doi:10.4103/0976-3147.188635

Tunkl, C., Paudel, R., Thapa, L., Tunkl, P., Jalan, P., Chandra, A., Belson, S., Gajurel, B. P., Haji-Begli, N., Bajaj, S., Golenia, J., Wick, W., Hacke, W., & Gumbinger, C. (2023). Are digital social media campaigns the key to raise stroke awareness in low-and middle-income countries? A study of feasibility and cost-effectiveness in Nepal. *PLOS ONE, 18*(9), e0291392. doi:10.1371/journal.pone.0291392

Vincos Blog (2023). World map of social networks. *Vincos – il blog di Vincenzo Cosenza.* https://vincos.it/world-map-of-social-networks/ (accessed 1 October 2025).

World Health Organization (2019). Afghanistan: enforcing bans on tobacco advertising, promotion and sponsorship. *World Health Organization – Regional Office for the Eastern Mediterranean*. http://www.emro.who.int/tfi/news/tobacco-control-in-afghanistan-enforcing-bans-on-tobacco-advertising-promotion-and-sponsorship.html (accessed 1 October 2025).

World Health Organization (2021). WHO report on the global tobacco epidemic 2021: addressing new and emerging products. https://www.who.int/publications/i/item/9789240032095 (accessed 1 October 2025).

World Health Organization (2025). Health workforce. https://www.who.int/health-topics/health-workforce (accessed 29 October 2025).

World Population Review (2025). Social media users by country 2025. *Worldpopulationreview.Com*. https://worldpopulationreview.com/country-rankings/social-media-users-by-country (accessed 29 October 2025).

CHAPTER 12

DELIVERY OF INTERVENTIONS ON SOCIAL MEDIA

Elizabeth Dennard[1], Yulin Hswen[1,2], and Thu T. Nguyen[1]
[1]Department of Epidemiology and Biostatistics, School of Public Health, University of Maryland, College Park, MD, USA
[2]The Artificial Intelligence Interdisciplinary Institute at Maryland (AIM), College of Computer, Mathematical, and Natural Sciences (CMNS), College Park, MD, USA

Overview

Social media platforms offer extensive opportunities to implement public health interventions by facilitating communication that transcends physical and geographic barriers. These platforms not only enable the dissemination of information but also support the collection of rich, user-generated data that can inform and enhance intervention strategies. Importantly, social media offers a means to engage hard-to-reach communities, including individuals who face stigma and discrimination based on identity characteristics (sexual orientation, gender identity, race, and ethnicity). This chapter offers an overview of interventions deployed through social media across diverse public health domains, including mental health, physical activity and nutrition, and HIV-related risk behaviors and knowledge.

LEARNING OBJECTIVES

1. **Understand the role of social media platforms in facilitating the implementation of public health interventions, particularly for hard-to-reach communities**
2. **Highlight public health topics in which social media-based interventions have been employed**
3. **Present an overview of opportunities and challenges in implementing public health interventions on social media**

Key Concepts/Main Topics

Social Media Platforms and User Demographics

Social media platforms attract a diverse and expansive user base, making them a powerful tool for implementing public health interventions. Functioning as virtual spaces, these platforms support two-way communication through discussion forums, social networks, multimedia sharing, and messaging systems. Notable platforms include Meta (formerly Facebook), Instagram, X (formerly Twitter), TikTok, LinkedIn, Pinterest, and WhatsApp. Each platform hosts diverse users whose engagement is shaped by a distinct distribution of social determinants of health and demographic characteristics such as age, gender, education level, race, ethnicity, and income.

For instance, in 2023, Meta had over 245 million users in the United States, with the largest share (24.2%) aged 25–34 and a majority identifying as female (53.8%; Dixon, 2024). Similarly, Instagram users skew female and tend to have higher educational attainment, with the majority having some college education or higher. X users also tend to have higher income and educational attainment (Gottfried 2024). Other platforms include Pinterest, TikTok, LinkedIn, WhatsApp, and Snapchat, of which accounts for approximately 30% of U.S. adults as users. While Meta remains the most widely used platform among U.S. adults overall and ranks as the third most trafficked website globally (Hitlin et al. 2019), younger U.S. adults are more likely to use Instagram, Snapchat, and TikTok (Gottfried 2024). These platforms support both quantitative and qualitative data collection through user-generated content such as videos, images, reactions, posts, comments, and messages. Furthermore, they facilitate the implementation of public health interventions by reaching diverse audiences that may be difficult to engage with due to physical, geographic, or language barriers.

Public Health Topics and Interventions

Numerous interventions have been implemented across social media platforms, addressing topics such as mental health, physical activity and nutrition, and HIV testing and risk awareness. Documented mental health interventions include closed platforms that provide evidence-based support through cognitive behavioral therapy (CBT), web-based psychoeducation tools that support shared decision-making and empower study participants to discuss quality of care with mental health providers, and peer-support forums. These interventions aim to improve outcomes such as perceived stress, social support, and disease-related distress. Nutrition and physical activity-focused interventions have leveraged social networking features on phone apps and platforms like Facebook and Instagram. These include discussion forums, resource centers, education modules, web-based rewards, and digital food diaries, all linked to behavioral outcomes among study participants. Documented HIV-related interventions utilize platforms such as MiCHAT, Facebook, Grindr, MSM, YouTube, Twitter, QQ, Jack'd, Scruff, A4A, and Radar to promote HIV testing and prevention strategies. These initiatives also aim to reduce substance use and unprotected sexual activity.

Mental Health

Social Media-Based Interventions and Depression

Social media platforms are increasingly being used to deliver mental health interventions among adolescents and young adults. A scoping review by Kruzan et al. (2022) evaluated empirical evidence on social media-based interventions aimed at improving mental health outcomes among individuals aged 10–26. Young adults experience disproportionately high rates of mental health conditions compared to other age groups, but often use fewer mental health services due to financial constraints, perceived stigma, medical mistrust, and preferences for self-management of mental health conditions (Kruzan et al. 2022). While previous scoping and systematic reviews have evaluated the efficacy of web-based digital interventions across public health topics, relatively few have explored the specific role of social media platforms in delivering mental health interventions to young adults.

Kruzan et al. (2022) identified 15 unique studies that met the inclusion criteria, each assessing the feasibility of mental health interventions among study participants. All studies included validated outcome measures for depression and anxiety. Additional indicators of well-being included perceived stress, quality of life, positive youth development, social support, and loneliness. The intervention strategies typically featured combinations of psychoeducation tools, peer support, and cognitive-behavioral therapy. Psychoeducation tools and skill-based content focused on providing educational information about mental health conditions, coping strategies, and self-management skills while also encouraging dialogue between study participants. The majority of studies incorporated peer or expert support and community-based interventions, fostering virtual spaces where participants could connect, share personal experiences, and offer mutual support. Peer support can provide a sense of belonging and reduce feelings of isolation, which are common symptoms among young adults living with anxiety and depression. Most studies utilized social media platforms to deliver psychoeducation tools and skills-based content to promote social support.

Several interventions incorporated therapeutic approaches, including CBT, positive psychology, and strength-based practices. These therapies often involve working with a mental health professional to recognize negative thinking patterns, develop stress management strategies, and improve mental health outcomes (Mayo Clinic 2019; Cleveland Clinic 2022). However, intervention delivery varied across studies and did not always conform to a single treatment approach. Social media platforms are increasingly being used by young adults who experience a range of mental health outcomes. Given the widespread use of social media, these platforms serve as a resource for delivering more accessible mental health interventions. Additionally, integrating mental health interventions into social media has the potential to reach hard-to-reach communities, especially those who may be hesitant to seek treatment due to barriers related to geographic location, socioeconomic status, or fear of stigma.

Social Media Interventions and Schizophrenia

Among individuals living with schizophrenia spectrum disorders, social media-based interventions have been shown to improve positive psychotic symptoms, enhance peer support, increase social connectedness, reduce depressive symptoms, support medication adherence, and lower rates of hospital admissions (Alvarez-Jimenez et al. 2014). Välimäki et al. (2016) conducted the first systematic review and meta-analysis to evaluate social media interventions aimed at supporting mental health and well-being among individuals with schizophrenia in the United States. Outcomes assessed included symptoms of schizophrenia spectrum disorders, knowledge about implemented schizophrenia instruments, recovery, quality of life, perceived empowerment, social support, and stress levels. The review identified only two publications that met the inclusion criteria: one implementing the Schizophrenia Online Access to Resources (SOAR; Rotondi et al. 2010) and the other using a peer-support listserv and bulletin board (Kaplan et al. 2011). The study developed online listservs and bulletin boards to allow participants to communicate anonymously via email (Välimäki et al. 2016). Additionally, intervention groups used online peer-support forums, while those in the control groups received treatment as usual.

Previous research supports the use of online peer-support forums and other online mental health interventions to reduce the isolation among individuals living with schizophrenia (Highton-Williamson et al. 2015). However, after comparing findings across included studies, individuals in treatment groups reported more symptoms of anxiety and psychological distress. A randomized control trial by Kaplan et al. (2011) examined the impact of unmoderated peer support on the well-being of individuals living with psychiatric disabilities. Three hundred study participants diagnosed with either a schizophrenia spectrum disorder or an affective disorder were randomized into one of three groups: experimental internet peer support via a listserv, experimental internet peer support via a bulletin board, or a control condition with no peer support. Findings from this study suggest that individuals in the treatment groups (listserv and bulletin board peer support) experienced higher levels of self-management and quality of life compared to those in the control group (no peer support). Interestingly, participants who reported more positive experiences (social connection, visibility, etc.) within peer-support forums also reported higher levels of psychological distress than those who encountered more negative online experiences (e.g., isolation and harassment). Many clinicians fear that engaging in online peer support without professional moderation may heighten psychological distress among individuals living with schizophrenia spectrum disorders compared to the general population. Ultimately, these studies suggest that the impact of social media-based interventions on schizophrenia spectrum disorders is mixed and largely unexplored across the literature. This data gap highlights the need for further investigation to explore the long-term effects of social media on mental health outcomes, particularly among hard-to-reach communities.

Online Intervention Development to Treat Social Anxiety

Social anxiety disorder (SAD) is recognized as one of the most prevalent anxiety disorders globally, with a reported lifetime prevalence of approximately 13% (Olson 2021). Social anxiety has been documented as a risk factor for poorer premorbid functioning, depression, paranoia, suicidal ideation, and reduced quality of life, particularly among individuals also experiencing psychosis (American Psychiatric Association 2013). While CBT is recommended as an effective form of treatment for SAD coupled with psychosis, its focus tends to revolve around reducing psychotic symptoms and not treating affective comorbidities linked to social anxiety (McEnery et al. 2019). Moreover, only two randomized controlled trials to date have evaluated the clinical effectiveness of CBT for the treatment of social anxiety and psychosis. To address this gap, McEnery et al. (2019) developed an online social cognitive behavioral intervention, EMBRACE, designed to treat social anxiety symptoms among individuals experiencing first-episode psychosis. EMBRACE provided clinical content online to study participants with four distinct modules: (1) psychoeducational modules that explain therapeutic principles; (2) therapeutic comics designed to maximize engagement; (3) behavioral experiments addressing social anxiety symptomatology; and (4) interactive discussion forums to foster interaction and peer engagement.

Comparable findings across the literature suggest that in the first year of psychosis, approximately 30% of young adults aged 18–35 experience symptoms of SAD. Despite this, no prior studies had explicitly examined the treatment of social anxiety symptoms in the context of first-episode psychosis. This data gap is concerning, given the empirical evidence supporting the implementation of early intervention to reduce social anxiety disorder symptoms. McEnery aimed to address this limitation by developing EMBRACE to treat documented symptoms, including shame, perceptions of lower social rank, and paranoia, among young adults with first-episode psychosis. The EMBRACE intervention is a novel approach incorporating therapeutic comics and moderation models to maintain peer support and strengthen problem-solving skills among study participants. EMBRACE provides users with opportunities to test cognitive assumptions about treatment within a safe online environment.

Physical Activity and Nutrition

Social Media Interventions for Nutrition Education

A systematic review by Welch et al. (2016) assessed the effects of interactive social media interventions on behavior change. The review synthesized 11 unique systematic reviews and found mixed effects of social media interventions on lifestyle-related outcomes, including healthy attitudes and behaviors, weight loss, physical activity, and dietary patterns. In contrast, a more recent scoping review by Kulandaivelu et al. (2023) found that social media interventions improve nutrition outcomes among adolescents. Adolescence represents a crucial period for developing healthy eating habits, cooking skills, and self-efficacy, with social media serving as a tool to strengthen these skills. Kulandaivelu et al. (2023) reviewed 28 unique studies, including 25 interventions, that met the inclusion criteria. These studies assessed the characteristics, feasibility, and effectiveness of social media-based nutrition education interventions among adolescents aged 10–18. The most frequently used platforms were researcher-developed websites with embedded social networking features ($n = 10$), followed by Facebook ($n = 8$), mobile phone apps ($n = 4$), Instagram ($n = 2$), and an unspecified social networking service ($n = 1$). Researcher-developed platforms typically included discussion forums, chat functions, resource centers, games, and education modules.

While intervention engagement varied across relevant publications, many interventions demonstrated significant improvements in dietary behaviors, suggesting that high engagement is not always necessary for effectiveness. Key factors contributing to successful outcomes included tailoring interventions to user needs, encouraging peer support, involving family members, and fostering community engagement. Notably, community-based interventions yielded better nutrition outcomes compared to individual-based interventions due to intervention acceptability among study participants (Kulandaivelu et al. 2023). Overall, social media interventions for adolescent nutrition are effective, well-received, and well-documented across the literature. However, future research should consider enhancing peer support and customizing interventions for hard-to-reach populations to make nutrition education more accessible. Critical research areas include study participant engagement, intervention adherence, and the long-term effects of implemented interventions. Ultimately, this review highlights the importance of peer support and user-centered design in social media-based nutrition education.

Social Media Interventions on Physical Activity and Dietary Behaviors

Social media has been documented as a powerful tool to facilitate healthy diet-related behaviors and physical activity engagement. However, limited guidance exists for researchers, clinicians, or policymakers on how to responsibly implement social media interventions across public health topics. Additionally, there is a lack of robust empirical evidence on how these interventions can promote healthy dietary behaviors and physical activity among hard-to-reach communities. A systematic review by Goodyear et al. (2021) aimed to update the current evidence on social media interventions for physical activity and dietary behaviors. The study examined intervention characteristics and assessed differences in outcomes across diverse populations. The authors identified 18 unique studies, including randomized control trials ($n = 4$), nonrandomized control trials ($n = 5$), noncontrolled trials ($n = 3$), mixed methods ($n = 3$), and cross-sectional studies ($n = 3$), with the majority of target populations including young adult women ranging from 18 to 35 years of age. Facebook emerged as the most commonly used platform for intervention implementation ($n = 12$). Other platforms included X, Reddit, WeChat, Instagram, and a combination of multiple platforms. These platforms leveraged features such as image sharing, group chats, group challenges, and rewards. Overall, the interventions demonstrated positive effects on physical activity levels, food intake, body composition, and body weight across publications. Goodyear et al. (2021) emphasized the utility of gamification strategies (e.g., group challenges and rewards for behavior change), image sharing, and multimodal applications in enhancing participant motivation and retention. These strategies represent promising avenues for future intervention design, especially for programs aiming to foster sustained lifestyle change through digital media.

HIV Testing and Risk Knowledge

Social Media Interventions to Promote HIV Testing

Social media platforms have been documented as effective tools for promoting HIV risk knowledge and testing by disseminating HIV-related information, reducing stigma, fostering peer support, and connecting hard-to-reach communities with testing services. Additionally, social media-based interventions can foster user interactivity, facilitate two-way content sharing, and increase user engagement. Cao et al. (2017) conducted a systematic review to examine the effectiveness of social media interventions in promoting HIV testing, linkage to healthcare services, treatment adherence, and HIV care retention among populations living with HIV. Key populations in this systematic review included men who have sex with men (MSM), transgender individuals, people who inject drugs (PWID), and sex workers. The authors identified 26 publications that implemented diverse interventions across the following social media platforms: Facebook ($n = 15$), Grindr ($n = 10$), YouTube ($n = 1$), X ($n = 3$), QQ ($n = 1$), Gaydar ($n = 3$), Jack'd ($n = 1$), Scruff ($n = 2$), A4A ($n = 1$), and Radar ($n = 1$). The majority of studies focused on HIV testing ($n = 21$), while others explored HIV testing and linkage to healthcare services ($n = 4$) and antiretroviral therapy adherence ($n = 1$). Additionally, interventions were used to build online communities and peer support to encourage HIV testing and adherence ($n = 10$), provide testing services ($n = 9$), disseminate HIV information ($n = 9$), and develop intervention materials ($n = 1$). Findings from this review indicated that social media interventions were effective in increasing HIV testing rates, particularly among MSM in high-income countries. The review highlights the need for additional research to assess the effectiveness of these platforms in implementing HIV-specific interventions for vulnerable populations living with HIV in low- and middle-income countries.

Social Media Interventions to Reduce HIV Risk

In addition to promoting testing, social media platforms have been used to reduce HIV-risk behaviors. Lelutiu-Weinberger et al. (2015) conducted a quasi-experimental study (without a control group) to examine the acceptability and efficacy of a social media-based intervention. This intervention provided anonymous sessions with licensed therapists using the Facebook chat feature to reduce HIV-risk behaviors among young men who have sex with men (YMSM) in the United States. Primary behavioral outcomes included condomless anal sex encounters with a casual partner and the number of days involving drug use within a 30-day period. At baseline, all participants reported engaging in condomless anal sex within the previous 30 days, with an average of 7.63 encounters (SD = 16.95). The average number of such encounters under the influence of drugs and alcohol was 5.05 (SD = 16.07). Participants also reported an average of 9.44 (SD = 7.22) heavy drinking days and 5.07 (SD = 6.28) drug-use days within the same timeframe (Lelutiu-Weinberger et al. 2015). Psychosocial outcomes included gay-related and HIV stigma, anxiety, depression, motivation, self-efficacy, and HIV-related sexual health knowledge. Findings from this study indicated that intervention participation was associated with reduced drug use, alcohol consumption, and the number of sexual encounters, including condomless anal sex. Additionally, intervention participation increased HIV-related risk knowledge at the three-month follow-up. These findings underscore the potential of social media platforms to deliver targeted, confidential, and scalable behavioral interventions for HIV prevention.

Opportunities and Pitfalls

Opportunities

Enhanced Access to Hard-to-Reach Communities

Social media platforms have the potential to break down traditional barriers associated with psychological, physical, and geographic constraints, enabling access to populations historically underrepresented in epidemiological research. Platforms such as TikTok, Instagram, and WhatsApp are particularly effective in engaging communities marginalized by sexual orientation, gender identity, and racial or ethnic background. For example, the integration of mental health interventions into social media platforms has expanded access to therapeutic resources for individuals experiencing depression, schizophrenia spectrum disorders, and anxiety. Additionally, given the widespread use of social media, these platforms have the ability to deliver more accessible interventions on a range of public health topics. Ultimately, they facilitate the collection of data in environments where users feel comfortable expressing their thoughts and behaviors, thereby improving the inclusivity and representativeness of public health data.

Organic Data Environments for Analysis

Social media platforms serve as unique spaces where individuals can share their experiences, beliefs, and behaviors with fewer filters than in formal research settings. These unstructured interactions offer valuable insights into societal trends and individual behaviors among those living with health conditions. For example, social media platforms have been documented as powerful tools to promote HIV risk knowledge by reducing stigma and fostering real-time peer support. Unlike traditional survey methods, social media enables continuous observation and the identification of behavioral shifts as they unfold, enabling more dynamic responses to emerging trends.

Real-Time Intervention Delivery

The real-time nature of social media supports the timely dissemination of public health interventions. For instance, during crises, such as the rapid spread of misinformation or sudden shifts in health-related behaviors, interventions can be tailored and deployed more quickly than through traditional media. This immediacy not only enhances the reach of the interventions but also ensures that public health messaging remains relevant to evolving population needs.

Support for Personalized Interventions

The granularity of social media data allows for the development of highly personalized public health interventions. By leveraging sentiment analysis and advanced artificial intelligence (AI) techniques, researchers can identify and respond to the emotional states and preferences of users. For example, targeted campaigns can be adjusted in tone and content based on real-time feedback from specific communities, thereby increasing their effectiveness, engagement, and uptake. This adaptability ensures that public health interventions resonate more deeply with intended audiences.

Pitfalls

Digital Inequities and Accessibility Gaps

Despite the expansive reach of social media, significant disparities in digital access and literacy remain. Populations in rural areas, low-income communities, and older adults may face challenges in accessing or navigating digital platforms and tools. As a result, these populations may be excluded from social media-based interventions, further widening the digital divide. Bridging these gaps requires complementary strategies, such as community-based outreach and the development of low-technology solutions, to ensure equitable access to public health initiatives.

Ethical and Privacy Concerns

The use of user-generated data for public health purposes raises complex ethical challenges, including issues of informed consent, data security, and data misuse. Users may perceive public health surveillance as invasive, potentially eroding trust in researchers and platforms. To uphold ethical standards, researchers must ensure that data are anonymized and used transparently. Clear communication about the purposes of data collection and benefits is essential to maintaining trust and safeguarding participant rights.

Propagation of Misinformation

The brevity and virality of content on platforms such as TikTok and X can lead to oversimplification or distortion of complex health topics, increasing the risk of misinterpretation and misinformation. Combating this requires robust content moderation systems, proactive fact-checking, and collaboration with platform administrators to identify and remove harmful content while amplifying credible sources. Public health interventions can also be designed to correct misinformation and promote media literacy.

Overgeneralization of Populations

Data collected from social media can reflect selection biases, such as the overrepresentation of vocal demographic groups or the underreporting of marginalized voices. Algorithms trained on such data may perpetuate inequities by prioritizing content aligned with engagement metrics rather than addressing unmet community health needs. For instance, dominant voices may skew perceptions of community needs, leading to the development of interventions that fail to address pressing health disparities. To promote inclusivity, researchers should consider strategies such as weighting data to account for underrepresented groups and developing algorithmic fairness to ensure that social media interventions reflect the needs of diverse and underserved populations.

KEY POINTS AND TAKEAWAYS

- **Social media facilitates the delivery of public health interventions across diverse platforms and audiences.**
  Social media platforms offer unique advantages in reaching populations that are often excluded from traditional public health efforts due to geographic isolation, stigma, or socioeconomic constraints. Their accessibility, anonymity, and widespread use enable the delivery of interventions to marginalized communities, including LGBTQ+ individuals, racial and ethnic minorities, and those with limited access to in-person care. By fostering inclusive and interactive digital spaces, social media facilitates more equitable engagement in public health interventions.

- **Social media-based interventions can promote health for all and reduce the impact of negative health outcomes.**
  Public health interventions delivered via social media have addressed a wide range of topics, including mental health (e.g., depression, schizophrenia, and social anxiety), physical activity and nutrition, and HIV testing and risk reduction. These interventions have been implemented on platforms such as Facebook, Instagram, TikTok, and Grindr to promote behavior change, provide peer support, and disseminate health information. The evidence shows positive outcomes in areas such as stress reduction, improved social support, healthier behaviors, and increased testing rates, particularly among adolescents, young adults, and MSM populations.

Conclusion

As digital landscapes continue to reshape human interaction, social media platforms have rapidly evolved into powerful channels for delivering public health interventions. They broaden access, foster inclusion, and enable real-time, tailored engagement with diverse and often hard-to-reach populations. From mental health to HIV prevention, these platforms support interventions that are not only scalable but also responsive to community needs. However, realizing their full potential requires careful navigation of challenges such as digital inequities, privacy concerns, and the spread of misinformation. By designing interventions ethically, ensuring they are accessible, and amplifying marginalized voices, social media can serve not merely as a communication tool but as a catalyst for advancing health for all.

References

Alvarez-Jimenez, M., Alcazar-Corcoles, M. A., González-Blanch, C., Bendall, S., McGorry, P. D., & Gleeson, J. F. (2014). Online, social media and mobile technologies for psychosis treatment: a systematic review on novel user-led interventions. *Schizophrenia Research, 156*(1), 96–106. doi:10.1016/j.schres.2014.03.021

American Psychiatric Association. (2013). Diagnostic and statistical manual of mental disorders. *Diagnostic and Statistical Manual of Mental Disorders*, 5(5). 10.1176/appi.books.9780890425596

Cao, B., Gupta, S., Wang, J., Hightow-Weidman, L. B., Muessig, K. E., Tang, W., Pan, S., Pendse, R., & Tucker, J. D. (2017). Social media interventions to promote HIV testing, linkage, adherence, and retention: systematic review and meta-analysis. *Journal of Medical Internet Research, 19*(11), e394. doi:10.2196/jmir.7997

Cleveland Clinic. (2022). Cognitive behavioral therapy (CBT). Cleveland Clinic; Cleveland Clinic. https://my.clevelandclinic.org/health/treatments/21208-cognitive-behavioral-therapy-cbt

Mayo Clinic. (2019). *Cognitive Behavioral Therapy*. Mayoclinic.org; Mayo Clinic. https://www.mayoclinic.org/tests-procedures/cognitive-behavioral-therapy/about/pac-20384610

Dixon, S. J. (2024). *U.S. Meta audience distribution by age and gender* 2022. Statista. https://www.statista.com/statistics/1319311/us-meta-audience-by-age-and-gender/

Goodyear, V. A., Wood, G., Skinner, B., & Thompson, J. L. (2021). The effect of social media interventions on physical activity and dietary behaviours in young people and adults: a systematic review. *International Journal of Behavioral Nutrition and Physical Activity, 18*(1), 72. doi:10.1186/s12966-021-01138-3

Gottfried, J. (2024). *Americans' social media use.* Pew Research Center. https://www.pewresearch.org/internet/2024/01/31/americans-social-media-use/

Highton-Williamson, E., Priebe, S., & Giacco, D. (2015). Online social networking in people with psychosis: A systematic review. *International Journal of Social Psychiatry, 61*(1), 92–101. doi:10.1177/0020764014556392

Hitlin, P., Rainie, L., & Olmstead, K. (2019). *Facebook Algorithms and Personal Data.* Pew Research Center: Internet, Science & Tech; Pew Research Center: Internet, Science & Tech. https://www.pewresearch.org/internet/2019/01/16/facebook-algorithms-and-personal-data/

Kaplan, K., Salzer, M. S., Solomon, P., Brusilovskiy, E., & Cousounis, P. (2011). Internet peer support for individuals with psychiatric disabilities: A randomized controlled trial. *Social Science & Medicine, 72*(1), 54–62. doi:10.1016/j.socscimed.2010.09.037

Kruzan, K. P., Williams, K. D. A., Meyerhoff, J., Yoo, D. W., O'Dwyer, L. C., De Choudhury, M., & Mohr, D. C. (2022). Social media-based interventions for adolescent and young adult mental health: A scoping review. *Internet Interventions, 30,* 100578. doi:10.1016/j.invent.2022.100578

Kulandaivelu, Y., Hamilton, J., Banerjee, A., Gruzd, A., Patel, B., & Stinson, J. (2023). Social media interventions for nutrition education among adolescents: scoping review. *JMIR Pediatrics and Parenting, 6*(1), e36132. doi:10.2196/36132

Larsen, K. (2024). Facebook (Meta) Statistics for Marketers. Kristian Larsen. https://www.kristian-larsen.com/info/facebook-meta-statistics/

Lelutiu-Weinberger, C., Pachankis, J. E., Gamarel, K. E., Surace, A., Golub, S. A., & Parsons, J. T. (2015). Feasibility, Acceptability, and Preliminary Efficacy of a Live-Chat Social Media Intervention to Reduce HIV Risk Among Young Men Who Have Sex With Men. *AIDS and Behavior, 19*(7), 1214–1227. doi:10.1007/s10461-014-0911-z

McEnery, C., Lim, M. H., Knowles, A., Rice, S., Gleeson, J., Howell, S., Russon, P., Miles, C., D'Alfonso, S., & Alvarez-Jimenez, M. (2019). Development of a Moderated Online Intervention to Treat Social Anxiety in First-Episode Psychosis. *Frontiers in Psychiatry, 10.* doi:10.3389/fpsyt.2019.00581

Olson, C. M. (2021). Familial factors in the development of social anxiety disorder. *Journal of Psychosocial Nursing and Mental Health Services, 59*(7), 23–34. doi:10.3928/02793695-20210219-01

Rotondi, A. J., Anderson, C. M., Haas, G. L., Eack, S. M., Spring, M. B., Ganguli, R., Newhill, C., & Rosenstock, J. (2010). Web-Based Psychoeducational Intervention for Persons With Schizophrenia and Their Supporters: One-Year Outcomes. *Psychiatric Services, 61*(11), 1099–1105. doi:10.1176/ps.2010.61.11.1099

Shaw, J. M., Mitchell, C. A., Welch, A. J., & Williamson, M. J. (2015). Social media used as a health intervention in adolescent health: a systematic review of the literature. *DIGITAL HEALTH, 1,* 205520761558839. doi:10.1177/2055207615588395

Välimäki, M., Athanasopoulou, C., Lahti, M., & Adams, C. E. (2016). Effectiveness of social media interventions for people with schizophrenia: a systematic review and meta-analysis. *Journal of Medical Internet Research, 18*(4), e92. doi:10.2196/jmir.5385

Welch, V., Petkovic, J., Pardo, J., Rader, T., & Tugwell, P. (2016). Interactive social media interventions to promote health equity: an overview of reviews. *Health Promotion and Chronic Disease Prevention in Canada : Research, Policy and Practice, 36*(4), 63–75. https://www.ncbi.nlm.nih.gov/pmc/articles/PMC4964231/

CHAPTER 13

USE OF AI, PREDICTIVE MODELS, AND SYNTHETIC DATA

Yulin Hswen[1], Thu T. Nguyen[2], Xiaoya Tang[3], Tolga Tasdizen[3], Pankaj Dipankar[4], and Quynh C. Nguyen[4]

[1]The Artificial Intelligence Interdisciplinary Institute at Maryland (AIM), College of Computer, Mathematical, and Natural Sciences (CMNS), Department of Epidemiology and Biostatistics, School of Public Health, University of Maryland, College Park, MD, USA

[2]Department of Epidemiology and Biostatistics, School of Public Health, University of Maryland, College Park, MD, USA

[3]Department of Electrical and Computer Engineering, University of Utah, Salt Lake City, UT, USA

[4]National Institute of Nursing Research (NINR), National Institutes of Health (NIH), Bethesda, MD, USA

LEARNING OBJECTIVES

1. Describe the opportunities and limitations of synthetic data and artificial intelligence (AI) in health research
2. Explain how generative AI can support or hinder public health communication, particularly in the context of social media content
3. Evaluate the role of foundational vision models, such as Vision Transformers, in analyzing large-scale visual datasets to study the built environment
4. Assess the implications of applying AI-based visual analysis for understanding associations between neighborhood conditions and population health outcomes

Overview

Synthetic data, defined as data artificially generated to reflect the statistical patterns and structures of real-world datasets, has gained increasing relevance in health research. Its utility lies in addressing challenges such as the protection of individual privacy, the underrepresentation of marginalized communities, and the scarcity of high-quality data. Synthetic data are now being explored for broader applications, including the analysis and potential generation of social media content.

The extension of synthetic data methodologies to social media contexts, however, introduces a range of ethical complexities. In contrast to structured datasets such as electronic health records or satellite imagery, social media content captures dynamic and subjective human experiences, encompassing users' thoughts, emotions, behaviors, and interactions. The deployment of generative artificial intelligence (AI) to simulate social media posts may inadvertently distort or misrepresent real user perspectives. Such distortions risk amplifying existing biases or undermining the perceived legitimacy of the data, thereby raising concerns about the reliability of subsequent analyses.

Nevertheless, AI technologies offer promising avenues for advancing public health research and communication. Recent deep learning models, such as Vision Transformers (ViTs; Dosovitskiy et al. 2021), are particularly well-suited for analyzing large-scale visual datasets, including imagery from platforms like Google Street View or Instagram. In these applications, AI serves not as a replacement for human expression but as an analytical tool that enhances the ability to interpret large-scale visual information. Moreover, when applied ethically and in collaboration with public agencies such as the Centers for Disease Control and Prevention (CDC), generative AI can support the development of targeted health messaging. These messages, crafted with transparency and adapted to the communication norms of various digital platforms, can inform the public about pressing health issues such as substance use or infectious disease outbreaks.

This chapter critically examines the opportunities and limitations associated with the use of synthetic data and AI in the context of social media and online visual data. An included case study demonstrating the application of foundational vision models to Google Street View imagery illustrates how these tools can yield insight into the built environment and its associations with population health outcomes.

Synthetic Data for Health Research

The use of synthetic data offers several advantages, including the protection of sensitive information, enhanced data accessibility for collaborative research, and the mitigation of dataset imbalances by augmenting data for underrepresented populations. In the context of health research, synthetic data generated through generative AI refers to artificially constructed datasets designed to augment dataset size and emulate the statistical properties and structural features of real-world data without disclosing specific individual's information. Leveraging models such as generative diffusion models (Ho et al. 2020; Rombach et al. 2022; Yang et al. 2024), and large language models (Brown et al. 2020; Touvron et al. 2023), researchers generate synthetic yet realistic outputs such as clinical images, text, and structured health records that preserve privacy while enabling robust analyses (Cao et al. 2023; Croitoru et al. 2023) https://www.nature.com/articles/s44222-024-00245-7. For instance, a generative model may be employed to stimulate electronic health records that reflect real patient trends while minimizing patient identities. This approach allows researchers to develop and test machine learning models in data-scarce settings or where privacy is a major concern.

Synthetic Voices, Misinformation, and Representation

Generative AI possesses the capacity to produce social media content at scale, a capability that presents both opportunities and challenges. A key concern involves the generation and dissemination of synthetic content that mimics human-authored communication but lacks an authentic human origin. This phenomenon can contribute to "bot-like" behaviors, wherein AI-generated accounts circulate fabricated messages that resemble authentic human communication (Pan et al. 2025).

The use of generative AI to propagate particular narratives introduces the risk of feedback loops in which systems generate increasingly refined content based on their own prior outputs. In some cases, this can result in the amplification of unintended messages or the emergence of synthetic ideas, concepts, or claims that gain traction not through genuine discourse but through algorithmically driven repetition and amplification. Such dynamics, if unregulated, may distort the informational landscape as a product of artificial generation rather than authentic public sentiment. Moreover, substituting authentic voices with synthetic ones may reduce the richness and diversity of human expression. Synthetic narratives cannot capture the nuance, cultural specificity, or emotional resonance embedded in lived experience.

In the absence of effective oversight, social media platforms may become increasingly saturated with AI-generated content, leading to a decline in public trust and greater difficulty distinguishing genuine expression from artificial simulation. These trends pose significant implications for democratic dialogue, evidence-based policymaking, and public health messaging. To safeguard the integrity of digital communication, it is essential to establish clear transparency protocols, invest in robust AI-content detection tools, and develop ethical standards for the deployment of generative AI across social media platforms.

AI for Social Media Public Health Communication

Despite the risks associated with synthetic content, generative AI holds significant promise as a tool for enhancing public health communication. The creation of tailored messages that resonate across diverse populations and languages remains a persistent challenge in health outreach. AI can assist by producing adaptable content in multiple modalities, such as text, imagery, audio, and video, aligned with specific cultural and contextual needs. For example, AI can support the development of antiracist messaging that actively counters discriminatory discourse or contribute to the design of antismoking campaigns that are linguistically accessible and culturally relevant. By adjusting language, tone, and format based on user engagement and platform dynamics, AI-generated content can help ensure that public health messages remain timely and responsive to evolving public concerns.

Governmental agencies, nonprofit organizations, hospitals, and local health departments can leverage generative AI to create context-specific messages, provided there is clear disclosure that the content originates from an AI system. Transparency is essential to ensure that audiences understand these messages are not from individuals but are instead produced by or on behalf of institutions through verified organizational accounts. For instance, an environmental organization could use generative AI to create informative and accessible content explaining climate change in relatable terms, fostering greater understanding without alienating the public. This approach offers a scalable and adaptable means of strengthening health and environmental communication, particularly for organizations with limited resources for content creation across multiple platforms.

AI in Visual Data Analysis

AI holds substantial promise in the analysis of social media image data such as photos, memes, or other forms of large-scale visual datasets such as Google Street View. These visual data sources can offer valuable insights into the built environment, including indicators of urban infrastructure, green space availability, and neighborhood-level socioeconomic conditions. Recent advancements in foundational vision models, particularly pretrained Vision Transformers (ViTs), enable the analysis of such imagery at scale without the need for extensive manual annotation, as they are capable of learning rich, generalizable representations from large unlabeled datasets. ViTs, which are trained using self-supervised learning techniques (Chen et al. 2020; He et al. 2020; Caron et al. 2021), demonstrate an ability to generalize across diverse geographic contexts (Haas et al. 2023). Unlike traditional convolutional neural networks (CNNs), which are inherently biased toward capturing local spatial patterns (Raghu et al. 2022; Khan et al. 2022), ViTs leverage an "attention mechanism" that allows the model to consider all image patches simultaneously, facilitating a more global and holistic understanding of the visual content. This enables the model to capture relationships between distant components of a scene, such as the spatial arrangement of buildings, green spaces, roads, and other contextual elements. For example, while a CNN might identify individual visual features (e.g., a tree, a sidewalk, or a building facade) in isolation, a Vision Transformer can interpret how these elements co-occur and interact within the broader urban landscape. This holistic perspective is particularly advantageous for analyzing complex scenes captured in street-level imagery, where the spatial configuration of features may convey information relevant to health outcomes, environmental quality, or accessibility (http://matter.as/). Empirical studies have demonstrated that ViTs outperform CNNs on a variety of computer vision tasks, including image classification and semantic segmentation, particularly when applied to large, high-quality datasets. These advancements in AI, particularly ViTs, have enabled new applications in analyzing large-scale visual datasets. One such application is Google Street View imagery, which offers rich, street-level perspectives of the built environment. The following case study illustrates how foundational vision models can extract public health-relevant features from this imagery, enabling scalable analysis of neighborhood conditions and associated health outcomes.

CASE STUDY 1. ASSESSING THE BUILT ENVIRONMENT WITH IMAGE ANALYSIS–AN APPLIED EXAMPLE USING GOOGLE STREET VIEW

While traditionally perceived as a navigational tool, Google Maps, and its visual extension, Google Street View (GSV), has evolved into a hybrid platform that exhibits characteristics of a social media ecosystem. Beyond facilitating spatial orientation, it now serves as a repository of user-generated content: photos, reviews, ratings, and localized knowledge that collectively offer insight into how individuals experience and interact with their environments (Parkes-Nield 2021; Peischl et al. 2023).

In particular, GSV offers high-resolution, panoramic imagery of neighborhoods across the globe. This imagery is often embedded with spontaneous and ambient depictions of daily life, reminiscent of visual storytelling on platforms such as Instagram or TikTok. However, unlike traditional social media, the content on GSV is not curated for personal branding or algorithmic visibility. Rather, it emerges organically through user uploads of locations, meals, destinations, and personal evaluations. As Peischl et al. (2023) notes, Google Maps can function as a "refuge from algorithms," offering content that is unfiltered, asynchronous, and deeply rooted in physical space.

In addition to mapping functionality, Google Maps has developed into a subtle but powerful social infrastructure. Users maintain profiles, contribute reviews and photos, follow others, and receive updates tailored to their location and interests. These features support local discovery and interaction, positioning the platform as a networked system of user-driven knowledge exchange (Parkes-Nield 2021). GSV further extends this infrastructure by encouraging users to contribute imagery from areas where automated systems (e.g., Street View Vehicles) cannot operate, such as rural or inaccessible regions. This crowdsourced participation helps maintain and expand the platform's reach.

Moreover, users are not only contributing images but also helping determine which images best represent a place. User engagement metrics, such as views and click frequency, influence which images are featured most prominently on location profiles. In this way, GSV functions as a dynamic, crowdsourced visual archive of the built environment. For public health researchers, this archive presents a novel and underutilized data source. In contrast to traditional social platforms that prioritize textual or emotional content, GSV imagery captures spatial and environmental attributes such as green space, infrastructure quality, and housing types, which are directly linked to the study of social determinants of health. When paired with health data, this imagery enables spatial analysis of how neighborhood characteristics relate to outcomes, including obesity, chronic disease, pollution exposure, and health inequities.

This case study explores how recent advancements in computer vision can be applied to large-scale GSV imagery to derive insights relevant to public health and urban planning. It focuses on the evolution of modeling approaches, from convolutional neural networks to ViTs, and examines the implications of using GSV as a socially layered visual platform in spatial and social epidemiology.

Early work in this domain includes efforts by Nguyen et al. (2019), who applied CNNs to classify built environment features using GSV imagery. CNNs are multilayered neural networks commonly used in image classification, object recognition, and analyzing

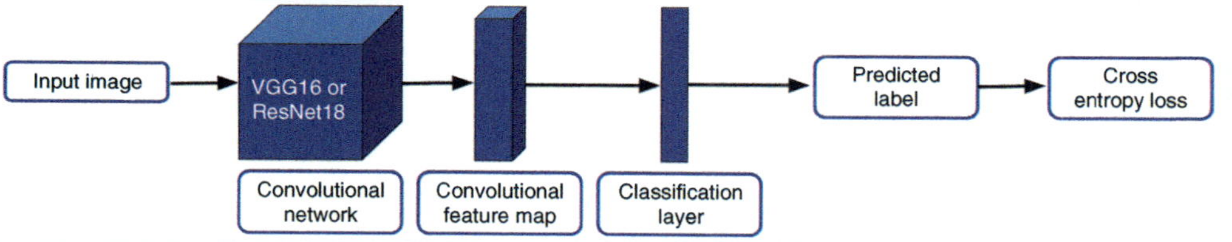

Figure 13.1 Convolutional neural networks. The classification layer maps features to classes found in ImageNet.
Source: Yue et al., 2022 / MDPI / CC BY 4.0.

structured arrays of data (Liu 2018). These models extract and transform features from images through a hierarchical process, with each successive layer learning more complex representations.

To optimize model performance on downstream tasks, an ImageNet-pretrained CNN model can be fine-tuned (i.e., parameter weights adjusted) using a smaller amount of training data from the targeted task (Hentschel et al. 2016). ImageNet is a large database comprising over 14 million annotated images across 22,000 categories (Krizhevsky et al. 2017). Through a technique known as transfer learning, Nguyen and colleagues fine-tuned these pretrained models, specifically VGG16 and ResNet, on a smaller set of manually labeled GSV images (Krizhevsky et al. 2017). Approximately 10,000 GSV images were annotated to identify key built environment characteristics such as green space, presence of crosswalks, housing type (e.g., single vs. multifamily), chain link fences, and utility wires. The fine-tuned models achieved high accuracy levels, ranging from 85% to 95%, depending on the feature of interest (Figure 13.1; Yue et al. 2022).

In addition to this classification-based approach, the researchers employed a "direct method," wherein GSV images were used as inputs and health indicators, such as obesity rates at the census tract level, served as outputs (Krizhevsky et al. 2017). This approach enabled the model to identify correlations between visible environmental features and health outcomes without explicitly labeling the images for specific features. Disease prevalence at the census tract level provided a supervisory signal for the model to learn predictive visual patterns associated with health risks (Figure 13.2: Jarvanmardi et al. 2020).

To improve model robustness, the researchers supplemented GSV data with images from Flickr, a user-generated photo-sharing platform (Alirezaei et al. 2023). Flickr images introduced variation in angle, lighting, and composition, which helped the model generalize better, as GSV images often follow a limited, uniform pattern (taken from car-mounted cameras on roadways). By learning from the diversity in Flickr photos, the model became more flexible and capable of interpreting different visual contexts that may exist in areas not fully captured by GSV.

As the project scaled to a national level, encompassing over 160 million GSV images, Nguyen and colleagues encountered a common machine learning challenge: poor generalizability across geographies. For example, models trained on imagery from cities such as Boston or Chicago performed poorly when applied to areas with markedly different architectural and environmental features, such as Hawaii. This phenomenon, known as "domain shift," highlighted the limitations of traditional supervised learning approaches that rely on labeled data from a narrow set of locations.

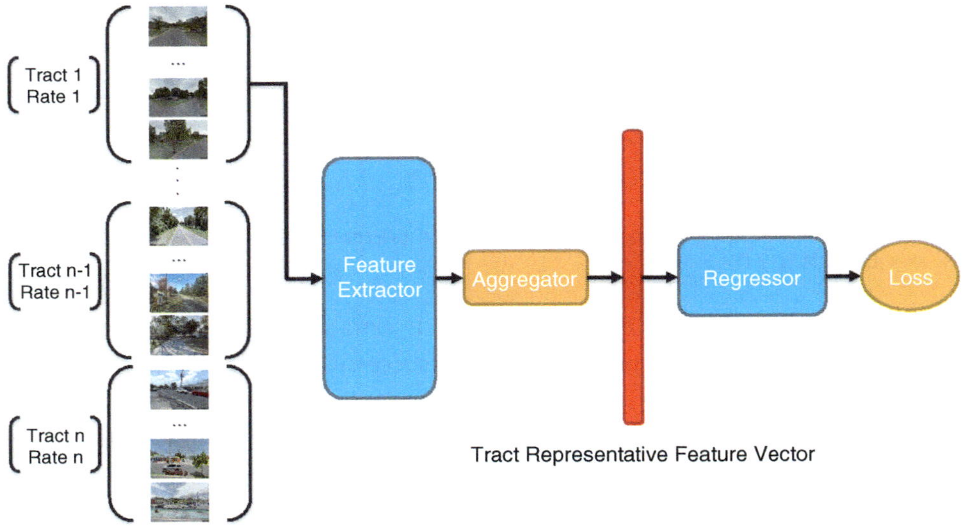

Figure 13.2 Direct method census tract level regression. Obesity rates for 19,707 tracts. Coefficient of determination $R^2 = 0.63$.
Source: Javanmardi, 2020 / IEEE / CC BY 4.0.

To address these limitations, the team adopted Vision Transformers. These models belong to a broader category of foundational models and are trained using self-supervised learning. These models, unlike CNNs that primarily capture local image features, employ attention mechanisms that allow them to model long-range dependencies across entire images. Among the prominent self-supervised learning (SSL) techniques are masking-based methods, such as Masked Autoencoders (He et al. 2021), which train models to reconstruct missing parts of images, and contrastive learning (Chen et al. 2020), which trains models by comparing pairs of images. During training, contrastive learning exposes models to image pairs: one image is a slightly augmented version of the other (positive pair), while the other is drawn from a different image (negative pair). By learning to bring representations of positive pairs closer together and push negative pairs apart in the feature space, the model teaches itself to understand patterns and features in images—without the need for human-annotated labels.

This self-supervised approach enabled the development of a generalized, scalable model that could predict environmental risks or health outcomes directly from visual data. By reducing reliance on labeled training data and increasing the ability to capture diverse geographic contexts, ViTs represent a promising advancement for public health and urban research applications. Moreover, such foundational models can be extended to analyze visual content from other sources, including social media platforms where image-based communication plays a central role in shaping perceptions and behaviors. In sum, GSV and other user-contributed image datasets represent valuable, yet underutilized, resources for understanding the built environment and its implications for population health. The integration of foundational vision models offers opportunities for scalable, interpretable, and geographically robust analyses, opening new possibilities for interdisciplinary collaboration across computer science, epidemiology, and urban planning.

Opportunities and Pitfalls

Opportunities

Scalable Visual Analysis

Self-supervised and semi-supervised learning represents a transformative advancement in the ability to interpret visual data without extensive human labeling (Liu et al. 2021). While these models still require some fine-tuning and minimal labeling, they demand far less supervision compared to traditional approaches because they leverage the structure within the data itself to create predictive tasks. Only minimal fine-tuning or light supervision is needed for downstream tasks, making the approach more scalable and efficient, especially when large, labeled datasets are not available. Vision Transformers trained using this method can detect complex built environment features such as fencing, roads, green cover, or indicators of infrastructure degradation. As a result, built environment indicators can now be extracted at scale, providing more comprehensive and spatial data to inform urban planning, housing policy, and neighborhood-level health risk assessments. The automation of this process supports faster and more adaptive public health surveillance that reflects evolving community conditions.

Democratizing Spatial Health Research

One of the most promising outcomes of this research is the development of a reusable pretrained model for street-level imagery analysis. By training on over 160 million unlabeled images from diverse geographic contexts within the United States, this foundation model serves as a flexible and accessible tool for researchers across disciplines. It can be applied to questions in urban health, environmental justice, and chronic disease prevention without the need for extensive computational infrastructure or advanced machine learning proficiency. This democratization of spatial analysis empowers institutions with limited resources to participate in high-resolution research and fosters cross-sector collaborations between academia, public agencies, and community organizations. It represents an important step toward equitable access to high-resolution, data-driven public health tools.

Pitfalls

Bias in AI Outputs and Spatial Representation

Despite their technical sophistication, foundational models are susceptible to encoding and perpetuating biases present in their training data. In the case of Google Street View, geographic coverage and image quality vary widely, often reflecting the structural inequalities inherent in infrastructure development and surveillance. Urban areas with higher socioeconomic status tend to be more frequently updated and more richly represented, while lower-income communities, rural regions, and less accessible areas may be underrepresented or missing. This leads to an overrepresentation of well-resourced areas and increases the risk of biased model outputs that overlook historically marginalized communities. For instance, if a model is trained primarily on high-resolution data from affluent neighborhoods, it may learn to associate features such as tree-lined streets or well-maintained sidewalks with positive health outcomes. As a result, it may fail to recognize or even exclude similar or alternative features in under-resourced areas simply because those features are not captured in the data. This exclusion reflects systemic neglect in data collection, not the absence of meaningful environmental predictors, ultimately misrepresenting the health behaviors and outcomes of marginalized communities. Moreover, when data from low-resource communities are missing or underrepresented, generative AI cannot meaningfully fill those gaps. As a result, models trained on such data may inform policies or interventions that do not align with the actual needs, risks, or environmental contexts of these populations. Without deliberate corrective strategies, these biases can lead to flawed conclusions and inequitable policy decisions.

Overfitting and Limited Generalizability Across Diverse Built Environments

Although Vision Transformers trained on large-scale image datasets offer improved performance over earlier convolutional neural networks, they still face significant challenges when applied to heterogeneous environments. One of the core assumptions in machine learning is that the training and testing data are drawn from similar probability distributions. This assumption is frequently violated in spatial analyses where architectural features, street layouts, vegetation, and cultural elements vary widely between regions. Without mechanisms to adapt to regional variation or incorporate localized feedback, models risk providing inaccurate or misleading results when deployed outside their original training contexts.

Loss of Interpretability in Black Box Models

A trade-off in the application of some AI models is the tension between predictive performance and interpretability. For example, models that use obesity rates as labels learn to associate certain visual patterns with health outcomes but do not reveal the specific environmental characteristics driving these associations. While these models may achieve high accuracy metrics, they operate as black boxes, offering little insight into the causal or mediating pathways that connect built environment features to health. This lack of transparency poses challenges for public health practitioners, urban planners, and community members who require actionable, explainable insights to guide policy or allocate resources. For instance, specific features including green space, walkability, and signs of disrepair may function as intermediate variables that help explain *why* or *how* a place might influence health. For black box AI models to contribute meaningfully to population health, efforts must be made to balance predictive power with interpretability through model design, visualization tools, and integration with domain-specific knowledge.

KEY POINTS AND TAKEAWAYS

- **Synthetic data has valuable use cases but requires contextual boundaries.** Synthetic data can improve privacy and representation, particularly for structured datasets such as electronic health records or built environment imagery. However, applying synthetic data to social media content raises ethical concerns due to the personal and authentic nature of user-generated expression.
- **Machine learning models enable scalable built environment analysis.** Models trained on large-scale visual datasets, such as Google Street View, can efficiently identify features such as greenery, housing type, and infrastructure quality, supporting nationwide spatial epidemiology studies.
- **Generative AI offers potential for adaptive public health communication.** Generative AI can help public health organizations craft tailored, platform-specific messaging across multiple formats, including text, imagery, and video. These tools are especially useful in multilingual or culturally diverse settings, provided the messages are transparent about their AI origin and are ethically deployed.
- **Bias and generalization limitations must be monitored.** Even with large-scale training, foundational models can replicate geographic and demographic biases. Domain shifts across regions can reduce model accuracy, underscoring the need for context-specific validation and adaptation.
- **Interpretability is essential for policy translation and community trust.** While deep learning models can predict outcomes effectively, maintaining explainability through intermediate variables enhances usability and the ability to inform actionable public health policies.
- **Ethics and transparency are central to AI integration in health.** As these technologies continue to advance, careful attention must be given to responsible use, transparency in data provenance, and the societal implications of automation in research and communication. Cross-sector collaboration and oversight are essential to ensure equitable outcomes.
- **AI has the power to democratize public health tools.** Pretrained models and synthetic datasets can reduce technical barriers for researchers and institutions with limited resources, enabling broader participation in high-resolution public health research.

Conclusion

The use of synthetic data and AI in health research must balance innovation with responsibility. Synthetic data can help protect privacy and fill data gaps, but future work should establish clear ethical standards to ensure it does not distort authentic voices or misrepresent communities. New foundation and vision models demonstrate the potential of AI to integrate complex datasets and conduct multimodal analysis with image, video, and text that can advance our understanding of how the built environment impacts population outcomes. Yet their future success depends on improving generalizability across diverse regions, addressing biases in data coverage, and making models more interpretable for policy and practice. In the near term, researchers can take practical steps such as validating models across multiple geographic settings, pairing synthetic data with real-world data for quality checks, and collaborating with communities to ensure outputs reflect lived experience. Policymakers and researchers should also prioritize transparency in how AI-generated findings are communicated so that results can be trusted and applied effectively. By combining these immediate actions with a longer-term commitment to accountability, collaboration, and improving health for all, AI models can evolve into trusted resources that advance population health and support more inclusive, data-driven decision-making.

References

Alirezaei, M., Nguyen, Q. C., Whitaker, R., & Tasdizen, T. (2023). Multi-task classification for improved health outcome prediction based on environmental indicators. *IEEE Access: Practical Innovations, Open Solutions, 11*, 73330–73339. doi:10.1109/access.2023.3295777

Brown, T. B., Mann, B., Ryder, N., Subbiah, M., Kaplan, J., Dhariwal, P., Neelakantan, A., Shyam, P., Sastry, G., Askell, A., Agarwal, S., Herbert-Voss, A., Krueger, G., Henighan, T., Child, R., Ramesh, A., Ziegler, D. M., Wu, J., Winter, C., ... Amodei, D. (2020). Language models are few-shot learners (No. arXiv:2005.14165). *arXiv*. doi:10.48550/arXiv.2005.14165

Cao, H., Tan, C., Gao, Z., Xu, Y., Chen, G., Heng, P.-A., & Li, S. Z. (2023). A survey on generative diffusion model (No. arXiv:2209.02646). *arXiv*. doi:10.48550/arXiv.2209.02646

Caron, M., Touvron, H., Misra, I., Jégou, H., Mairal, J., Bojanowski, P., & Joulin, A. (2021). Emerging properties in self-supervised vision transformers. 9650–9660. https://openaccess.thecvf.com/content/ICCV2021/html/Caron_Emerging_Properties_in_Self-Supervised_Vision_Transformers_ICCV_2021_paper.html (accessed 15 October 2025).

Chen, T., Kornblith, S., Norouzi, M., & Hinton, G. (2020). A simple framework for contrastive learning of visual representations. In *Proceedings of the 37th International Conference on Machine Learning*, pp. 1597–1607. https://proceedings.mlr.press/v119/chen20j.html.

Croitoru, F.-A., Hondru, V., Ionescu, R. T., & Shah, M. (2023). Diffusion models in vision: a survey. *IEEE Transactions on Pattern Analysis and Machine Intelligence, 45*(9), 10850–10869. doi:10.1109/TPAMI.2023.3261988

Dosovitskiy, A., Beyer, L., Kolesnikov, A., Weissenborn, D., Zhai, X., Unterthiner, T., Dehghani, M., Minderer, M., Heigold, G., Gelly, S., Uszkoreit, J., & Houlsby, N. (2021). An image is worth 16x16 words: transformers for image recognition at scale. (No. arXiv:2010.11929). *arXiv*. doi:10.48550/arXiv.2010.11929

Haas, L., Alberti, S., & Skreta, M. (2023). Learning generalized zero-shot learners for open-domain image geolocalization (No. arXiv:2302.00275). *arXiv*. doi:10.48550/arXiv.2302.00275

He, K., Fan, H., Wu, Y., Xie, S., & Girshick, R. (2020). Momentum contrast for unsupervised visual representation learning (No. arXiv:1911.05722). *arXiv*. doi:10.48550/arXiv.1911.05722

He, K., Chen, X., Xie, S., Li, Y., Dollár, P., & Girshick, R. (2021). Masked autoencoders are scalable vision learners (No. arXiv:2111.06377). *arXiv*. doi:10.48550/arXiv.2111.06377

Hentschel, C., Wiradarma, T.P., and Sack, H. (2016). Fine tuning CNNS with scarce training data — Adapting imagenet to art epoch classification. In *2016 IEEE International Conference on Image Processing (ICIP)*, pp. 3693–3697. 10.1109/ICIP.2016.7533049.

Ho, J., Jain, A., & Abbeel, P. (2020). Denoising diffusion probabilistic models. *Advances in Neural Information Processing Systems, 33*, 6840–6851. https://proceedings.neurips.cc/paper/2020/hash/4c5bcfec8584af0d967f1ab10179ca4b-Abstract.html

Javanmardi, M., Huang, D., Dwivedi, P., Khanna, S., Brunisholz, K., Whitaker, R., Nguyen, Q., & Tasdizen, T. (2020). Analyzing associations between chronic disease prevalence and neighborhood quality through Google street view images. *IEEE Access, 8*, 6407–6416. doi:10.1109/ACCESS.2019.2960010

Khan, S., Naseer, M., Hayat, M., Zamir, S. W., Khan, F. S., & Shah, M. (2022). Transformers in vision: a survey. *ACM Computing Surveys, 54*(10s), 1–41. doi:10.1145/3505244

Krizhevsky, A., Sutskever, I., & Hinton, G. E. (2017). ImageNet classification with deep convolutional neural networks. *Communications of the ACM, 60*(6), 84–90. doi:10.1145/3065386

Liu, Y. H. (2018). Feature extraction and image recognition with convolutional neural networks. *Journal of Physics: Conference Series, 1087*, 062032. doi:10.1088/1742-6596/1087/6/062032

Liu, X., Zhang, F., Hou, Z., Wang, Z., Mian, L., Zhang, J., & Tang, J. (2021). Self-supervised learning: generative or contrastive (No. arXiv:2006.08218). *arXiv*. doi:10.48550/arXiv.2006.08218

Nguyen, Q. C., Khanna, S., Dwivedi, P., Huang, D., Huang, Y., Tasdizen, T., Brunisholz, K. D., Li, F., Gorman, W., Nguyen, T. T., & Jiang, C. (2019). Using Google Street View to examine associations between built environment characteristics and U.S. health outcomes. *Preventive Medicine Reports, 14*, 100859. doi:10.1016/j.pmedr.2019.100859

Pan, L., Wang, C.-Y., Zhou, F., & Lü, L. (2025). Complexity of social media in the era of generative AI. *National Science Review, 12*(1), nwae323. doi:10.1093/nsr/nwae323

Parkes-Nield, S. (2021). Can calendar customs engender stewardship of our natural environment? An investigation into real-world and fictional calendar customs in the UK and their potential for environmental engagement. *Green Letters, 25*(3), 252–265. doi:10.1080/14688417.2021.2023029

Peischl, J., Aikin, K. C., McDonald, B. C., Harkins, C., Middlebrook, A. M., Langford, A. O., ... Brown, S. S. (2023). Quantifying anomalies of air pollutants in 9 US cities during 2020 due to COVID-19 lockdowns and wildfires based on decadal trends. *Elem Sci Anth, 11*(1), 00029.

Raghu, M., Unterthiner, T., Kornblith, S., Zhang, C., & Dosovitskiy, A. (2022). Do vision transformers see like convolutional neural networks? (No. arXiv: 2108.08810). *arXiv*. doi:10.48550/arXiv.2108.08810

Rombach, R., Blattmann, A., Lorenz, D., Esser, P., & Ommer, B. (2022). High-resolution image synthesis with latent diffusion models (No. arXiv:2112.10752). *arXiv*. doi:10.48550/arXiv.2112.10752

Touvron, H., Lavril, T., Izacard, G., Martinet, X., Lachaux, M. A., Lacroix, T., ... Lample, G. (2023). Llama: open and efficient foundation language models. *arXiv preprint arXiv:2302.13971.*

Yang, L., Zhang, Z., Song, Y., Hong, S., Xu, R., Zhao, Y., Zhang, W., Cui, B., & Yang, M.-H. (2024). Diffusion models: a comprehensive survey of methods and applications. *ACM Computing Surveys, 56*(4), 1–39. doi:10.1145/3626235

Yue, X., Antonietti, A., Alirezaei, M., Tasdizen, T., Li, D., Nguyen, L., Mane, H., Sun, A., Hu, M., Whitaker, R. T., & Nguyen, Q. C. (2022). Using convolutional neural networks to derive neighborhood built environments from Google Street View images and examine their associations with health outcomes. *International Journal of Environmental Research and Public Health, 19*(19), 12095. doi:10.3390/ijerph191912095

CHAPTER 14

PUTTING LESSONS INTO ACTION FOR RESEARCHERS, POLICYMAKERS, AND THE COMMUNITY

Thu T. Nguyen[1], Shaniece Criss[3], Heran Mane[1], Yulin Hswen[2], Penchala Sai Priya Mullaputi[1], and Quynh C. Nguyen[4]

[1]Department of Epidemiology and Biostatistics, School of Public Health, University of Maryland, College Park, MD, USA

[2]The Artificial Intelligence Interdisciplinary Institute at Maryland (AIM), College of Computer, Mathematical, and Natural Sciences (CMNS), School of Public Health University of Maryland, College Park, MD, USA

[3]Department of Health Sciences, Furman University, Greenville, SC, USA

[4]National Institute of Nursing Research (NINR), National Institutes of Health (NIH), Bethesda, MD, USA

Overview

Empirical evidence from social media analyses offers valuable guidance for identifying emerging trends and topics in public health research. For example, spikes in hate speech, the proliferation of misinformation, and increased mentions of symptoms linked to infectious diseases may highlight the need for further investigation and intervention. Social media research provides a valuable evidence base to inform policies and resource allocation by identifying prevalent needs, beliefs, and attitudes around health issues, or by evaluating the impact of specific programs. Social media can also be leveraged to assess the implementation and real-time impact of public health policies, programs, and treatments by capturing public sentiment and behavioral response as they are implemented. This timely feedback loop allows researchers to assess the impact of exposures and interventions and identify unintended consequences. By analyzing patterns in conversations and behaviors on social media, stakeholders can quickly adapt strategies to

LEARNING OBJECTIVES

1. Provide an overview of key messages from this book
2. Share lessons learned
3. Offer future directions

enhance intervention effectiveness and address emerging concerns, making evaluation more responsive to the needs of diverse populations.

Beyond monitoring, social media serves as a platform for public health interventions and a powerful amplifier for extending the reach of offline initiatives. It supports participant recruitment, facilitates information dissemination, and fosters communication and support among community members. The growing influence of digital content creators and the collective strength of online communities signal that increasing attention and investment will be directed toward these spaces. As social media becomes increasingly central to public engagement, it remains crucial to study its dynamics, address its potential harms, and harness its vast potential to drive positive social impact and improve population health. This chapter reflects on lessons learned by the coauthors in navigating the social media environment. It also offers recommendations for future directions in this rapidly evolving field.

Lessons Learned

The complexity of modern societies requires versatile and interdisciplinary approaches to promote public health. In this book, we demonstrate how insights gleaned from social media can help researchers and public health officials address health inequities. Social media provides a vast, ever-changing landscape of data that allows researchers to better understand interconnected factors, such as systemic racism, socioeconomic status, and environmental conditions that could lead to adverse health outcomes. Access to social media data allows researchers to develop better strategies to mitigate existing risk factors and subsequent adverse events in real time.

Effectively addressing health disparities demands research methods capable of capturing these intricate relationships beyond simple statistics, leading to more targeted and culturally competent interventions. We describe the rapid evolution and history of social media, offering guidance on how to carefully design research that examines public health topics through a social media lens. We outline key considerations on how to acquire and apply rich social media data and navigate the important and constantly evolving ethical considerations that must remain central to the research.

We further highlight quantitative and qualitative methods, including artificial intelligence (AI)-generated synthetic data and predictive models that leverage social media to investigate issues such as identity-based discrimination and a wide range of health topics, from chronic conditions to emerging public health challenges. From these diverse applications, we draw key takeaways about the opportunities that social media offers for real-time surveillance, direct public engagement, and cost-effective data collection, as well as the limitations and ethical considerations that accompany its use in public health research.

The Opportunities Are Endless, and the Limitations Are Real

The opportunities and limitations of social media research are equally vast. This duality captures the quintessence of the digital public square, especially in the realm of public health. Social media and other online forums present great potential for improving public health outcomes. This technology offers unprecedented access to real-time and historical conversations, allowing researchers to study social phenomena that shape health behaviors and outcomes. For example, researchers can explore drivers of vaccine hesitancy, detect and predict health outbreaks, and analyze public discussions of new medications. Social media can also be used to connect health professionals to the population at large for participant recruitment, advocacy, and large-scale data collection.

On the other hand, these same platforms are constrained by practical and ethical considerations. While they can serve as essential channels for informing communities and countering disinformation, they can also propagate misinformation, amplifying harmful narratives and biases that undermine public health. The dichotomous nature of social media as both a tool for empowerment and a vector of risk underscores the need for a balanced, critical approach in leveraging it for health research and interventions.

Start Simple and Build from There

Our research began with sentiment analysis of race-related social media posts, with the goal of measuring and investigating the impact of the social environment on health. We delved into mixed-methods research to understand the nuance of the meanings of social media posts. As we gained experience and developed additional expertise, we incorporated more sophisticated analytic techniques, including multimodal models capable of detecting both hate and anti-hateful content across image and text modalities. As we continued on this research path, we explored both risk and protective factors and developed a greater conceptual understanding of the influence of social context on public health. We began to delve more deeply into cultural racism and structural stigma as foundational forces that shape risk and opportunity and drive policy.

Over time, the research expanded to examine social media experiences and exposures of various marginalized communities, including the unhoused, immigrants, and gender and sexual minorities, and incorporated an intersectional lens to better understand how multiple intersecting social identities impact health outcomes. Starting with simple models and a focused scope allowed us to build a methodological and theoretical foundation. This approach proved especially useful in a newly emerging field where established guidelines are often lacking.

Prioritize the Research Question

In an era where technologies and analytic methods are advancing rapidly, it is easy for researchers, particularly those new to the field, to become focused on the methodological novelty rather than the core purpose of their work. Throughout our research, consistently centering the research question, the overarching goals, and the populations of interest has been essential in guiding decisions about methodology, data, and interpretation. As emphasized in the previous section, advanced methods should be employed when they are well-justified and address critical data gaps in existing knowledge. However, in many cases, simpler models often remain more interpretable, resource-efficient, and allow findings to be more easily compared with prior studies.

For example, in our cross-platform, decade-long analysis of public sentiment related to immigration discourse, we aimed to understand how conversations evolved over time and across platforms. To address this question, we employed accessible and interpretable methods, using support vector machines (SVMs) for classifying sentiment at the post level and average sentiment scores to examine patterns at both the keyword and geographic levels. These approaches were selected not for their novelty but because they aligned closely with our research objectives and provided insights that were both clear and actionable. When methodological choices are driven more by novelty than by research relevance, findings may become difficult to interpret, replicate, or apply to real-world contexts, particularly in public health, where actionable insights are critical. In contrast, methods grounded in the research question are more likely to produce findings that are timely, relevant, and useful. Prioritizing the research question also means considering the end users of the research, such as policymakers, practitioners, and community organizations, and selecting analytic strategies that make results accessible, interpretable, and applicable in practice.

The Virtual Ivory Tower

While social media has gained a lot of popularity as an efficacious tool for various research questions and for informing communities, this approach has also garnered criticism. Researchers have long been accused of being detached from the real-life implications of their work. Similarly, social media researchers have been faulted for living in "Cyber Ivory Towers," where they risk overlooking the practical consequences of their studies and the effects their work may have on the populations they investigate.

The ability to leverage big data for high-level comprehension of various topics is extremely valuable. However, by adopting mixed methods such as incorporating community or stakeholder input, researchers can further enhance the relevance and accuracy of their studies. Engaging more directly with the people and issues being examined allows for more nuanced insights and helps reduce misinterpretation and biases.

Future research should continue to leverage the efficiency and breadth of big data sources such as social media data, while adding the necessary depth and grounding of human-centered methods to produce more comprehensive and responsible studies.

Teamwork

Conducting this research would not have been possible without interdisciplinary collaboration. Data scientists played a critical role in collecting, processing, and analyzing social media data, while epidemiologists contributed to the development of study design, methodological decisions, and interpretation of results. In some cases, such as the application of multilevel models designed for intersectional analysis, we brought in new collaborators with specialized expertise to support more advanced methods. Building a team with a wide range of expertise and experiences facilitates the application of a variety of methods. This pluralistic approach enabled us to address complex research questions in a more comprehensive and robust manner than any single method could achieve alone.

Our projects and publications were enriched by layering diverse perspectives, including those from community members. For example, when creating the keyword list of race and ethnicity terms used to collect race-related discussions on social media, the team reviewed prior research, consulted public databases, and engaged with scholars whose research focuses on specific racial and ethnic populations. Similarly, during our qualitative work on experiences of racism during pregnancy and birthing, we held regular meetings with a community advisory board. This board included mothers with lived experience of preterm birth, frontline health and social service providers, and representatives from community-based organizations. Their input was essential in shaping both the data collection and the interpretation of findings. This collaborative process not only made the research more enriching but also allowed us to build a community of scholars and experts who could guide us through a range of research challenges and projects.

Participating in both formal and informal networking spaces also proved valuable. Attending academic conferences and workshops enabled us to present our findings, receive critical feedback, and stay informed on emerging methodologies. Networking provided opportunities for project collaboration, sharing of technical resources and expertise, and professional growth.

Adaptability

While research is continually evolving across all fields, the pace of change in social media data research is especially rapid. Platforms emerge and fade, analytic methods continue to evolve, and platform policies are regularly revised. For example, modifications to content moderation policies can significantly affect the visibility and nature of content encountered by users, and it is important to track and investigate the implications of these changes. While these changes can be challenging, they also provide opportunities for reflection and adaptation. Some of our most impactful studies emerged from unexpected events and shifting circumstances. The coauthors of this book began this research with the collection and analysis of Twitter data, taking advantage of the publicly available application programming interface (API), which allowed access to a collection of random 1% samples. Twitter also offered an Academic Track API, granting researchers affiliated with academic institutions no-cost access to historical data. However, in 2023, Twitter was rebranded as X, and both the public and the Research Academic Track APIs were discontinued. Anticipating this shift, our research team collected as much Twitter data as possible before access ended and subsequently expanded efforts to explore other platforms. We broadened our technical capacities and knowledge base to collect, clean, and analyze data from Facebook, Instagram, Bluesky, Reddit, and YouTube.

Although platform popularity and data accessibility may fluctuate, the importance of studying these spaces remains undiminished. Social media is no longer merely a communication tool; it is where people form identities, build relationships, engage in public discourse, and express both personal and collective beliefs. To understand human behavior and society today, we must understand what happens online.

The fast-paced nature of these environments means researchers must contend with constantly evolving topics, trends, language, and lingo—making the study of online discourse and its impacts more complex. Researchers must continuously remain attuned to this rapidly morphing landscape, which bridges the physical and digital worlds.

Additionally, researchers must consider differences in how users engage with various platforms and recognize the distinctions between them. Modes of information dissemination have evolved from text-based communication to the incorporation of images, video, and virtual environments. With the advent of AI technologies, researchers will benefit from developing a comprehensive understanding of emerging platforms, their features, and their implications for target audiences.

Longitudinal data collection across platforms has improved our ability to track public discourse cycles, including changes in interest, beliefs, and discussions. Remaining open to emerging events and responding in real time has been a valuable lesson. This flexibility takes full advantage of one of social media's greatest strengths—that data are constantly created, generated, and engaged with on the platform. As the digital terrain transforms, our research must adapt alongside it—remaining committed to promoting health for marginalized communities and open to new forms of data that reflect the complexity of modern life.

Centering Ethics and Authenticity in Social Media Research

Central to the future of social media research lies ethical responsibility: to prioritize people over data. Behind every post, tweet, or comment are real individuals expressing emotions, beliefs, and lived experiences. Unlike curated survey data or structured clinical records, social media content emerges organically and often reflects marginalized perspectives absent from institutional datasets. These voices must be treated with respect, interpreted with care, and protected from harm.

Conclusion and Future Directions

Social media has become a dominant ecosystem where individuals spend a significant amount of their time, shaping their daily interactions, perceptions, and behaviors. As a digital space that permeates nearly every aspect of life—from social connection and news consumption to health information and entertainment—social media holds immense influence over both individual and collective thinking. Understanding how people engage within these platforms is essential for developing responsive public health strategies, addressing societal challenges, and leveraging digital technologies for positive societal change.

The future of social media research is inherently multimodal. New generations of users are gravitating toward platforms that prioritize visual and ephemeral content—platforms such as TikTok, Instagram Reels, YouTube Shorts, and others, continuing to emerge. This shift requires researchers to develop tools and frameworks capable of analyzing diverse data modalities, from facial expressions and tone of voice to visual symbolism and editing style.

While research tools and platforms advance, we must remain vigilant about the persistent harms that accompany them. Misinformation, hate speech, and the algorithmic amplification of harmful content continue to pose significant threats to society. At the same time, it is crucial that advancements in social media and AI serve not only advantaged groups but also those historically marginalized or excluded from public discourse and health systems. As AI-based tools become more prevalent, researchers must remain attentive to potential biases introduced at every stage of the analytic pipeline, from model training on incomplete or biased data to the uncritical application of model outputs. For example, a model may produce biased outcomes if trained on data lacking sufficient heterogeneity, and applying such models without examining differential impacts can inadvertently reinforce inequities. Analyzing social media content for indicators of criminal behavior or drug use, while valuable for public health surveillance, may unintentionally perpetuate stigma against certain communities.

In investigating health disparities, it is critical to consider individual, social, and structural drivers of health. Moreover, integrating community voices throughout the research process from design to interpretation can enhance both the validity and impact of findings.

Moving forward, flexibility, collaboration, and health promotion must remain at the center of social media research. Sustaining a commitment to interdisciplinary teamwork and community engagement has enabled us to ask more relevant questions, employ inclusive methods, and generate findings that are both actionable and socially relevant. By continuing to explore the potential of social media, we strive to advance research that supports health and responds meaningfully to the needs of communities in a digitally connected world.